NOTES FROM A NARROW RIDGE: RELIGION AND BIOETHICS

NOTES FROM A NARROW RIDGE: RELIGION AND BIOETHICS

DENA S. DAVIS
AND
LAURIE ZOLOTH

WITH A FOREWORD BY MARTIN E. MARTY

University Publishing Group
Hagerstown, Maryland

University Publishing Group, Inc.
Hagerstown, Maryland 21740
1-800-654-8188

ISBN (cloth):   1-55572-077-3
ISBN (paper):   1-55572-052-8

Photo credit—William C. Walsh made the photograph on the front cover,
"Alpine-glow on Mount Whitney at Sunrise," taken in the Alabama Hills
above Movie Flat in Lone Pine, California, on October 18, 1997, with a
Nikon FG camera, using a Tamron 28-70 Tele-macro lens, and Kodak Select
Elite Chrome asa 200 film. Copyright © 1999 by W.C. Walsh; it is used with
his kind permission.

For my parents, Freda and Milton Rubin.
—Dena S. Davis

For my grandparents, Julia and Nathan Cohen, who taught a
Judaism of the deepest faith and spoke of R. Akiba,
and Esther Zoloth, who taught a Judaism of the deepest rebellion,
and mentioned Emma Goldman.
—Laurie Zoloth

I have occasionally described my standpoint to my friends as the "narrow ridge." I wanted by this to express that I did not rest on the broad upland of a system that includes a series of sure statements about the absolute, but on a narrow rocky ridge between the gulfs where there is no sureness of expressible knowledge, but the certainty of meeting what remains undisclosed.

—Martin Buber

Contents

Foreword

Martin E. Marty

Most of us carry around portable metaphors and put them to work on favored causes. Thus the editors have summoned the authors in this volume to provide perspective on "religion and bioethics" by joining them on a narrow ridge. Jewish philosopher and theologian Martin Buber provided them with that image, and it works. Rather than anticipate by condensing all the variations of their theme, I will try to provide perspective on their perspectives by reaching into my tote bag of metaphors and offering a match.

This one is from W.H. Auden's long "New Year Letter (1 January 1940)," a set of rhymed polysyllabic couplets addressed to his friend Elizabeth Mayer. The "we" of his letter includes more than the poet and his correspondent. Readers and the citizenry at large as an implied audience are to make their way into the wartime decade with them. Auden at one point uses the mountain-hiking image that attracted Buber and our editors. The poet pauses to look around, but finds no sure footing:

So, perched upon the sharp *arête*,
Where if we do not move we fall,
Yet movement is heretical,
Since over its ironic rocks
No route is truly orthodox.[1]

Almost 60 years ago, when I first read that poem, I had to look up *arête* and found it to mean "a narrow ridge," from a French word for a fishbone or a spine. It has stayed with me ever since as the appropriate metaphor for the terrain on which late-modern walkers walk and have their being.

They, "we," Auden and Mayer and their readers and the readers of this book, are not the first people to walk or climb. To move from metaphor to present reality in one quick leap, from ridge to ridge as it were, we must note the obvious: people in recent decades are not the first to have thought about or practiced "religion and bioethics." As far as history reaches and then beyond it, back to the evidence that prehistoric graves have left us, people have sought to endow their joys and their sorrows, their successes and failures, their lives and their deaths-to-be, with meaning. On the course of that life they have encountered ills, evils, and threats to healthy bodily existence. They have had to make choices and decisions about human care. When they did so, those who wanted to be good and do good practiced something that today we might call bioethics.

The difference between *all,* or almost all, of the thens and now is that most of those people then did some of their walking on flat terrain and broad plains among many signposts and landmarks. They tended to live with people who thought about ultimate reality pretty much as they did. Usually one set of powers proposed one set of symbols in a network that webbed the private meanings together. Of course, there were polities that we would call pluralist. Ancient Greece and Rome were full of competing altars. But people could live within their diasporas and find their own symbol systems intact and protectable.

Such is not the case in the epoch called modern. Mass media of communication, if nothing else, intrude on all intactnesses and remove most protections. It is true that in this period, as before, there tend to be some connecting symbols. Governments, commercial forces, academies, vogue philosophies, and interest groups tend to generate systems that either attract the witting and the unwitting or are virtually forced upon them. Thus the authors in this book assume that something they might call "post-Enlightenment secular rationality" had come to dominate late-modern bioethics. What the fashioners of that informal but effective and encroaching system did not notice was that they too were not on firm, flat, solid philosophical ground. It turns out, as the essays in this book make clear, that they were perched upon a sharp *arête* of their own or, rather, of their fathers'—and it was almost always fathers'—invention.

In order to make ethical decisions about anything "bio-," these modern academics determined that "in the original position," as some philosophers among us like to say, all parties must at least implicitly agree to make their ethical moves employing nothing but this "secular rationality." To do so, it was thought and claimed, would put them on firm ground, and they could walk in relative agreement or disagreement on its plain as they debated issues of life and death.

Among the fashioners, however, was a set of thinkers called theologians or theological ethicists. They did much of their moving and perching on narrow and sharp ridges called seminaries and divinity schools. Some of the authors in this book celebrate those anticipators of the present situation. They reasoned—and, let it be clear, they were reasoners who also inhabited the culture determined by secular rationality and made use of its understandings, so far as they went—that such rationality was not by itself sufficient. It needed supplementation, correlation with other approaches, and the examination of its presuppositions.

So it was that these pioneer bioethicists suggested, in broad scope, that ethical decision had to include other instruments than mere secular rationality "in the original position." Among these were narrative, tradition, memory, community, affection, and hope. These other instruments helped provide some sort of access to orders of reality that went and go by various code names: the transcendent, the sacred, the spiritual, the wholistic.

They did not find a plain or stay still. These bioethicists in some cases themselves lost patience or faith or position, and some of them moved into secular academies or medical institutions where their distinctive voices were muffled or they were simply outnumbered or outshouted. But today, as the following pages make clear, there is in this variety of institutions, and among the public at large, a new openness to resuming the climb at places and in ways that allow for fresh perspectives, including the religious and the theological.

It would be nice to assure readers that if they follow the route picked up and advanced by the authors of this book they will find a new plain. It would be pleasing to advertise that a new agreed-upon symbol system and formal set of meanings would now be available, and everyone could rest or at least could feel assured that they were on solid footing.

No, it wouldn't. It wouldn't be nice or good because such assurances and advertisements would not do justice to reality. And bioethics will not prosper or be of use if it loses touch with reality. The reality is that, in the midst of the pluralisms and relativisms, the enterprises and innovations, the technological breakthroughs and political desperations that make up the late-modern condition, they were only moving us to new ridges, new *arêtes*. And instead of providing encompassing philosophies or systematic theologies, they offer us, as the first word of the title says appropriately, "Notes."

Fine. Mountain climbers who come across bottled notes that suggest ways ahead, or report on false trails to be avoided, welcome what they find. In the pursuit of health and medicine today, new patients, new peoples, new procedures, some of them perplexing and others full of promise, are ahead. Facing them, "if we do not move we fall," it will be clear that "movement is heretical." The authors may draw upon old orthodoxies and pay respect to finders of old routes. No one is invited or allowed to stop along the way, to sit still, to rest on their climbing laurels, or be content with inherited perspectives. "No route is truly orthodox."

If not orthodox, however, they are still routes. And those of us—all of us—who are impelled to the fields implied by bioethics will find reason to welcome these notes along the way on the narrow ridge where religion and bioethics come together to form, not a plain, but a sharp *arête*. The only place to be.

NOTES

1. E. Mendelson, ed., *W.H. Auden: Collected Poems* (New York: Random House, 1976).

Acknowledgments

We have not opened a book in our lives that does not indicate the extraordinary debt that editors owe their contributors. This one is, of course, no exception. The notes for this book began in hallway conversations and back-row comments at conferences in bioethics, emerged fully in panels on the topic, and have become the wonderful articles that you hold in your hand. None of this could have been possible without the careful scholarship of the authors in this book, all of whom have written passionately about the subject at the very heart of their professional lives. We thank them for this work, and for the commitment that animates the field of bioethics. We are privileged and honored by their commitment to this project.

This book came into being because Leslie LeBlanc approached us after a session at an American Association for Bioethics meeting and asked us if we would turn that session into this volume. We are so pleased to have worked with her and with April McNamee over the years of production. University Publishing Group and *The Journal of Clinical Ethics* have long been a home for serious reflection on the role and meaning of religion in the field of bioethics, and we are grateful for such steadfast support. Leslie is far more than an editor—she is a colleague and a friend, whose intellectual contribution pushes the discourse forward, and whose warmth and humor allow it to flourish. We thank Norman Quist, the publisher, and stauch supporter of this project from the start, who suggested the applicability of Buber's use of the narrow ridge in addressing the issues connecting bioethics and religion.

We also wish to thank our families, especially our children: Andrew Jesse (DSD) and Matthew, Noah, Benjamin, Joshua, and Sarah (LZ) for understanding and cheerleading.

Many thanks to William C. Walsh, who made the photograph that appears on the front cover, "Alpine-glow on Mount Whitney at Sunrise," taken in the Alabama Hills above Movie Flat in Lone Pine, California, on October 18, 1997.

Finally, we wish to thank our teachers, many of whom honor us with their contributions to this book, and our students.

I have learned much from my teachers, more from my friends, and from my students, most of all.
        —Rabbi Hanina, Babylonian Talmud, Ta'anith, 7a.

Introduction

Dena S. Davis

This volume began life in 1993 as a panel discussion at the first meeting of the American Association of Bioethics. The title, as I recall, was "The Role of Religious Studies in Bioethics," and the members included four of the authors represented in the book. Laurie Zoloth and I presided jointly; Steve Lammers and Tom Shannon participated. To our surprise and delight, the room was packed, and not only with other scholars of religion. Many people in the interdisciplinary field of bioethics were genuinely curious about how we fit in, what we had to offer, whether and why our influence was waning, and if that was a good or a bad thing.

We created this book to address those questions. We asked some of the most thoughtful practitioners in the field to reflect on their role(s) in the endeavor we call bioethics, given the following factors:

- the interdisciplinary nature of the fields of bioethics and of religious studies
- the challenge to religion by philosophy for ownership of the keys to the values shop
- the ambiguous status of any claims to religious or ethical truths in our post-modern era.

We asked contributors to think about what someone with training and scholarship in religious studies brings to the bioethics enterprise. What can they offer that is not already offered by philosophy or anthropology? Do they think they have anything special to say about swimming in this pluralistic world in which doctor, patient, nurse, and ethicist may each come from a different religious tradition? As H. Tristram Engelhardt, Jr. asks in the opening paragraph of chapter 6, "After all, philosophical bioethics analyzes issues, clarifies arguments, and assesses justifications for claims. What more could one want? What more would one need and why?"

In the 1960s, the decade in which bioethics began to emerge as a separate field, no one would have thought to ask these questions. Without scholars of religious studies, bioethics itself would hardly have existed. Scholars of religion were in at the creation. Joseph Fletcher's *Morals and Medicine* (1954) and Paul Ramsey's *The Patient as Person* (1970) are widely regarded as founding documents.[1] Daniel Callahan, in a brief history of bioethics, sees these two theologians as the bookends of American bioethics, which ultimately chose a middle course between "the Joseph Fletcher route of totally blessing everything that came along, or the Paul Ramsey route of seeming to reject everything."[2] Although one trembles to make a list of founding fathers lest someone be left out, everyone conversant with the early days of bioethics would include such names as James Childress, John Fletcher, James Gustafson, Stanley Hauerwas, Albert Jonsen, Richard McCormick, Warren Reich, Robert Veatch, and LeRoy Walters—all trained in some aspect of religious ethics. Later, as the male hegemony began to break down, Lisa Cahill, Beverly Harrison, Karen Lebacqz, and other women entered the field. A more recent phenomenon is the contribution of Jewish studies scholars such as Elliott Dorff, David Novak, and Laurie Zoloth. Islamicists such as Abdul-Aziz Sacherdina are also contributing to the field of bioethics.

As I write in 1999 however, it is clear that we need to take stock and make explicit our claim to a unique contribution to bioethics. First, the proliferation and reorganization of professional societies, with their concomitant subcategories of interest groups, tends to spotlight people's professional pedigrees. Second, philosophy, by sheer numbers, threatens to overwhelm the contribution of religious studies to bioethics. Third, the age of self-styled bioethicists ("have values, will travel") is giving way to an era of credentials and a perceived need, at least by some, to delineate what combinations of degrees and experience are the minimum criteria for calling oneself a bioethicist.

It is an interesting point that at least four of the contributors to this volume (including myself) might well not be recognized by the casual reader of bioethics as coming from a religious studies background. Since my own view of academic disciplines is omnivorous and eclectic, I do not find that disturbing, but sometimes find it puzzling. James Gustafson, in a famous essay in 1978, criticized religious ethicists who fail to make explicit the religious grounding of their positions, and said, "They will either have to become moral philosophers with a special interest in 'religious' texts and arguments, or become theologians," with overt grounding in specific theological perspectives and methodologies.[3] Some contributors to this volume would situate themselves on one side of Gustafson's forced choice, some on the other; many would deny the validity of the dichotomy. (I have always thought it interesting, in this context, that James F. Childress and Tom L. Beauchamp, in their introduction to the first edition of their groundbreaking *Principles of Biomedical Ethics*, make something of their differing allegiances to deontological versus utilitarian theories of ethics, but fail to even mention that one is a religious ethicist—or at least has his degree in that discipline—while the other is a philosopher.)[4] But those of us who are comfortable functioning—at least some of the time—as moral philosophers with a special interest and expertise in religious texts and arguments (or religious behaviors and "sensibilities," to use Ronald Green's term) then must face the challenge of the moral philosophers. Is our training in moral philosophy as rigorous and complete as theirs, with our knowledge of religion a "value-added" dimension (to borrow Thomas A. Shannon's vocabulary)? Or is our training and perspective fundamentally different? If the latter, do we merit Gustafson's jibe that "an ethicist is a former theologian who does not have the professional credentials of a moral philosopher"?[5] And if these distinctions matter, are they important only when we are operating at the level of "deep theory," or do they also make a difference at the more practical level—for example, when choosing people to serve on local hospital ethics committees or selecting members of national commissions?

In some sense, religion and bioethics are inseparable. Religion, after all, deals with "life, death, and the meaning of everything," to quote *The Hitchhiker's Guide to the Galaxy.* Part of religion's continuing appeal is that it is a powerful maker of meaning when things go awry—when babies are born deformed, when couples prove infertile, when people die too young. It is entirely appropriate that many of the chapters in this collection focus at least partly on the clinical experience. Clinical bioethics, as Courtney Campbell notes in chapter 2, "is beset with a reality that is not acknowledged in its fullness by academics—namely, the continued reminders of human finitude and mortality." This reality is the very stuff of religion. As Laurie Zoloth reminds us: "Hence, in the clinical world, where much has gone astray—where we are already dealing with the outskirts of the expectable, controllable world—we are confronted with both the force and the pluralities of religious explanatory narrative. In fact, it is precisely at the moment of crisis in the clinic that there is the utter recognition that the medical gesture (even the dramas of reproductive technology) is actually a gesture concerning death. This is a moment that Americans see as their most religious, a moment when what is at stake is the relationship between the self and God."[6]

Religious studies have never been able totally to escape into symbolic abstraction, a constant temptation for philosophy. K. Danner Clouser has said that many philosophers disdained bioethics as something "unworthy of the higher calling of philosophy—unworthy because bioethics was seen as a mechanic's job of merely applying the intellectual masterpieces of real philosophers to practical and mundane problems, and real philosophers, after all, do not traffic in the mundane."[7] Although the connections between religious studies and theology and between scholars and practitioners (often the same people wearing slightly different hats) have often been confusing and even conflicted,[8] they have also been an invaluable tether to reality. After all, physicians and clergy are old companions, meeting from time immemorial over the beds of the ill and the dying, well aware that the boundaries of their respective portfolios are porous indeed. Christian bioethicist Stanley Hauerwas explains, "As a theologian I have been drawn to medicine because it provides the issues where we might see again what difference Christian convictions or their absence might have for how we live."[9]

For religious studies, bioethics began with the sticky issues that arise at the bedside or in the confessional. Thomas A. Shannon notes in chapter 7 that many religious orders held regular case conferences very like our current practice in bioethics. In religious bioethics, we are still aware that the clergy and seminary professors who make up part of our professional ranks will be taking home a message that may eventually trickle down and influence how a rabbi counsels a member of her congregation or how an imam interprets the Koran. Thus, the problem Claude Welch identified in his 1971 report on graduate education in religion, where he described the field as "a science divided between the community of faith and the secular academy," has its positive aspects.[10] One could also describe the field as enriched by people who move between the community of faith and the secular academy; part of that enrichment is the connection to preaching and pastoral activities that are tied ineluctably to events, often medical events, in actual people's lives.

The distinction between theology and religious studies is too complex and contentious an issue to take up here with any adequacy. It used to be said that theology is the study of a single faith while religious studies looks at many,[11] but that is obviously incorrect; theologians may engage in interfaith dialogue, and rigorously scientific scholars may spend their careers analyzing only one faith tradition. Nor should we tolerate the rather silly nomenclature by which "comparative religion" becomes a code name for academic objectivity. (Indeed, the traditional distinction between "objective" and "subjective" ways of studying something can be attempted today only to a background chorus of postmodernist giggles. This contemporary view may also have put the kibosh on that handy dichotomy: normative versus descriptive.) A useful approach is suggested by Michael Slusser:

> The distinctive questions which the theologian asks of reality are, "What should we believe, what should we do, and why?" The "should" points to the critical character of the inquiry: a decision as to truth or falsity, doing or not doing, is the goal, and the theologian must be prepared to act on it whether or not it matches his or her preconceptions. The "we" points to the communal character, that the theologian's inquiry tries to serve a community of which he or she is a part. . . . In contrast, religious studies . . . studies religion and religious traditions without asking, "Should we believe and do this?" and in fact without asking "Should they or anyone believe and do this?" Such questions, the really interesting questions to theologians, are considered improper and beyond the purview of religious studies, and the scholar of religion is expected to bracket personal and communal religious commitments.[12]

The existence, in one and the same discipline (often, in one and the same department) of scholars who do and those who do not ask the "should" questions has given rise to a good deal of friction and arguably even incoherence, but it has also guaranteed that the "should" questions are not allowed to disappear. Bioethics, of course, also asks "should" questions, because it is a field of inquiry in which scholars from a host of disciplines come together to train their gaze upon practical problems and human tragedies in which choices need to be made. And because the questions asked in bioethics are those asked in religious studies and theology as well—should we prolong life in the face of great physical pain? Should we legalize abortion? Should we encourage infertile couples to use cloning as a way to have a child?—there is a natural affinity of the one for the other.

Religious studies, at least part of the time, has a built-in constituency that philosophy lacks. To take an example, Cynthia Cohen, a senior fellow at the Kennedy Institute of Ethics who is a member of the Standing Commission on National Concerns of the Protestant Episcopal Church, recently published a paper on suicide from the perspective of that tradition.[13] Although her conclusions bind no one, they do speak with special force to a particular community, which shares a narrative and attempts to live by certain values and which will at least take note of her report even if it rejects her conclusions. There is no such natural constituency for philosophy (although philosophers can create such constituencies by getting appointed to commissions or as advisors to professional organizations).

We hope the constituency for this book includes scholars within and without religious studies—as well as everyone concerned with bioethics, its interdisciplinary character, and its internal and external conversations. The contributors to this volume all "do" bioethics, and they all come from the home discipline of religious studies.

In chapter 1, I repeat a challenge originally articulated in a 1994 article in *The Journal of Clinical Ethics*. I sketch out some tasks of religious scholars who choose to write on bioethics, and argue that at least one task, that of accurate description and analysis of *behavior* of religious adherents, particularly when it does not comport with the precepts stated by religious authorities, is going undone.

In chapter 2, Courtney S. Campbell explores the different contexts in which the role of bioethics must be pursued, examining variously pedagogical, clinical, institutional, community, civil, and policy bioethics. Ronald A. Carson describes himself in chapter 3 as a practitioner of "problematic theology [that] eschews apologetics and instead joins practitioners of other humanities disciplines in sorting through experience and trying to make livable sense of it." That almost sounds like a definition of bioethics itself.

Using as his example the current controversy over human cloning, and drawing upon his experiences as a member of the National Bioethics Advisory Commission (NBAC), James F. Childress asks in chapter 4 about "the proper role for religious convictions in the formulation of bioethical public policy in a liberal, pluralistic democracy." In chapter 5, Dolores L. Christie examines what religion offers—a community, a set of attitudes, a location vis-à-vis the sacred—in relation to the tasks of bioethics, including finding solutions to concrete dilemmas and making public policy, and she looks critically at some stumbling blocks to the dialogue between religion and bioethics.

In chapter 6, H. Tristram Engelhardt, Jr. asserts that "the role of religious studies in bioethics depends crucially on the role, experience, and meaning of religion in bioethics," and assesses the possibilities for and implications of "a bioethics grounded in the revelation of a transcendent God." Thomas A. Shannon speaks in chapter 7 of religion and bioethics as a "value-added" discussion that can offer additional resources as bioethics moves away from an overemphasis on the individual to a greater focus on social justice. Stephen E. Lammers, on the other hand, criticizes religious bioethicists (chapter 8) for not doing more to move the field in the direction of social justice issues, especially issues of access to medical care. Further, Lammers critiques the history of bioethics, which can be understood primarily as "the attempt to think out the implications of making choice the central datum in medical care." One implication of this centrality of choice is that religion, too, is seen as one more choice that a patient might make, rather than as a commitment or covenant to which the patient is called.

Ronald M. Green, in chapter 9, is responsive to this challenge when he posits a "bioethical sensibility" that includes a tradition's teaching and texts, but also its economic, social, and cultural history. Michael M. Mendiola argues in chapter 10 for the special contribution religious ethics can make at the public policy level. Taking John Robertson as her sparring partner, Karen Lebacqz asserts in chapter 11 that there is no way to keep religious convictions out of public policy making in bioethics, for those convictions "determine the very questions we ask and the assumptions that undergird our answers." She goes on to argue that "sectarian voices are necessary for public policy making precisely because they will lift up concerns that are neglected by the majority voice."

Laurence J. O'Connell and Martin E. Marty (chapter 12) see bioethics and religion as coming together more fruitfully in recent years, after an earlier relationship marked by "specialization and misunderstanding." They also point to the current interest in alternative and holistic healing as evidence of the public's continuing interest in a connection between medicine and spirituality. In chapter 13, Daniel P. Sulmasy argues that all theories of bioethics, whether categorized as religious or philosophical, depend on an underlying *mythos* or story about the meaning of human life. Thus, to distinguish between religious and nonreligious moral theories, or to privilege some and marginalize others, is based on a profound misconception about the ethical project itself.

In chapter 14, Laurie Zoloth revisits her original response to my article, and goes on to explore how Jewish ethics, in particular, is "a conversion point" in an ongoing discourse about the place of "God talk" in the discipline of bioethics.

Today's bioethicists seem to be in a self-reflective mood, sparked perhaps by the coming millennium, by a massive reorganization of competing professional societies into the new American Society for Bioethics and Humanities, by the ongoing debate about credentialing, and by the proliferation of graduate-level programs in bioethics. As part of this reflective process, we in religious studies are asking: Who are we? What do we know? What can we contribute? We hope this volume will be a useful and provocative part of that process.

NOTES

1. J.F. Fletcher, *Morals and Medicine* (Princeton, N.J.: Princeton University Press, 1954); P. Ramsey, *The Patient as Person* (New Haven, Conn.: Yale University Press, 1970).

2. D. Callahan, "Why America Accepted Bioethics," in "The Birth of Bioethics" (special supplement), ed. A.R. Jonsen, *Hastings Center Report* 23, no. 6 (1993): S8-S9.

3. J.M. Gustafson, "Theology Confronts Technology and the Life Sciences," *Commonweal* 105 (1978): 386-92, p. 392.

4. T.L. Beauchamp and J.F. Childress, *Principles of Biomedical Ethics* (New York: Oxford University Press, 1979), 40.

5. See note 3 above, p. 386.

6. See chapter 14 of this volume, p. 257.

7. K. Danner Clouser, "Bioethics and Philosophy" in "The Birth of Bioethics" (special supplement), ed. A.R. Jonsen, *Hastings Center Report* 23, no. 6 (1993): S10-S11.

8. D.G. Hart, "The Troubled Soul of the Academy: American Learning and the Problem of Religious Studies," in *Religion and American Culture*, ed. G. Marsden (San Diego, Calif.: Harcourt, Brace, Jovanovich, 1990), 49-61.

9. S. Hauerwas, "Why I Am Neither a Communitarian Nor a Medical Ethicist," in "The Birth of Bioethics" (special supplement), ed. A.R. Jonsen, *Hastings Center Report* 23, no. 6 (1993): S9-S10.

10. C. Welch, quoted in Hart, see note 8 above, p. 65.

11. Michael Slusser quotes Arvind Sharma as attributing this view to Ray Hart. See M. Slusser, "Theology and Religious Studies: A Reply to Bulletin 26/4," *Council of Societies for the Study of Religion Bulletin* 27, no. 1 (1998): 9.

12. Ibid.

13. C.C. Cohen, "Christian Perspectives on Assisted Suicide and Euthanasia: The Anglican Tradition," in *Physician-Assisted Suicide: Expanding the Debate*, ed. M.P. Battin, R. Rhodes, and A. Silvers (New York: Routledge, 1998), 334-46.

1

It Ain't Necessarily So: Clinicians, Bioethics, and Religious Studies

Dena S. Davis

INTRODUCTION

The central tenet of the bioethics movement has been the importance of understanding and respecting patients' values. This focus on values is crucial to virtually every area of discussion in bioethics, including informed consent, so-called compliance, and decision making with and for the terminally ill. As a result of the bioethics movement, the emphasis on multiculturalism in all areas of American life, and the increased visibility of disciplines such as medical anthropology and sociology, there is a growing awareness that healthcare providers need to be knowledgeable about the religious and cultural values of the people they treat.[1] If only for this reason, religious ethics scholars will always have an important role in the interdisciplinary enterprise of bioethics.

What are clinicians looking for from scholars of religious ethics? Put from another perspective, how can scholars of religion be useful to clinicians who are dealing with actual patients? Religious studies scholars were instrumental in the founding of bioethics,[2] but despite debate among the scholars themselves as to what they ought to be doing, there has not been much dialogue between scholars and clinicians. This chapter posits some ways that religious ethics scholars can meet the needs of clinicians. It argues that the clinicians' needs should translate into goals for at least some religious ethics scholars, or at least some of those who contribute regularly to the field of bioethics. It demonstrates how poorly religious ethics scholars are meeting those needs at the present time and suggests some paths for improvement.

Perhaps the most important need that clinicians have of religion scholars is for them to describe religiously motivated behavior and values as they relate to bioethics issues. Although in our current debates in bioethics we tend to employ a deliberately secular vocabulary,[3] patients are likely to be significantly influenced by their own religious backgrounds and beliefs when they make decisions. It hardly needs saying that the stuff of bioethics—life and death, the definition of personhood, the meaning of suffering—goes to the very core of religious belief. Furthermore, in many religious traditions, most obviously the Roman Catholic, church leaders have attempted to codify the correct responses for believers who are faced with such dilemmas as infertility, an unexpected pregnancy, or a family member in a persistent vegetative state. Thus, a clinician who wishes to be sensitive to a patient's values must have some awareness of the patient's religious beliefs (or lack thereof). That was difficult enough for dear old Marcus Welby. But today, in a typical American city, a clinician might treat patients who are Catholic, Protestant, Hindu, Jewish, or Muslim—all in the course of one day. And even these terms are crude categories that mask a tremendous variety; an Irish Catholic whose family has been here for generations may have a constellation of beliefs and practices that is very different from that of a recent immigrant from El Salvador. And what about a Korean Baptist, a Vietnamese Catholic, or a Ugandan Jehovah's Witness?

The busy clinician hardly has time to get a doctorate in comparative religious ethics, and usually must rely on the religious studies "presence" in bioethics journals, reference works such as *The Encyclopedia of Bioethics*,[4] and various panels, presentations, and workshops. Scholars of religious ethics should keep in mind the following four goals when addressing an audience of clinicians:

1. Religious ethicists[5] should explain the role and function of religious beliefs in the lives of individuals and in the culture as a whole.
2. Religious ethicists should explain how a specific religion wrestles with a moral issue and describe the religion's current teaching.
3. Religious ethicists should describe how real people actually believe and act.

4. Religious ethicists, like all scholars, must employ their expertise in a helpful and honest manner.

Of course, not every presentation can or should fulfill all of these goals.

GOAL 1

Religious ethicists should explain the role and function of religious beliefs in the lives of individuals and in the culture as a whole. If a person says that he is Lutheran and a ballet dancer, and that he grew up in North Dakota and now lives in Chicago, how might one expect his religion, culture, and experience to influence his health-related behaviors and values? What might he mean by saying he is Lutheran? Does he mean that he goes to a Lutheran church weekly and teaches in the Sunday school, or that he was raised Lutheran but is now irreligious, or that he is a faithful churchgoer for the companionship and the music but has no interest in doctrine and gets all his ideas about issues in bioethics from the *New York Times*? Obviously, religious ethics cannot give clinicians these answers, but it can suggest a set of questions—a way of thinking about religion and the roles it plays in people's lives—that will be helpful to the clinician trying to build a picture of the patient and the patient's values.

GOAL 2

Religious ethicists should explain how a specific religion wrestles with a moral issue and describe the religion's current teaching. For example, in an essay a religious ethicist might explain how the Roman Catholic church uses scripture, tradition, secular disciplines, and contemporary experience to arrive at its official teachings on a specific issue, what authority the church assumes when speaking to the faithful on this issue, and how much room exists for dissent and change.[6] Although this type of essay is the one most commonly found in bioethics literature, it is the least useful to the clinician. Clinicians might consult such an essay to help them think about their own religious values, such as whether it is permissible for a clinician as a Catholic to work in a hospital that performs abortions. Or, out of intellectual curiosity, someone might pursue the question of why official Catholic teaching prohibits the use of oral contraceptives while Orthodox Jewish teaching permits it. But most clinicians primarily are interested in people's actual behavior and beliefs, not in the official set of behaviors and beliefs that religious authorities would like their constituents to have.

GOAL 3

Religious ethicists should describe how real people actually believe and act. James Wind wrote, "Religion's first contribution . . . is to furnish a more accurate view of the human beings whom we encounter in the secular worlds of the academy, health care, and public policy."[7] We are now moving into the province of the anthropology and sociology of religion. Without some understanding of theology and religious ethics, however, mere description will not take us very far. For example, we know that the abortion rate among Catholic women in America is 38 percent higher than among Protestant women, relative to their respective proportions in the U.S. population.[8] But the meaning and inner experience of those abortions will differ according to whether the woman is a devout Catholic or evangelical Protestant whose religion condemns abortion, a liberal Protestant whose religion permits it, or perhaps a "lapsed" Catholic who is still struggling to come to terms with the tradition she has left.

By any standard, Americans are the most religious people in the industrial West.[9] However, the mix of religious belief and practice works out differently for each person, and the clinician's goal is to understand the individual patient standing before him or her. Often, the patient's attitudes reflect a mixture of religious teachings and reactions against the teachings. David Lodge's novel, *Souls and Bodies*, about young Catholics in the 1950s, contains a perfect example of this. Beset by the pressures of sexual desire, incomes that cannot expand as fast as their families, and the church's ban on all forms of "artificial contraception," the young married couples make their own compromises. Violet, after one child and one miscarriage, decides to "go on the pill," despite the fact that she believes that she has "effectively excommunicated herself." Having placed herself out of the Catholic community, at least in her own mind, she finds herself more open to crossing other boundaries, including having oral sex with her husband. Eventually, mutual masturbation and oral sex become their preferred and only forms of lovemaking. One night her husband remarks that if this is all they are going to do, she might as well stop taking the pill. "If I wasn't on the Pill, I wouldn't be doing it," she replies.[10] This woman's choice of contraceptive is still very much driven by church teaching, but hardly in the predictable direction. A sensitive physician, trying to understand this patient, must have a rudimentary knowledge of Roman Catholic teaching—but also so much more. To begin with, the physician must understand why someone who disobeys church teaching, and thus defines herself out of the church, may still feel every inch a Catholic. The physician who is a Unitarian, an agnostic, or a Reform Jew, may have trouble understanding the hold that church teachings have over Violet even when she opposes them.

Scholars of religious studies serve clinicians poorly in large part because they ignore the third goal, and then compound the problem by pretending that the third goal is subsumed in the second. The unspoken premise is that if one knows the religious teaching, one knows people's behavior as well. We fail to make clear the differences between the ideal and the real or between theory and practice; we tend to speak entirely in the language of theory and analysis, ignoring actual behavior. Furthermore, we often give preference to the orthodox perspective on an issue without regard to how widely it is accepted by members of that religious tradition.[11]

To illustrate these points, let me draw a picture of a hypothetical young woman, a composite of many of the students to whom I taught bioethics at the University of Iowa. This woman, let's call her Gwen, has just graduated from medical school and accepted a residency in obstetrics and gynecology (ob/gyn) in New York City. She grew up in Iowa and took her undergraduate and medical degrees there. She is very bright and open to new ideas but limited in her exposure to members of religious and racial minorities. That is one of the reasons she has elected to do her residency in New York.

Gwen knows that respecting patients' values is not only good ethics but good medicine as well. If their values are ignored, patients are less likely to follow the prescribed regimen, return for follow-up, and so on. So Gwen figures that she should do a little reading on Jewish attitudes toward such issues as contraception and abortion. (Judaism serves as the example here, but the same critique could apply to other traditions as well.)

Where would Gwen turn for some information? Let's think a little more about Gwen and the questions that she might ask. Gwen is not a student of religion; she probably majored in the sciences. She may be aware that Judaism has four branches, but she probably does not know what that means. She also has not framed her questions with the precision of a religious studies scholar; she just knows that she is going to be treating a lot of Jewish people and that the issues that routinely arise in an ob/gyn practice are often those that religious groups feel strongly about. If pressed to formulate her questions, she would respond something like, "What attitudes do Jews have toward contraception, abortion, and so on, and what am I likely to run into in the patients I treat?"

So Gwen is looking for basic introductory information. I see her going to an obvious source—*The Encyclopedia of Bioethics.*[12] This is an indispensable resource and the first place to which I send students looking for introductory material. The *Encyclopedia* defines itself as "a reference work . . . that gather[s] together . . . what is known about the questions of bioethics, the data from which they arise, a full range of responses to them, and the principles and values that account for those responses" (p. xvi).

What does Gwen find, and why is it problematic? She finds seven articles on Judaism—one a general overview and the others focused on specific issues. But these articles, and the composite picture they present, are seriously deficient. First, she finds little or no discussion of how the writers perceive their work or what question(s) the authors are attempting to address. Second, as an inquiring reader without the expertise to read between the lines, Gwen gets a picture of a Judaism that can only be described as a fantasy world. There are almost no similarities between the views set forth by the authors and the behaviors and attitudes of most Jewish people. In respect to this second point, Gwen almost would have been better off had she done no reading at all. These points are discussed in order.

First, what is the purpose of the article? Let's imagine that Gwen looks up the essay entitled "Abortion: Jewish Perspectives," in the *Encyclopedia.* The essay, written by Talmudic authority David Feldman, begins, "The abortion question in Talmudic law begins for some with an examination of the fetus' legal status" (p. 5). Hmm. If the answer is Talmudic, what is the question? Why does Feldman, or the editors, assume that the typical reader who wants to know something about Jews and abortion is interested primarily in Talmud? Gwen could have a couple of responses to this article. She could be put off at the outset by the unexplained connection between her inquiry into the attitudes of Jewish patients that she is likely to meet and the Talmudic discussion that she finds here. But let's give her more credit than that. Say she reads the article and is quite intrigued. "I get it," she thinks. "When asking about Jews, the answer is Talmudic. I guess that means that I can infer their

behavior and attitudes from the Talmudic precepts Feldman explains."
Nothing could be further from the truth, but how is Gwen to know
that? Nothing in Feldman's article or in the cross-references or bibliog-
raphy that follow it suggests that the answer to the question could be
descriptive—that is, that it might paint a picture of how Jews in America
and elsewhere think and behave around the abortion question.

Second, to the extent that it is possible to infer anything about contemporary Jewish attitudes and behavior from the articles Gwen has
looked at, what picture is given and how does it comport with reality?
For most clinicians, this is probably the most important issue. In Gwen's
case, she almost would have done better to have read nothing at all. If we
compare the pronouncements made in the *Encyclopedia* with actual Jewish behavior in the United States and Israel, we find the discontinuity to
be striking.

For example, in the *Encyclopedia*, Feldman states: "Abortion for
'population control' is repugnant to the Jewish mind. Abortion for economic reasons is also not admissible" (p. 8). Jakobovits claims: "There is
general agreement on requiring [abortion] to save the mother's life and
on forbidding it for purely social or economic reasons" (p. 793). In reality, among Israeli Jews, there are more abortions than live births.[13] In the
United States, in a 1989 survey 75 percent of Jews—more than double
the percentage of non-Jews—responded "yes" when asked, "Suppose your
unmarried teenage daughter told you she was pregnant and intended to
have an abortion. Would you support her decision to have an abortion?"[14]

Also in the *Encyclopedia*, Jakobovits grades the various methods of
birth control, from most to least acceptable: (1) the pill or the intrauter-
ine device (IUD) (if not an abortifacient); (2) female sterilization; (3) post-
coital douche; (4) cervical cap; (5) spermicides; (6) diaphragm; (7) IUD as
an abortifacient; (8) condom, "to be used only in extreme cases of acute
danger and if other means are unavailable or unacceptable" (p. 800) Male
sterilization is not even ranked on the list, as the author asserts that it is
never acceptable as a contraceptive measure but permitted "only if urgently necessary as a therapeutic measure" (p. 800). In reality, Jews seem
to choose contraceptives in near opposition to the dictates of Jewish law.
The diaphragm is the method of choice, closely followed by the condom.
The pill is somewhere in the middle, and sterilization is also popular
(used by 18 percent of females and 13 percent of males).[15]

How are we to understand the abyss that separates the written material from the reality of Jewish life? These authors do not understand that
their writing should be descriptive; they assume that, by reporting what

the most respected Orthodox rabbis have written, they have told readers all that they need to know.

This misunderstanding appears to pervade *The Journal of Clinical Ethics (JCE)* as well. *JCE* holds itself out as a resource for health professionals seeking practical responses to clinical issues, but its articles on Jewish topics, which could have been so helpful to the practitioner, are mired in the same problems described above. Fred Rosner and Benjamin Freedman, two authors who have written about Judaism in *JCE*, do explain at the outset that they are interested in applying Jewish law to contemporary issues. However, Gwen would face the same confusion and misleading statements in *JCE* that she found in the *Encyclopedia*. For example, in an article on social issues related to the human immunodeficiency virus (HIV) "from the perspective of Jewish law and values," Freedman informs readers that "male homosexual activity" is "sinful" in "rabbinic Judaism."[16] Quite correct. But because he does not define "rabbinic Judaism," Gwen may not understand that he roughly means "Talmudic Judaism" by this, and she certainly will not find out from Freedman that homosexuality is not considered sinful or a bar to ordination in Reform Judaism.

Another misleading article is Rosner's "Screening for Tay-Sachs Disease: A Note of Caution."[17] This is precisely the sort of essay that one hopes for from *JCE*. A practical discussion aimed at doctors and genetic counselors, it describes a New York City premarital screening program and purports to explain the background of religion and culture against which this disease needs to be understood. Unfortunately, Rosner obfuscates as much as he helps. Rosner includes only pronouncements by Orthodox rabbis—but the unwary reader may not realize this. Readers are not told what percentage of Jews are Orthodox, nor are they told what Jewish people really do. Readers are left with the strong impression that few if any Jews—certainly not religious Jews—would engage in amniocentesis and abortion to avert the birth of a baby with Tay-Sachs. In fact, when I made inquiries of the Tay-Sachs screening program at Montreal's Children's Hospital, a program that has been in existence for 20 years, I discovered that every Jewish woman with an at-risk pregnancy had availed herself of amniocentesis, and every fetus discovered to have Tay-Sachs had been aborted. I assume that this is typical of behavior in the United States as well.

I do not want to depict Gwen as so naïve that she would arrive in New York with the tranquil certainty that her Jewish patients will eschew condoms and male sterilization, practice abortion only to safeguard the health of the mother, and so on. But has she learned anything useful from her odyssey through bioethics? Arguably not—unless it is to appreciate the message that Sportin' Life sings in *Porgy and Bess,* "It Ain't Necessarily So."

GOAL 4

Religious ethicists, like all scholars, must employ their expertise in a helpful and honest manner. Precisely because bioethics is an interdisciplinary enterprise, it is crucial that all of us present our arguments and findings in ways that make our agendas clear.

Scholars of religion who are engaged in interdisciplinary endeavors need to pay attention to some basic pedagogical issues. When teaching students or conducting workshops, they may identify with certain views but must be careful to point to the existence of other perspectives. They should apply the same ethics to colleagues. To present one school of thought within a diverse religious tradition as if it equaled the entire tradition is dishonest. It is also disempowering, because it makes it much more difficult for nonexperts to pursue their own line of inquiry. As a scholar of law and religion, I am unable to evaluate the material I read by my colleagues in such areas as neurology or economics. If they are limiting their purview in order to privilege a particular point of view, they need to say so up front. Furthermore, editors have an obligation to invite a wide range of perspectives, even if this requires them to go beyond the obvious names and faces. Andrew Greeley, for example, is probably the reigning expert on the behavior and beliefs of American Catholics (including in his writings a fascinating discussion of how they are able to reject church teaching on the issues of contraception, divorce, and premarital sex, while accepting it on the issue of nuclear power).[18] Surely his writing, or comparable works, should be appearing in journals like *JCE*.

Renee Fox has written about the tentative and tenuous relations between bioethics and the social sciences.[19] This is unfortunate (and surprising) with respect to the sociology of medicine. It is equally sad with respect to the anthropology and sociology of religion, strong disciplines with an important contribution to make to bioethics. Editors and conference coordinators who invite anthropologists and sociologists of religion to play a greater role in the bioethics endeavor will provide an invaluable service to clinicians and patients.

NOTES

1. P. Marshall, "Anthropology and Bioethics," *Medical Anthropology Quarterly* 6 (1992): 49-73; J.C. Barker, "Cultural Diversity—Changing the Context of Medical Practice," *Western Journal of Medicine* 157 (1992): 248-54; J. Klessig, "The Effect of Values and Culture on Life-Support Decisions," *Western Journal of Medicine* 157 (1992): 316-22.

2. A.R. Jonsen, "Forward," in *A Matter of Principles? Ferment in U.S. Bioethics*, ed. E.R. DuBose, R.P. Hamel, and L.J. O'Connell (Valley Forge, Penn.: Trinity Press International, 1993), ix-xvii.

3. R.C. Fox, "The Entry of Bioethics into the 1990s," in *A Matter of Principles?* Ibid., p. 53.

4. W.T. Reich, ed., *The Encyclopedia of Bioethics*, 2nd. ed. (New York: Simon & Schuster Macmillan, 1995).

5. I adopt this term for the sake of brevity. I do not mean to imply that scholars of religious ethics are necessarily religious themselves.

6. M.A. Farley, "An Ethic for Same-Sex Relations," in *A Challenge to Love: Gay and Lesbian Catholics in the Church*, ed. R. Nugent (New York: Crossroad Publishing, 1984), 93-106.

7. J.P. Wind, "What Can Religion Offer Bioethics?" *Hastings Center Report* 20, no. 4 (1990): 18-20.

8. S.K. Henshaw and J. Silverman, "The Characteristics and Prior Contraceptive Use of U.S. Abortion Patients," *Family Planning Perspectives* 20, no. 4 (1988): 158-68.

9. K.D. Wald, *Religion and Politics in the United States* (New York: St. Martin's Press, 1987).

10. D. Lodge, *Souls and Bodies* (New York: William Morrow, 1982), 155.

11. To some extent, this confusion mirrors an identity crisis within the field itself, as it grows from its historical roots in theology and moral theology (approached from within a faith perspective) to make room for the "objective" or "scientific" study of religion that is often called "religious studies" or "history of religions." See D.G. Hart, "The Troubled Soul of the Academy: American Learning and the Problem of Religious Studies," in *Religion and American Culture*, ed. G. Marsden (San Diego, Calif.: Harcourt, Brace, Jovanovich, 1990), 49-77. Most bioethicists are not quite sure what to call their religious studies colleagues, settling variously on "theologians," "religious ethicists," and the very misleading "religionist," which I assume is an attempt to make the name parallel with "anthropologist" and "sociologist."

12. W.T. Reich, ed., *The Encyclopedia of Bioethics* (New York: Free Press, 1978). All subsequent references to the *Encyclopedia* are to the 1978 edition. When I wrote this chapter, the revised edition had not been published (see note 4 above). For a review of the second edition with respect to some of these issues, see D.S. Davis, "The Jewish Tradition in the *Encylopedia of Bioethics,*" in *Reli-*

gious Studies Review 22, no. 4 (1996): 282-4.

13. E. Dorff, "Choose Life: A Jewish Perspective on Medical Ethics," *University Papers*, vol. 4, no. 1 (Los Angeles: University of Judaism, 1985).

14. S. Cohen, *The Dimensions of Jewish Liberalism* (New York: American Jewish Committee, 1989), 45.

15. C. Goldshieder and W.D. Mosher, "Patterns of Contraceptive Use in the United States: The Importance of Religious Factors," *Studies in Family Planning* 22 (1991): 102-15.

16. B. Freedman, "An Analysis of Some Social Issues Related to HIV Disease from the Perspective of Jewish Law and Values," *The Journal of Clinical Ethics* 1, no. 1 (1990): 45-9.

17. F. Rosner, "Screening for Tay-Sachs Disease: A Note of Caution," *The Journal of Clinical Ethics* 2, no. 4 (1991): 251-2.

18. A. Greeley, "Sex and Authority," in *American Catholics Since the Council: An Unauthorized Report* (Chicago: Thomas More Press, 1985).

19. R. Fox, "The Evolution of American Bioethics," in *Social Science Perspectives on Medical Ethics,* ed. G. Weisz (Philadelphia: University of Pennsylvania Press, 1991), 201-17.

2

Bearing Witness:
Religious Resistance and Meaning

Courtney S. Campbell

INTRODUCTION

In his thoughtful discussion of the role of religion in American public culture, Stephen L. Carter describes religious traditions as "autonomous communities of resistance and as independent sources of meaning."[1] This essay formulates and critically examines some of the implications of this interpretation of religion within the culture of bioethics. Although the concept of bioethics needs more specific qualification, as delineated below, this analysis draws primarily on two recent examples—debates over physician-assisted suicide and over human cloning—in which the contribution of religious thought to a bioethics question was contested and controversial. Despite these controversies, it is incumbent upon religious communities to "bear witness" and affirm precisely the kind of resistance and independence suggested by Carter.

PROFESSIONAL BIOETHICS:
RELIGIOUS BIOETHICS IN A PHILOSOPHICAL WORLD

For a good portion of the past two decades, the question of the relationship between religion and bioethics has largely been pursued from within the relatively safe havens of the academy. The discussion has been carried out among scholars trained in religious studies and their theological counterparts; it also occurs in professional journals and literature and at interdisciplinary academic meetings and conferences. In these professional contexts, the contribution of religious perspectives to bioethical reflection can be vigorously challenged. The discussion that follows briefly reviews and responds to some challenges to taking religious views seriously as presented by philosophical bioethicists.

One philosophical critique is that religious perspectives and arguments in bioethics borrow intellectual legitimacy and credibility from questions they purport to answer. Thus, religious traditions may be portrayed as offering "answers" to deep substantive questions about the meaning of suffering, or answers to practical questions such as the morality of abortion. The problem, at least in the philosophical view, is that the "questions" that religion attends to may not be terribly significant in the first place, and the "answers" turn out to be inextricable from broader metaphysical assumptions and particular traditions that are largely inaccessible, perhaps even incomprehensible, to the general public.

Now, there is no doubt some validity to this first criticism. Debates about birth control, for example, may seem trivial to persons outside a religious community. Even on the ultimate questions of life—such as human nature, the purpose of suffering, and death—religious thought can be tentative and intellectually exasperating. Yet, in general, this criticism radically misrepresents the character of religious scholarship in bioethics. In large measure, religious scholars seek to bear witness to the necessity of attending to basic questions of human purpose and meaning as part of the agenda of bioethics. And these questions can be embedded in debates even about birth control, which turn on understandings about issues such as human relationships, sexuality, and embodiment. These kinds of substantive questions, as the examples of assisted suicide and human cloning discussed later in the chapter suggest, are systematically ignored or marginalized by philosophical and policy-oriented bioethics. In response to this first critique, James M. Gustafson asserts: "Theology [and religious studies] might not provide answers you like to accept, but it can force questions you ought to be aware of."[2]

A second critique offered by philosophical bioethicists is that religious arguments and perspectives derive intellectual legitimacy and credibility from the limits of scientific discovery. That is to say, the deity of the Abrahamic religious traditions is a "God of the gaps"—for example, an explanation of the holes in scientific research about the origins of human life. Insofar as these gaps remain, and understanding them is central to many issues in bioethics, religious views presume to have bioethical relevance.

Certainly, religious studies scholars and theologians are sensitive to, and critical of, a "God of the gaps" approach to bioethics, particularly in the realms of reproductive technologies and genetics research. However, the philosophical criticism pits religion and science as adversaries in a manner that is simply unfair and unwarranted. Many of the Abrahamic traditions see the new knowledge about biological organisms revealed by scientific study not as a threat but as a witness to the wondrous complexity and gift of creation. There are religious motivations for the scientific quest, and not simply religious obstacles. Many within religious communities would agree with the perspective of Francis Collins, current head of the Human Genome Project: "For the scientist who is also a Christian, science is a form of worship. It is an uncovering of the incredible, awesome beauty of God's creation."[3] Without denying some significant differences, it is a careless oversimplification to see religious communities and scholars as engaged in a rearguard effort to save space for God in a secular world. Religious scholars can and do bear witness to the integrity and contributions of scientific research in shaping a comprehensive and adequate religious bioethics.

A third philosophical critique of religious argumentation in bioethics is that it tends to borrow selectively from authoritative sources—whether formative narratives, texts, or practices. Although this objection raises interesting questions of hermeneutical interpretation and authority, it sets the bar of consistency and coherence untenably high for even philosophical ethics to meet. We would rightly think it arbitrary to dismiss the wealth of philosophical and ethical insight from Aristotle on the basis of his biases about the nature of women. Similarly, the valuable contributions that Kant has made to philosophical reasoning, and to bioethics particularly, should not be discarded simply because Kant took an idiosyncratic view on tooth transplantation and considered it a form of self-murder. Part of what it means to be in a living moral tradition is to engage in interpretation, selection, and application of relevant historical materials—an approach that Michael Walzer has designated the "interpretative" path in moral philosophy.[4] This interpretative mode of ethics is perhaps a task that philosophical bioethicists should be more self-reflective about, and that scholars in religious studies should be prepared to bear witness to and explicate with respect to the traditions they study.

For all the searching substantiveness of these philosophical critiques, not a great deal of practical import has been at stake in how these issues have been resolved. This relative practical insignificance of professional bioethics stands in marked contrast to other contexts of bioethics in which religious studies and religious thought does have a relevant practical dimension. The sections that follow identify and discuss some of these contexts and provide examples to illustrate religious traditions as communities of resistance and independent meaning.

PEDAGOGICAL BIOETHICS

A first context in which the question of the relation between religious studies and bioethics discourse is often broached is in the classroom—what is designated as *pedagogical bioethics*. Scholars in religious studies confront a significant obstacle in teaching bioethics, because bioethics teaching anthologies exclude or marginalize religious thought. A current and otherwise useful text advocates "sidestepping religion" in order to conduct ethical argument. A religious approach to ethics, it is claimed, is "certain to produce a breakdown in communication and then a standoff," a situation that can be readily demonstrated by numerous historical examples.[5]

Indeed, with very few exceptions,[6] the principal teaching texts for courses in bioethics contain minimal materials from religious traditions that would lend themselves to religious studies scholarship. At best, an anthology may include a selection from a papal encyclical (for example, on a topic such as reproductive technology) to provide a contrasting perspective to a standard secular argument. This approach, however, gives a misleading impression to students about the nature of ethical dialogue within religious traditions and communities and overlooks the pluralism that exists among religious traditions on many issues in bioethics.

Thus, pedagogical bioethics is structured on the pretense that religion and religious studies are largely ethically irrelevant. Conversely, students with religious convictions come to see bioethics as primarily about procedure, and otherwise substantively shallow and spiritually hollow. In my teaching career, I have found that it requires considerable courage for a student to appeal to a religious value in the classroom setting. Students with substantive religious convictions are all too often silent in class; if they do venture an opinion, it is done so hesitantly—even apologetically—out of concern for offending the sentiments of nonreligious persons in the class. Sometimes, the issue *forces* the expression of a religious claim, most frequently when the value or sanctity of life is challenged by arguments about abortion, suicide, or euthanasia. This constricted classroom conversation (it cannot be called dialogue) is also misleading for students, for it can readily be concluded that religion is best kept out of civic discourse, that it is only a source of moral conflict (not moral contribution or resolution), and that religious arguments invariably support a form of vitalism.

Although the peers of students with religious views often state that they respect the opinions of classmates with religiously grounded positions, they tend to see religion as a form of coercion and thus are suspicious about the imposition of religious views. It thus turns out that religion can easily be a conversation stopper, rather than an invitation to deeper discussion in the classroom setting. This classroom scenario is often replicated at the level of public discourse about bioethics.

It might be countered that religious discourse is in one respect at the core of pedagogical bioethics, for language that comes readily to all students is that of "playing God." This phrase does not have great significance when used in the classroom; it typically is invoked as an indiscriminate shorthand description for what is occurring in a very complex situation requiring a decision about life or death, or in genetic questions. As Allen Verhey has commented of this phrase more generally, it "invokes a perspective," but, unless this perspective is critically and discriminately used, its moral substance is diluted and vacuous.[7]

It is nonetheless possible for teachers to use such moments of discursive dissonance to bring the insights and issues of religious studies into pedagogical bioethics. An appeal to playing God invites deeper reflection on both the notions of "play" and of "God," reflection that is necessary to give content to the normative force the phrase is presumed to have. More generally, teachers should emphasize at the outset of their courses that bioethics is necessarily an interdisciplinary enterprise that encompasses perspectives beyond those that may be represented in the textbook. In so doing, teachers should make an effort to have an open and welcoming classroom environment, rather than one in which, as one student put it, "God is made to hide in a corner" and some students, especially those with religious values, feel intimidated or defensive about voicing their convictions.

This open and inclusive environment can be fostered by using methods of religious reasoning and argumentation in a way that furthers the general purposes of teaching ethics. Daniel Callahan's influential essay on the subject identifies five basic goals in ethics teaching: (1) recognizing ethical issues, (2) stimulating moral imagination, (3) developing critical and analytical skills, (4) cultivating moral responsibility, and (5) tolerating moral conflict and ambiguity.[8] Religious narratives have been commonly used in the professional bioethics literature to help identify the ethical core of a situation. Religious methods of analogical reasoning not only can help students see an ethical issue in a different light, but also can enable the exercise of students' imaginative faculties. Religious communities can be portrayed as intermediate social institutions who do take substantive positions on many bioethical questions in what is otherwise a sea of cultural relativism. Teachers can encourage their students to study those viewpoints with the aim of illustrating the concept and meaning of moral responsibility.

If bioethics is understood not simply as an academic occupation by which intellectually minded persons engage in profound discourse with one another, but also as a social practice (namely teaching) involving deliberation upon profound *actions*—actions that reflect the meanings persons attach to their lives, relationships, and deaths—pedagogical bioethics will find in religious studies resources of moral wisdom and learning skills that are vital to the education of citizens.

CLINICAL BIOETHICS

Professional and pedagogical bioethics devotes attention to the study of actions and choices, but it is admittedly at some distance from the persons whose lives are directly affected by these actions. This limitation is one reason why the emergence of *clinical bioethics* over the past decade has been both necessary and significant. This form of bioethics emphasizes clinical interactions, primarily encounters between patients and professional caregivers, as the locus of ethical reflection in medical and nursing care. Other professionals, including academic bioethicists, may well be participants in clinical bioethics, through ethics rounds or consultations, but the relationship between patient and professional caregiver is the essential feature of ethical experience, action, and reflection. In this context, religious values may be relevant to ethical choices because of the religious convictions of either the patient or the professional; in both instances, religion is part of the moral matrix of clinical bioethics through the principle of respect for persons.

The potential for religious studies scholars to make a substantial contribution to bioethical deliberation may be greatest in this context although, as Stephen E. Lammers has observed, it is often not clear that this contribution comes from a person's role as scholar.[9] Nonetheless, bioethics scholarship, including that developed by persons in religious studies, has shown increasing sensitivity to the reality that persons experience ethical issues most significantly not through the grand policy quandaries posed in teaching anthologies, but rather by living with and through the anguish of patients, their families, and professionals in the clinical setting. Scholars in religious studies have, for example, contributed to the development of a series of short booklets by the Park Ridge Center designed to provide "accessible and practical information about the values and beliefs of different religious traditions" for an audience of nurses, physicians, chaplains, social workers, and administrators.[10] What is different and important about this scholarship is the audience and intended use. These are guides for practical decision making and caregiving, not treatises for academic debate. They also seek to avoid the generalizations academics can get away with about the position of such-and-such tradition by acknowledging the moral authority of the patient. The values identified in these practical resources as characteristic of a certain tradition are not intended to displace the religious views and convictions of the patient, but they can offer a supplementary guide.

One can acknowledge this kind of scholarly contribution and still ask whether professional and clinical bioethics function in their own insular and different worlds.[11] Clinical bioethics is beset with a reality that is not acknowledged in its fullness by academics—namely, the continued reminders of human finitude and mortality. In one respect, these features ought to make clinical bioethics very appealing to the scholar in religious studies, for a concern to articulate the purpose and meaning of these human experiences has been a core historical theme of religious communities. But the bedside is the place for compassionate human presence, not a scholarly presentation. The academic professional in the clinical setting risks the same mistake that Larry Churchill indicates befell the followers of Elisabeth Kubler-Ross—namely, the substitution of academic constructs and commentaries for the real "text," the stories of patients and their families as they engage in a narrative quest for meaning.[12] It is little surprise that Lammers (as does Churchill) commends *listening*, as well as humility and patience, for the professional bioethicist who ventures into the unfamiliar terrain of the clinic; these are valuable virtues for the moral life, but are not likely to bring tenure.

INSTITUTIONAL BIOETHICS

Institutional bioethics—whether in academic settings, such as institutional review boards (IRBs) or animal care committees, or in nonacademic settings, such as hospital ethics committees—is comprised of distinctive features amenable to study by scholars of religion. First, the ethical parameters of institutional bioethics are set out by an underlying institutional sense of mission. For example, when voters in the state of Oregon approved a ballot measure in 1994 to legalize physician-assisted suicide, a hospital ethics committee met for a special session to recommend institutional policy for terminally ill patients who requested such assistance in their deaths. The particular hospital—while now a major nonsectarian, community hospital—affirmed values in its institutional mission statement derived from its historical roots in the Episcopalian tradition. Thus, one level of the committee deliberations concerned whether a practice such as physician-assisted suicide could be accommodated within these formative values of the hospital, or whether the hospital's moral identity would be changed and its integrity compromised by facilitating participation in the practice. Not surprisingly, the committee members did not agree on the way to resolve this question. Some argued that assistance in suicide violated the hospital's core values (religious and otherwise) and thus should not be accommodated by the hospital; others agreed with that moral premise but held that this issue provided a rationale to revise the mission of the hospital, at least in its religious language; still others maintained that the core values would not be fundamentally threatened by institutional facilitation of the practice.

Kevin W. Wildes has developed an insightful discussion of the forms of institutional response to ethical issues that challenge institutional moral identity, with a particular focus on potential compromises of core religious values. He has sketched a typology of institutional responses along a continuum from acceptance of the controversial practice, to various forms of toleration, to nonparticipation, and finally to a "holy-war" approach.[13] The degree of institutional acceptance, toleration, or rejection is shaped in large measure by the underlying moral vision or mission of the institution; this moral identity may at times undergo modification in response to new developments in biomedicine.

Institutions, such as universities or hospitals, share with religious traditions the characteristic of embodying an intermediate community. It seems possible, as the example of Wildes's analysis suggests, for religious studies scholars to understand and interpret institutional responses to biomedical questions in patterns somewhat similar to the ongoing evolution of religious traditions and communities over time. Religious communities have their own implicit statements of purpose—some more focused on evangelization, others on social justice, others on inclusiveness, and so forth. Some developments in biomedicine challenge the fundamental values and convictions of a community (an example of this appears later in the chapter), and others may be perceived with relative indifference. Scholars of religion can draw on these similarities in a mutually reciprocal dialectic to illuminate what is transpiring in both the medical institution and the religious community.

In addition, religious studies scholars are well positioned to interpret institutional events in terms of analyses of power, disempowerment, and liberation.[14] Questions of ecclesiastical power and its abuse are certainly well documented in the history of the Western Christian church; it would be very surprising if similar patterns of power would not be disclosed in analyses of healthcare institutions. As one obvious parallel, misuse of institutional power inevitably leads to the imposition of harm on society's most vulnerable persons, whether they be religious minorities or the medically indigent. That historical parallel can provide normative support from within the religious traditions for a healthcare system rooted in justice and universal access.

Not all forms of institutional bioethics, of course, involve policy deliberation and formulation. Review of research protocols carried out by IRBs or animal care committees presumes an implicit settled consensus on the policy question (for example, it is morally permissible to engage in research on animals), and largely involves interpretation and application of the settled policy principles to the research study. Religious values may be descriptively studied in some behavioral research protocols, but they are characteristically not invoked as justifications or objections to the study. That is to say, the principles used to evaluate the study—such as fairness, informed consent, confidentiality, risks and benefits, or the imposition of pain and suffering—do not necessarily depend on religious backing, although they are not incompatible with basic religious claims about the treatment of persons or animals.

By contrast, case review by institutional ethics committees often is prompted by questions about how best to respect and accommodate religious convictions of the patient relative to the practice of ethical medicine. In some circumstances, a conflict at the level of clinical bioethics between patient (or family) and professional caregivers that cannot be resolved because of deep-rooted religious values is transformed into a question of institutional bioethics when a committee is requested to consult on the case or offer a prospective or retrospective review.[15] The hope is that an airing of the conflict before a broader deliberative body such as a committee will facilitate communication between the parties and help them clarify the medical, ethical, and religious values at stake—thus empowering the parties to resolve the conflict, rather than moving to the adversarial setting of a courtroom.

One well-known illustration of this process, and one that no-less reflects questions of institutional power, occurred in the case of Helga Wanglie, an elderly woman who was comatose and dependent upon a respirator. Believing that continued treatment constituted medical futility, her attending physicians asked Ms. Wanglie's husband to authorize removal of the respirator. Mr. Wanglie refused, citing religious values that had shaped their common life together and by which they wished to live and die. He believed that life and death are in the hands of God, and "physicians should not play God, [Ms. Wanglie] would not be better off dead, that removing her life support showed moral decay in our civilization, and that a miracle could occur."[16]

These are statements reflecting profound religious convictions, but it is understandable why they cannot be taken as normative for medical practice. They would consign medicine to either passivity or vitalism, either to avoid getting in the way of the natural processes of life or to forestall death for as long as is technologically possible. Indeed, such convictions are not terribly good theology, because they imply that the will of God is contingent on the current status of medical technology. Nonetheless, the conflict between this religious understanding of what was in Ms. Wanglie's best interest and what her caregivers deemed to be good medicine directed toward her best interest could not be resolved at the clinical level, and a hospital ethics committee review was requested. An issue in clinical bioethics was transformed into a question of institutional bioethics. Although in the case of Helga Wanglie, the conflict ultimately was appealed to the legal system, an ongoing challenge in both clinical and institutional bioethics is determining whether respect for and accommodation of religious beliefs and practices are compatible with the practice of ethical medicine.

COMMUNITY BIOETHICS

A context implicit in the above discussion is the community of which one is a member as a locus of bioethics reflection and action; this context is referred to here as *community bioethics*. The community here may be a particular religious community, or a broader community bound together by the ideal of citizenship.

James M. Gustafson has referred to religious traditions as "communities of moral discourse."[17] This designation has several implications.

Religious communities have historic traditions of reflection and practice on questions of health and medicine that can be formative in shaping the responses of believers to issues in bioethics. However, as discussed above relative to philosophical critiques of religious selectivity, these traditions and responses are communally retrieved, interpreted, disputed, and applied. One of the most common misconceptions of religious traditions is that ecclesiastical positions exercise a kind of preemptive moral tyranny on the values and practices of religious adherents. This "top-down" perception of religious ethics certainly does not hold for many issues in contemporary bioethics, whether regarding the beginnings of life or its endings. Rather, the exercise of genuine moral authority is communal rather than hierarchical. It is also the case that religious communities, in their ethics discourse and practices, can offer an alternative model of being and living to the general society.

Gustafson has been sharply critical of religious studies in the context of community bioethics, implying that there exists a conflict of commitment between the role of religious scholars in the academy and their responsiveness to the interests of particular religious communities.[18] Having participated in many bioethics workshops with religious communities, I believe Gustafson is mistaken in his argument. While believers seek to remain faithful to the value legacy of their tradition, there is substantial interest in seeking methods of interpreting these values in light of the developments of contemporary biomedicine and biomedical technology. It is in this process of communal retrieval, discernment, and interpretation that scholars in religious studies are vital moral resources for the community—not presenting answers but portraying a range of possibilities. These biomedical developments raise not only questions of "What should we do?" but, more fundamentally, "What does this development mean?" For example, how should one understand the moral significance and meaning of parenting in the wake of numerous innovations in reproductive technology? How should traditions of thought about the purpose of suffering be understood and revised in response to the medical goal of alleviating human suffering (even when suffering can be relieved only by taking life)? It is over questions of meaning about birth, parenting, identity, suffering, disability, and death that religious communities seem to embody a community of moral discourse.

Yet, citizens may also constitute communities of bioethics discourse in which religious values and ideas play a significant role. I have in mind here the "bottom-up" or "grassroots" forms of bioethics that go formally under the name of the health decisions movement. The goal of such movements, which were initiated in and have played an important policy role in Oregon,[19] is to empower citizens in their communities (not as isolated agents) with the skills and practical knowledge to assume responsibility for their own decisions regarding healthcare. Community bioethics is an exercise in participatory democracy, with citizens actively engaged in articulating and prioritizing personal and collective values about such matters as access to healthcare resources, choices at the end of life, or ownership of genetic information.

Although religious studies may not have a direct role to play in this setting, they can certainly contribute in indirect fashions. For several reasons, the values of religious traditions have equal standing with non-religious sources of values. They are acknowledged by the community as expressions of legitimate moral concerns in keeping with a civic ethos of tolerance of diversity. And although professional bioethicists may dispute the logical or necessary dependence of ethics on religion, within the communal context it is not disputed that many important values (such as compassion, dignity, and equality) are chronologically or historically dependent upon religious traditions, however much they may have become detached from those formative roots in the current era. Indeed, it is possible to discern in these community deliberations the presence of what R.N. Bellah once referred as a "civil religion"—that is, a shared sense of moral convictions among a vast majority of the citizenry.[20]

Community bioethics therefore presumes the relevance of religious traditions as a moral resource for communal deliberation and interpretation. Community bioethics does not necessarily focus on resolving the "hard cases" of quandary bioethics; rather it focuses on the effort to articulate the values that will bind citizens together in a common political and social life.

The chapter thus far has provided a brief sketch of five contexts of bioethics—professional, pedagogical, clinical, institutional, and communal. Each of these contexts have their own distinctive features as well as aspects that may overlap with other contexts. These distinctive features and similar foci need to be carefully understood in considering the influence of religious studies for "bioethics." The danger that often arises is that these contexts become so separated and compartmentalized that, for example, professional or academic bioethics and clinical bioethics occur in entirely different worlds.

Put another way, the question of the role of religious studies in contemporary bioethics contains a level of abstraction that belies its academic home.[21] That is an important part of the story of bioethics, but only a part. Absent a theory of bioethics that unifies the various contexts delineated above, an academic query cannot be taken as a complete or definitive discussion. Specific contexts in which the focus of attention is not intellectual debate—but practical decision making or the human search for meaning initiated by common human experiences of birth, life, and death—will necessarily give a different shape to both the question and the kinds of responses the question engenders.

These themes are illustrated and magnified in two final contexts of bioethics—what I will refer to as *civic bioethics* and *policy bioethics*. The discussion of these contexts is developed in some depth, drawing on recent social debates over the legalization of physician-assisted suicide and human cloning. It is within these macro settings of bioethics that the issues of relevance of religious studies and religious discourse are fully and publicly displayed. In these settings it is important that religious traditions bear witness to the values they embody and enact as communities of resistance and meaning.

CIVIC BIOETHICS

In *civic bioethics*, citizens are directly involved in the decision-making process to discuss and resolve a bioethical question, as distinguished from indirect participation through the legislative process. It thus reflects a step beyond, although it may be a logical extension of, what is contemplated in community bioethics, in which citizens determine what values would (or should) shape their common life together. In civic bioethics, citizens are engaged in the process of appealing to purportedly common values to persuade fellow citizens to adopt a particular position on an issue, the resolution of which typically occurs through the practice of voting.

These characteristics make civic bioethics a very rare occurrence. While public sentiments and preferences on controversial issues are often solicited to provide support for or against a particular proposal undergoing legislative scrutiny, it is quite another thing for the public to bypass the legislature altogether and make policy based on majority vote (or a majority of the minority that do vote). Similarly, while citizens' comments are commonly elicited by legislative or executive policy commissions, it is a different matter for citizens' comments to be decisive and beyond policy review.

Nonetheless, civic bioethics has been prominent regarding the most heated bioethics question of the 1990s, the legalization of physician-assisted suicide. Civic bioethics must necessarily operate within a certain amenable political structure—namely, one in which citizens have significant powers of self-legislation. Although many states in the United States do not give such powers to their citizens, the Pacific Coast states of California, Oregon, and Washington all provide for citizens to initiate ballot referendums that, if passed, can become statutory or constitutional law. It is thus not surprising that the most influential forums of civic bioethics on physician-assisted suicide have occurred in this region.

The emergence of civic bioethics is also attributable to the power and persuasiveness of persons who have experienced terminal illness, as well as to those who act as advocates on their behalf. The principle of self-determination has given legitimacy to the moral authority of the patient's voice in the debate over assisted suicide in a manner almost unparalleled in other realms of medicine. This is strikingly illustrated in the comment of the president of the Oregon Medical Association following that organization's adoption of a position of "neutrality" regarding a 1994 ballot initiative, the Oregon Death with Dignity Act, that aimed to legalize physicians' participation in the suicides of competent, terminally ill persons: "We need to hear from our patients on this. We need to hear from the people of Oregon what to do."[22] Civic bioethics is rare in part because most physicians and professional bodies are unwilling to grant patients (or voters) the authority to determine the standards of good medical practice.

In the context of physician-assisted suicide, civic bioethics thus builds on themes present in clinical bioethics, insofar as the morality of the relation between patient and physician is central to moral resolution. It also builds on communal bioethics, insofar as empowerment of citizens encompasses and facilitates empowerment of patients. The difference is that civic bioethics seeks not only to inform consciousness but also to bring about a change in law.

What is the place of religious studies and religion in civic bioethics? One unfortunate aspect of civic bioethics—albeit one in which it mirrors the general political landscape—is its incivility, including incivility toward religiously grounded opinions. The three examples that follow from the debates over legalized physician-assisted suicide in Washington and Oregon illustrate this incivility toward religion:

1. The 1994 announcement by the Oregon Catholic Conference that it intended to oppose and campaign against the passage of the Oregon Death with Dignity Act was viewed by proponents of the act as "promot[ing] Catholic religious doctrine by influ-

encing Oregon voters," and as "pushing [Catholic] religious doctrine on the rest of Oregonians."[23]

2.   The concluding paragraph of the Ninth Circuit Court's 1996 decision in *Compassion in Dying v. Washington* affirms: "Those who believe strongly that death must come without physician assistance are free to follow that creed. . . . They are not free, however, to force their views, their religious convictions, or their philosophies on all the other members of a democratic society, and to compel those whose values differ with theirs to die painful, protracted, and agonizing deaths."[24]

3.   A (successful) effort in the Oregon state legislature in 1997 to refer the Death with Dignity Act to the voters for a second vote symbolized to proponents of the act a legislative body held "hostage" to the "raw political power" of institutionalized religion.[25]

Now, surely some of this language is the kind of vitriolic incivility that passes for campaign rhetoric in American politics at the end of the millennium. However, not all of the language can be so portrayed, and certainly not when it is given a judicial imprimatur by a federal court. The common thread in these comments is that, in the context of civic bioethics, the expression of a religious opinion is an exercise of moral tyranny. The metaphors of "hostage-taking," "force," "compulsion," "pushing," and "raw power" used to convey the purported political influence of religion reflect a fear of religious views as morally intimidating and imperialistic. So pervasive is this attack on the freedom of religious expression that the circuit court opinion suggests that *any* position opposed to assistance in suicide is a religious position that is, a "creed." However misleading such a claim, what clearly does not follow is that the articulation of this creed is a form of force that justifies compulsion in the manner of death. The court, as well as the proponents of the Death with Dignity Act, have simply conflated the ethics of persuasion with the ethics of coercion in their efforts to dismiss religious argumentation from civic bioethics. That conflation is itself problematic in a democratic society.

Scholars in religious studies cannot retreat to the safe havens of the academy in the face of such incivility in civic bioethics. (Needless to say, the academy exhibits its own forms of intolerance toward religious expression.) The scholar can bear witness to the civic value of religion in three important ways. First, scholars can refute the misconceptions about religious discourse in a democratic society as an instrument of force.

Second, they should identify and dispute the transformation of civic discourse into uncivil emotivism. Third, they should be advocates for the principle of freedom of religious expression.

An appeal to a religious value (such as the sanctity of human life) or the expression of a position justified by religious values (such as Roman Catholic opposition to physician-assisted suicide) does not preclude thoughtful deliberation upon and acceptance or rejection of the value or position. Whether the religious position will be accepted or not depends not on the imposition of certain views, but on whether it will make a persuasive case to the audience of citizens. That, in turn, requires the religious argument to connect with values already embedded in social practices and accepted by the citizenry. It is ironic that, in the guise of seeking to preserve civic freedom, the circuit court decision insults the critical consciousness of citizens; the implication of views expressed by the court is that, when deliberating upon public matters, citizens can only swear obeisance when the "creed" is enunciated by a religious authority. It is, by contrast, essential to differentiate the expression of a position rooted in religious convictions from the imposition of that position on other citizens.

The scholar can also affirm solidarity with religious communities and citizens in general in bearing witness to the moral necessity in a democratic society of meaningful public discourse. In doing this they stand against the attempt to reduce civic discourse, including civic bioethics, to a realm of politicized emotivism or "raw power." This illegitimate discourse of power might be appropriate for the state of nature or a Leviathan, but it is contrary to the processes and ends of a democratic society. Religious communities can resist ethical emotivism best through offering reasoned and sustained arguments on the contested issue. Such arguments respect the autonomy of citizens by seeking to persuade rather than by manipulating or imposing a position, or by silencing alternative positions.

Religious communities must also resist efforts, implicitly endorsed by the Ninth Circuit Court, to dismiss or exclude religious argumentation from the realm of civic bioethics because they somehow constitute force or compulsion. This resistance involves bearing witness to the foundational freedom of religious expression. Just as expression of a religiously grounded opinion is distinguishable logically and in practice from its imposition, religious freedom does not necessarily imply establishmentarianism, or what Carter refers to as the "horror" of "the Christian nation."[26] Nonetheless, political or legal discourse that equates the expression of a religious position with its forcible imposition makes precisely this mistake. If these distinctions are not affirmed by political advocates or the courts, then religious communities and their adherents are deprived of a fundamental civil and human right. Scholars and communities must affirm and defend basic claims to freedom of religious expression in civic bioethics.

It is important to recognize that moves toward exclusion of religion from civil discourse are not confined to polarizing issues such as assisted suicide. In an insightful discussion, Kent Greenawalt maintains that, although it is entirely legitimate for religious adherents to consult their religious conscience and values in their personal deliberations on an issue of public importance, such values should not be directly cited in public discussion.[27] It is not clear, however, just how invoking a value such as the sanctity of human life and appealing to a specific biblical passage violates the ground rules of democratic discourse. Certainly, an appeal to a value with specific religious content and justification may not be an effective mode of persuasion; an audience may disagree with the value, its religious content, or its scriptural basis. However, the issue of what will be most ethically persuasive is a different question than whether an appeal that risks being unpersuasive should even have a place in civic discourse.

Religious communities also have a stake in resisting cultural deference to personal autonomy. This follows in part because of the nature of the religious life as necessarily communal and relational. While autonomy can be supported by religious positions, such as the theological anthropology of human beings as created in the image of God, autonomy is inextricably coupled with accountability. Accountability requires answering for one's actions to others in the community, or perhaps ultimately to God. This is a very different understanding of autonomy than is contemplated in the Oregon Death with Dignity Act, wherein a patient who requests assistance in suicide is not required to inform even family members of the decision. Accountability assumes the person is a responsible moral agent.

Religious resistance to asocial views of autonomy is important for another reason, one that concerns the moral status of social institutions and practices. One implication of the claim that, at least with respect to assistance in suicide, patients should dictate to physicians what is appropriate is that the social practice of medicine is denied any ongoing moral identity or integrity. The ideology of the market is to satisfy (and create) personal preferences, but it is ethically problematic that the purpose of medicine as a moral vocation is to cater to patients' autonomy. To be sure, insofar as a market ideology becomes ever more pervasive in contemporary medicine, as exemplified by the transformation of the physician-patient relationship into a provider-consumer relationship, then medicine will likewise assume the market interest in satisfying consumers' autonomy. Under this logic, medicine cannot say no to medically assisted suicide or voluntary euthanasia; for that matter, medicine will have lost the moral capacity to say no to any patient preference. As one intermediate community, religious communities and scholars can delineate the social stake in the ongoing moral viability of other intermediate communities, such as medicine.

Finally, religious communities can and should resist the tendency to ethical polarization and divisiveness. Put more constructively, they should infuse civility back into civic bioethics. This is best done by beginning ethical discourse not with points of difference but rather with areas of common ground and points of agreement. Despite polarizing rhetoric to the contrary, in the context of assisted suicide, there are several themes of commonality. There is first a shared commitment to enhance care at the end of life received by terminally ill patients, particularly the use of palliative measures. There is also agreement over the need to provide patients with more control over the dying process. This is not only basic to supporters of assisted suicide; it is at the foundation of such programs as hospice and such policies as advance directives, both of which have received strong support from many religious communities. In addition, a common conviction is that terminally ill patients should not have to walk through the valley of the shadow of death alone and abandoned. Rather, patients should experience the compassionate presence of others at the end of their life's journey. Finally, few oppose taking measures to enhance the dignity of the person in dying.

These are important, substantive commitments that are shared across the moral divide of assisted suicide. There are differences over the implications of these commitments, but there should be shared respect for these different implications and positions, so long as they are founded on ethical arguments and not on politicized emotivism. Respect for an opposing argument is itself a way to diffuse the polarization and instill civility into civic bioethics. Religious arguments that begin with what is shared, rather than what is divisive, can enable a constructive civic discourse even on very contentious issues.

Thus far, this discussion has concentrated on ways that religious traditions can be an embodied community of resistance in civic bioethics, and how arguments of religious studies scholars can help to bear such witness to society. The general purposes of moral resistance are to prevent a minimalistic morality that holds the only moral relation of any import to be that between the self and the state and to offer positions of moral substance for civic bioethics. But how do such communities bear witness to sources of meaning—for example, with respect to physician-assisted suicide?

While much of the debate over assisted suicide has focused on the scope and limits of personal choice, this is in many respects misleading. The question is rather about what constitutes a death with dignity, or a humane and dignified death. So, we must understand proponents of assisted suicide to be recommending (even though they have not understood their position as such) not merely a choice to die, but a choice to die in a particular way, or a choice that will bring on a death endowed with particular characteristics—namely, those summarized by the concept of dignity. However, it is not immediately clear that a dignified death requires or is achievable through the means of medical assistance in suicide. In short, civic bioethics discussion of assisted suicide involves a substantive inquiry about the meaning of dignity.

The concept of dignity is not exclusively a religious concept, but it has received sustained attention from religious scholars and traditions.[28] On the other hand, there has been a paucity of discussion of this concept by nonreligious writers, including those advocating for the political right to a dignified death. Indeed, the most popular book on death and dying during this decade of debate on assisted suicide, Sherwin Nuland's *How We Die*, maintains that the current perception of death with dignity is a comforting but illusionary myth. Nuland contends that the ideology of the dignified death creates expectations amongst the public that are carried into the setting of terminal illness by patients, families, and caregivers but are subsequently shattered and betrayed by the actual dying process. A central purpose in Nuland's book is to "demythologize" the dignified death through recounting the stories of actual dying processes and deaths in order to bring expectations and reality into some congruence.[29]

It is sometimes possible to infer an understanding of dignity from what is considered not to constitute dignity. The Ninth Circuit Court, for example, maintained that a person "has a strong liberty interest in choosing a dignified and humane death rather than being reduced at the end of his existence to a childlike state of helplessness, diapered, sedated, incontinent."[30] A dying state in which pain, dependency, or loss of control is present violates the ideal of dignity, and this violation constitutes "suffering." The approach in this respect suggests that dignity in dying is achieved not by the *freedom to choose* as much as it is by the *freedom from* certain physical, psychological, and social conditions that constitute dehumanization and suffering.[31]

It is important to recognize the legitimacy of these conditions—what might be called "negative conditions of dignity." Although dependency and dignity are not mutually exclusive, alleviating these negative conditions is a valid moral objective of medicine and, indeed, should be included in a discussion of the common moral concerns delineated above. Nonetheless, this does not offer a morally sufficient account of dignity in dying, and it is a responsibility of religious scholars and communities to bear witness to an account of the "positive conditions of dignity" based on the resources of their theological traditions and communal practices. Part of the religious claim must be that dignity is not something that is legally conferred during the dying process, but it is achieved and earned throughout an entire life. A dignified death is a mirror and reflection of a life lived with dignity—that is, a life directed by certain traits of character, dispositions, and virtues that give moral shape and substance to a person's identity and integrity. A religious account of dignity, therefore, will give primacy to authenticity of character and continuity in values, rather than to a choice made six months prior to death, as though dignity were a modern-day equivalent of deathbed grace.

A religious inquiry about the meaning of dignity in dying will also emphasize the necessity of compassionate human presence to the dying. We live our lives out in communities of various kinds, through which we are nurtured and give, in mutual reciprocity. It is incumbent that the dying know that the cords of compassion and community are stronger than the separation that death brings.

Insofar as dignity is a meaningful concept in dying, and not an illusionary myth, we cannot be satisfied with truncated accounts of dignity as the existence of a choice to die. Yet, that is largely what the civic and professional bioethics debate has evolved into during recent years. A dignified death will encompass both negative and positive conditions, some of which have been sketched above. Religious traditions, which have a historical concern with "dying well,"[32] are inescapably communities of meaning for civic bioethics.

POLICY BIOETHICS

Policy bioethics is much more familiar than civic bioethics as a method by which bioethical questions receive a policy resolution—through hearings by federal or state bioethics commissions—and recommendations for legislative enactment, or through case law. Policy bioethics builds upon many of the themes present in institutional and professional bioethics and typically has implications for clinical bioethics. The analysis that follows draws on the recent policy discussion of human cloning to illustrate and deepen the understanding presented thus far of the roles of religious scholars and religious traditions as communities that bear witness to resistance and meaning.

Shortly after the announcements in early 1997 of the somatic cell cloning of the sheep Dolly, President William Clinton announced a moratorium on federally funded human cloning research and asked for policy recommendations from the National Bioethics Advisory Commission (NBAC). In so doing, Clinton indicated that the prospects of human cloning raised profound questions not only of morality but also of spirituality. NBAC held public hearings on the issue at which speakers from various religious traditions gave testimony,[33] and invited a scholarly paper to examine theological discussion on human cloning from diverse religious communities. NBAC issued its recommendations to the president in June 1997 but, as of this writing, no federal legislation has been passed to permit, regulate, or prohibit human cloning.[34] The question explored here is the significance of religious voices in this policy process.

Given President Clinton's comments and the fact that the first testimony presented in the public hearings came from religious studies scholars, it may appear that religious voices were important in setting the ethical and policy agenda for human cloning. However, this impression is misleading. In meetings conducted before public hearings, NBAC commissioners adopted a policy methodology common to such deliberative bodies. This methodology was comprised largely of a commitment to the moral validity of scientific research that may promise human benefits (in particular, the enhancement of reproductive choices through cloning options) and to a consequentialist risk-benefit assessment (concerns about risks and safety ultimately led NBAC to support a provisional moratorium on human cloning research through somatic cell procedures).

This meant that religious thinkers who presented testimony to NBAC faced two significant obstacles. First, these scholars were frequently asked to formulate their perspectives and concerns on human cloning in language or concepts that could be readily conveyed and understood by persons outside their religious community or, in the parlance of professional bioethics, in "publicly accessible reasons." NBAC implicitly imposed a "standard of informed-citizen consciousness" on those present-ing religious issues and arguments. This is problematic inasmuch as no other presenters were asked to "translate" their testimony in such a fash-ion. Neither the scientists who presented very technical testimony on the scientific process of cloning nor the philosophers who relied on fic-tional scenarios to build a case for support of cloning were required to meet the informed-citizen standard. Moreover, the informed-citizen stan-dard was shaped by the policy methodology described above—a commit-ment to autonomy (scientific and reproductive) and to a consequentialist assessment of technological innovation. Thus, many eloquent and sub-stantive arguments offered by the religious thinkers ultimately had neg-ligible policy significance because they did not readily conform to the policy categories. Some scholars, for example, appealed to the common good of the society as a relevant, if not decisive consideration, in evaluat-ing research proposals. This is not an unreasonable appeal, given that NBAC was commissioned to engage in deliberation by, for, and of the people, but it clearly founders against a policy presumption in favor of freedom in scientific inquiry and in reproductive matters.

Second, NBAC seemed to value religious arguments primarily as an occasion for giving thoughtful voice to *objections* to human cloning re-search—that is, to the articulation of potential "risks." This is an argu-ment that cannot be compellingly made. Any such risks are speculative and in the future, and the only way to determine whether the risks are actual, present, and overriding is to give a green (or, at least, amber) light to research proposals.

If this example is illustrative, religious argumentation in policy bio-ethics must be conveyed in a very constricted moral world, meeting cer-tain standards shaped by largely secular moral categories. Scholars in religious studies and religious communities should resist this constric-tion of the policy world. This resistance will require a greater dialogue within and between religious communities than, to this point, has been forthcoming on the issue of human cloning. It means religious scholar-ship should be engaged in enhancing the scientific literacy of these com-munities and in the retrieval, interpretation, and application of those values deemed relevant to the policy issue. It also means being willing to participate in the policy process and democratic discourse, and enriching that discourse through appeals to moral values that cannot be subsumed under the principles of autonomy and utility. Such values may involve expositions of the nature and destiny of persons, the notion of human dignity as expressed in the concept of the image of God, or substantive perspectives on the meaning of parenthood and procreation that transcend the liberal notion that moral responsibilities are restricted to those relationships entered into by voluntary choice. In presenting such claims, religious argumentation is not only resisting the contraction of public bioethics, but also bearing witness to the human and communal meaning of the policy issue. Human cloning is an issue that warrants public deliberation, for example, precisely because it presents important challenges to human identity, personal integrity, and concepts of parenting.

NBAC did seek to solicit opinion on human cloning research from a broad range of religious perspectives and traditions, and invited information from traditions in addition to Catholic, Protestant, and Jewish thought that have been the standard religious fare for past advisory bodies. The quest for religious diversity and inclusiveness was reflected in both the verbal testimony and the scholarly study, and it resulted in commentary on human cloning from African-American, Buddhist, Hindu, Islamic, Native American, and Orthodox religious thinkers and scholars.[35] These minority religious traditions also offered voices of resistance and meaning, as illustrated in the three examples that follow.

1. A religious community will set a moral issue, even with something apparently breathtakingly new as somatic cell cloning in mammals, within a communal context and social history. Within African-American religious communities, for example, reports of successful cloning research were greeted with a high degree of distrust and moral suspicion. Such attitudes are made intelligible within the historical legacy of abuse and violation of African Americans by biomedical research. This history grounds moral resistance to new interventions in genetic or reproductive technology because of the potential to perpetuate past exploitation.

2. In contrast to a bioethics approach rooted in the principles of autonomy and utility, religious communities commonly use methods of analogy, story, and narrative. Some religious scholars in the Native American and Hindu traditions found it somewhat presumptuous, for example, that the sheep created through somatic cell cloning was heralded as a new creation. Many of the foundational creation narratives in these traditions portray the creation of humanity and other species from divine beings in a manner that appears very close to a cloning process. The creation narratives, it might be claimed, anticipate scientific devel-

opments, rather than offering anachronistic attitudes, and thereby shed an illuminating meaning on the significance of human attempts at cloning persons.

3. A communal claim of moral resistance and moral meaning can be discerned in a religious perspective on scientific research. This argument holds that promoting the freedom of scientific inquiry to pursue cloning can lead to a distortion of societal priorities. Funding and research allocated to cloning studies could mean diminished attention to chronic diseases that currently afflict African-Americans. And Buddhist and Hindu scholars expressed concern that cloning represented a misguided attempt to resolve issues of meaning, such as the concept of human nature or the purpose of parenting, through technological means.

It is not terribly surprising that cultural traditions and communities formulate, perceive, and resolve ethical problems in ways that are different than the standard accounts offered in professional bioethics. This has been a principal theme of the pioneering sociology of bioethics developed by Renee Fox and Judith Swazey, among others.[36] These particular religious voices offered a form of moral resistance to human cloning that resonates with deeply embedded cultural values about care for the voiceless and vulnerable, who are increasingly marginalized by market medicine. These voices also sharply disclose that concerns about meeting the desires of reproductive autonomy reflect a public bioethics carried on at a rather superficial level. Deeper issues of human meaning should also be heard for public bioethics to be genuinely inclusive. In this respect, it seems most unfortunate that these religious voices were omitted from the final NBAC report to the president.

It is nonetheless important that two of the NBAC recommendations for continuing public education involve the creation of analogues to "communities of moral discourse." These recommendations consist of a charge to the federal government and to other interested civic parties to (1) enhance the scientific literacy of citizens with respect to genetics and (2) encourage continued deliberation on the ethical and social implications of cloning technology, with a view to establishing sound public policy.[37] This is a striking illustration of the necessity of community bioethics as a supplement to informed public bioethics. Yet, NBAC did not commend an examination of the religious issues in human cloning in these communal efforts at ethical and scientific literacy. Those voices need to be heard in community bioethics for the reasons delineated above; as embodied communities in a democratic society, they have a right to moral expression in civic and public bioethics.

CONCLUSION

This chapter has sought to illustrate Carter's claim that religious traditions embody autonomous communities of resistance and independent sources of meaning, and to identify the ways scholars of religious studies can bear witness to resistance and meaning within the diverse cultures or contexts of bioethics. Much of this analysis has been critical of the ways that bioethics, especially civic and public bioethics, often excludes or fails to acknowledge the reality and importance of religious voices. However, in fairness, it must be stated that religious communities have often failed to live up to the ideal of a community of moral discourse when important bioethical issues have been in dispute.

In the face of new scientific and biomedical developments, some religious traditions may defer sustained moral discourse (or fail to respond to a federal commission's call for community bioethics) for a period of time in part because of a concern about becoming committed to a particular normative position with inadequate scientific information (as is the case with human cloning research). Some commentators risk becoming caricatures of religious reactionaries to innovative developments by invoking the slogan of "playing God" at the outset of proposed research. This can cause a loss of credibility precisely among those groups, such as scientists or policy makers, who are essential conversation partners in community or public bioethics.

Thus, deferring discourse until the scientific discussion, and even the ethical and policy discussion, has largely played itself out can be a course of ecclesiastical pragmatism. Moreover, this can give greater latitude to members of the community (physicians, patients, and so forth) to exercise personal moral autonomy. The difficulty, however, with sitting on the sidelines while a bioethics debate proceeds is that the ethical stance of a religious community can then only be reactive to a scientific *fait accompli*. Theological convictions are made to seem dependent on the progress of science and medical technology, rather than derived from historical theological claims or developed in dialogue with scientific advances.

Moreover, if religious voices do not emerge until the relative closure of the scientific and moral controversy, it can become very difficult to control the interpretation of silence and deference during the interim between the scientific breakthrough and the closure of the ethical and policy questions initiated by the breakthrough. Silence may be taken to mean indifference or endorsement. For example, Fox and Swazey's study of the religious context of the first artificial heart experiment could lead a reader to draw the mistaken conclusion that the religious community myopically celebrates technological achievements as revelations of the will of God, while neglecting the social and ethical implications of scientific and biomedical research.[38]

Hasty reactionarianism and sitting on the sidelines lead neither to good religious studies, communal reflection, nor good citizenship. The more responsible approach is for religious communities to take seriously their responsibility as communities of moral discourse, in which they bear witness to expressions of resistance and meaning in contemporary bioethics discussions. As was the case with the debate over human cloning research, these religious voices often require public articulation by scholars in religious studies. Given the general absence of science literacy among the public (particularly in regard to genetics and biotechnology) and the reticence of professional scientists to communicate their findings in public forums, religious communities can play a significant role in shaping the many cultures of bioethics by initiating this necessary bioethics dialogue among believers and among citizens.

NOTES

1. S.L. Carter, *The Culture of Disbelief: How American Law and Politics Trivialize Religious Devotion* (New York: Basic Books, 1993), 40.

2. J.M. Gustafson, "Theology Confronts Technology and the Life Sciences," *Commonweal* 105 (16 June 1978): 386-92.

3. F. Collins, "The Human Genome Project," in *Life at Risk: The Crises in Medical Ethics,* ed. R.D. Land and L.A. Moore (Nashville, Tenn.: Broadman & Holman, 1995), 100-13.

4. M. Walzer, *Interpretation and Social Criticism* (Cambridge, Mass.: Harvard University Press, 1987).

5. A. Ridley, *Beginning Bioethics* (New York: St. Martin's, 1998), 6-7.

6. S.E. Lammers and A. Verhey, ed., *On Moral Medicine: Theological Perspectives in Medical Ethics,* 2nd ed. (Grand Rapids, Mich.: William B. Eerdmans, 1998).

7. A. Verhey, "Playing God and Invoking a Perspective," *Journal of Medicine and Philosophy* 20 (1995): 347-64.

8. D. Callahan, "Goals in the Teaching of Ethics," in *Ethics Teaching in*

Higher Education, ed. D. Callahan and S. Bok (New York: Plenum, 1980), 61-74.

9. S.E. Lammers, "The Marginalization of Religious Voices in Bioethics," in *Religion and Medical Ethics: Looking Back, Looking Forward*, ed. A. Verhey (Grand Rapids, Mich.: William B. Eerdmans, 1996), 19-43.

10. For example, E.N. Dorff, *The Jewish Tradition: Religious Beliefs and Health Care Decisions* (Chicago: Park Ridge Center, 1996).

11. See note 1 above, p. 28.

12. L.R. Churchill, "The Human Experience of Dying: The Moral Primacy of Stories over Stages," *Soundings* 62 (1979): 24-37.

13. K.W. Wildes, "Institutional Integrity: Approval, Toleration and Holy War or 'Always True to You in My Fashion,' " *Journal of Medicine and Philosophy* 16, no. 2 (1991): 211-20.

14. A.V. Campbell, *Health as Liberation: Medicine, Theology, and the Quest for Justice* (Cleveland, Ohio: Pilgrim, 1995).

15. R. Macklin, "The Inner Workings of an Ethics Committee: Latest Battle over Jehovah Witnesses," *Hastings Center Report* 18, no. 1 (February-March 1988): 15-20.

16. S.H. Miles, "Informed Demand for Non-Beneficial Treatment," *New England Journal of Medicine* 325 (1991): 512-5.

17. J.M. Gustafson, *The Contributions of Theology to Medical Ethics* (Milwaukee, Wis.: Marquette University Press, 1975).

18. J.M. Gustafson, "Theology Confronts Technology and the Life Sciences," *Commonweal* 105 (16 June 1978): 386-92.

19. R. Crawshaw et al., "Oregon Health Decisions: An Experiment with Informed Community Consent," *Journal of the American Medical Association* 254, no. 22 (1985): 3213-6; Oregon Health Decisions and Oregon Hospice Association, *Request for Physician-Assisted Death: How Will You Vote?* (Portland, Ore.: Oregon Health Decisions, 1994).

20. R.N. Bellah, "Civil Religion in America," in *Secularization and the Protestant Prospect*, ed. J.F. Childress and D.B. Harned (Philadelphia: Westminster, 1970): 93-116.

21. See note 9 above, p. 22.

22. C.S. Campbell, "When Medicine Lost Its Moral Conscience: Oregon Measure 16," in *Arguing Euthanasia*, ed. J. Moreno (New York: Simon & Schuster, 1995), 147.

23. M. O'Keefe, "Catholic Church Plans to Fight Suicide Measure," *Oregonian*, 9 September 1994, A1; J. Long, "Churches Denounce Suicide Bill," *Oregonian*, 19 September 1994, B1.

24. *Compassion in Dying v. Washington*, 79 F.3d 790, at 839.

25. M. O'Keefe, "House Approves Asking for Repeal of Suicide Law," *Oregonian*, 14 May 1997, A18.

26. See note 1 above, pp. 83-101.

27. K. Greenawalt, *Religious Convictions and Political Choice* (New York:

Oxford University Press, 1988), 49-76.

28. P. Ramsey, "The Indignity of 'Death with Dignity,' " *Hastings Center Studies* 2 (May 1974): 47-62; L.R. Kass, "Averting One's Eyes, or Facing the Music? On Dignity and Death," *Hastings Center Studies* 2 (May 1974): 67-80.

29. S.L. Nuland, *How We Die: Reflections on Life's Final Chapter* (New York: Alfred A. Knopf, 1994), xiv-xvii, 263-9.

30. See note 24 above, p. 837.

31. C.S. Campbell, "Suffering, Compassion, and Dignity in Dying," *Duquesne Law Review* 35, no. 1 (1996): 109-24.

32. Bishops of the Oregon Catholic Conference and the Washington State Catholic Conference, *Living and Dying Well: A Pastoral Letter about the End of Life* (Portland, Ore.: Archdiocese of Portland in Oregon, 1991).

33. J.F. Childress, ed., "Religious and Ethics Perspectives on Human Cloning," *BioLaw* 2, no. 6 (June 1997): S99-S152.

34. National Bioethics Advisory Commission, *Cloning Human Beings* (Rockville, Md.: NBAC, 1997).

35. C.S. Campbell and J. Woolfrey, "Norms and Narratives: Religious Perspectives on the Human Cloning Controversy," *Journal of Biolaw and Business* 1, no. 3 (Spring 1998): 8-20.

36. R. Fox and J.P. Swazey, "Medical Morality Is Not Bioethics—Medical Ethics in China and the United States," *Perspectives in Biology and Medicine* 27, no. 3 (1984): 336-60.

37. See note 34 above, pp. 107-10.

38. R. Fox and J.P. Swazey, *Spare Parts: Organ Replacement in American Society* (New York: Oxford University Press, 1992): 162-9; C.S. Campbell, "Ecclesiology and Ethics: An LDS Response," in *Theological Developments in Bioethics: 1992-1994*, ed. B.A. Lustig (Dordrecht, The Netherlands: Kluwer Academic Publishers, 1997), 33-54.

3

Focusing on the Human Scene: Thoughts on Problematic Theology

Ronald A. Carson

Faith-working-through-love is a practice, "a prolongation of
the incarnation . . . among those in need" . . . .
—Paul Ramsey, *Basic Christian Ethics*

PROBLEMATIC THEOLOGY

I was brought up on the stories and songs of the Bible—the prophets
and the Psalms, the parables and the Sermon on the Mount. Only much
later did I gain critical perspective on what it meant to have been initiated into this way of viewing the world and thinking about life. By then
I was in divinity school, caught up in the social strife of the 1960s, moved
by the dedication of Black churches to the cause of civil rights, disaf-
fected by mainline Protestantism's general lack of commitment to racial
justice, and struggling to discern the relevance of faith to the events of
those turbulent times. It was the life and work of Dietrich Bonhoeffer,
the Lutheran theologian who was executed for participating in a plot to
kill Hitler, that spoke most clearly to me. I was especially drawn to his
understanding of faith as "participation in the suffering of God in the life
of the world"—an ethical rather than a ritual exercise of faith. William

Hamilton interpreted the participation that Bonhoeffer had lived and written about in a larger Lutheran context as indicative of a characteristically Protestant movement from the cloister to the world: "Of course, there is no specific event in Luther's life that can be so described, but the movement is there in his life nonetheless. . . . From cloister to world means from church, from place of protection and security, of order and beauty, to the bustling middle-class world of the new university, of politics, princes and peasants. Far more important than any particular ethical teaching of Luther is this fundamental ethical movement." In the world, faith is not recognizably ecclesial but "a being with or standing beside the neighbor . . . the man in need . . . and the bearer of the worldly Jesus."[1] With hindsight, I realized that taking up my calling as a theologian in the medical humanities marked a move into a secular setting in which the life story that had formed me, and that I was critically appropriating, was one story among others and had no place of privilege. But it was (and is) my way of making sense of things. It indelibly informs my work as a practitioner of problematic theology.

Some years ago William F. May distinguished problematics from systematics, one of Christian theology's central subdisciplines (in the Protestant tradition of which I was trained). Whereas systematic theology aims to systematize and defend propositional statements of faith arising from communities of faith, problematic theology eschews apologetics and instead joins practitioners of other humanities disciplines in sorting through experience and trying to make livable sense of it. In the mid-1980s, May accurately predicted that "in the setting of the humanities, it [theology] will probably focus on common human problems—such as birth, death, politics, human creativity, and destiny—which it shares with many other disciplines. . . . The theologian in the university, alongside the political scientist, the literary critic, and the psychologist, will attempt to throw whatever light he or she can on these problems. As such, theology will belong to that mix of disciplines in the humanities that focus on the human scene."[2] Although the term *problematic theology* did not catch on, the distinction May drew helps explain why religious thinkers, although their views did not otherwise resonate widely in the culture of late modernity, were prominent in the early evolution of modern moral inquiry into questions of medical ethics as the professionalized field of bioethics emerged.

FAITH AND CULTURE

In a prescient essay published in the mid-1960s, John B. Cobb, Jr. reflected on some reasons for the difficulties then being experienced by theologians in their dialogue with secular culture. Nineteenth-century, liberal Protestant theology had sought a synthesis between faith and culture. Early in the 20th century this view was vigorously contested by those who argued that the only way for faith to be true to itself was by rejecting culture. Dialectical theology insisted on the radical disjunction of faith and culture. Culture was understood to be the human realm, faith was of God, and God was Wholly Other. Faith looked to God, not culture, for sustenance. This was the argument. But in fact the dialectical theologians themselves took an active part in molding historical circumstances in their time.[3] And their experience from the end of World War I through the post-World War II years tempered the insistence on the separation of faith and culture so that, when the wind went out of the sails of dialectical theology, its legacy was that of a new openness to culture—an openness reflected in theological interest in medical ethics.[4]

This legacy of openness was promising but problematic. For as Cobb observed, the culture to which dialectical theology had turned its attention was "a culture for which God is dead. What does it mean for Christian theology to take this culture seriously?"[5] In Cobb's view, only one of two options was available. Either "accept and live the death of God" or "refuse the modern world . . . fence in . . . traditional faith, and seek to preserve it from the corrosion of the world outside."[6] Cobb considered both options desperate. He concluded: "It is no wonder that theologians find it difficult to speak relevantly in such a time."[7]

In his 1966 Bampton lectures on the fate of theism, Alasdair MacIntyre recounted a similar story from the vantage of moral philosophy. He noted that the role of theism in Victorian life had been conflict creating, with the result that Christian theology was central to public debates about important cultural questions. A half-century later in Europe and the United States, such debates, when they occurred at all, were culturally marginal. Indifference toward questions of faith and commitment was the rule. Troubled by this turn of events, MacIntyre made the following remark: "With religious issues absent from the scene we are distanced not just from thinkers like Sidgwick and Leslie Stephen but from George

Eliot and Tolstoy, too. Consequently, theologians as various as Dietrich Bonhoeffer, Rudolf Bultmann, and John Robinson in Europe; Paul Tillich, William Hamilton, and Paul van Buren in America, have attempted to restate Christian theology so that it will be a vital issue."[8]

MacIntyre characterized these attempts as "a search for a new response to the second crisis of theism, a response which will neither reject the Christian religion nor retreat into a self-enclosed set of formulas . . . nor attack contemporary secular culture in favor of self-conscious archaism. Neither Bertrand Russell nor Karl Barth nor T.S. Eliot, but . . . but what?"[9] On MacIntyre's account, the first crisis of theism, associated with 19th-century disputes over biological evolution and historical criticism of the New Testament, was epistemological. The second crisis, the one that continues to occupy Christian theologians today, is a moral crisis. The link between the two crises is "the fear that the loss of theistic belief would result in moral collapse."[10]

For MacIntyre, theism's fate was sealed and defenses of it doomed because language about God had become largely unintelligible in our secular culture. If theologians wish to engage in modern moral debates, they must eschew religious language. But the moral parlance of secular culture does not allow them to say anything distinctive. This is the dilemma as MacIntyre saw it. In order to understand, one must first believe; but belief is just what is in short supply. What theologians have to say may be unique and unintelligible, or intelligible and irrelevant ("evacuated . . . entirely of . . . theistic content" and thus lacking critical force), but never intelligible and illuminating.[11]

MacIntyre was looking for theological propositions and "biblical premises"—"the Bible's point of view" philosophically framed.[12] His way of conceiving theology's task was to ask: "What is the philosophy required for the exposition and application of the Bible in nonbiblical cultures?"[13] Surely this is mistaken. It is true that theologians avail themselves of a variety of intellectual means in their search for understanding and in their effort to make moral sense and use of what people hold dear. Philosophical reasoning is one such means, but only one among others. What is needed to do medical ethics theologically is not philosophy but, as MacIntyre himself later argued, an interpretive grasp of the manner in which morality is embedded in practices and of the ways in which communities of practice are guided by living traditions of thought and conduct.[14]

Although in the 1960s and 1970s MacIntyre misread theology's response to our current cultural condition, his diagnosis of that condition was accurate. We late moderns are in a moral muddle, not for epistemological reasons, but because we are spiritually adrift. It is not that we are faithless, and thus in need of moral prescriptions, but that we are having trouble understanding our moral sentiments and convictions well enough to live by them. Although problematic theology claims no monopoly, it is adept at interpreting moral practices.

FAITH WORKING THROUGH LOVE

For more than a decade prior to the emergence of bioethics as an applied philosophical ethics that took medicine and science as its subject matter, Christian theologians had been vigorously debating the relative importance of norms and contexts in moral life.[15] When it was published in 1966, Joseph Fletcher's *Situation Ethics: The New Morality* created considerable controversy, not only in academic theological circles, but also among a broad lay readership.[16] Conceived as a corrective to what Fletcher considered "the basic legalism of classical Christian ethics . . . situation ethics . . . holds flatly that there is only one principle, love, without any prefabricated recipes for what it means in practice, and that *all other* so called principles or maxims are relative to particular, concrete situations!"[17] Fletcher's situationism[18] was in the mainstream of Protestant ethics in the central importance it accorded individual conscience. But for all its insistence on the sufficiency of love as a moral guide, situation ethics was curiously unsituated.[19] "Love is the only universal," and the work of ethics is "to find *absolute love's relative course*" in the situation at hand.[20] How to chart this course was, however, not spelled out. Situation ethics was more polemic than position. It was a timely reminder that, because circumstances matter greatly in moral deliberation, responsible action cannot be achieved in unreflective adherence to abstract norms. Ironically, universal love is just such an abstraction. Fletcher left it up to each loving individual to decide the right thing to do in every new situation.[21]

Paul Ramsey's work offered a principled alternative to situation ethics. Throughout the 1960s, Ramsey had been in search of "unexceptionable rules" of conduct by which to take one's bearings while traversing the "wasteland of utility."[22] That search yielded a rearticulation of the *law* of love as the fundamental norm of conduct in the Christian tradition.

The language of law is not much in evidence in Protestant moral discourse. Love as liberty, as forgiveness, as freedom from the law, is the characteristically Protestant understanding. The antinomian view often attributed to Protestant moralists is, however, without foundation. Luther's sharp distinction between law and gospel, for example, is sometimes taken to be tantamount to a separation of law and love. But for Luther, whereas faith was a gift and as such unachievable by human effort, love was an active virtue lived out in the lives of the faithful under the law. To Roman Catholic moralists following Aquinas, natural law was a conception of human good toward which human nature tends by reason and conscience, unaided by divine guidance. And, regarding natural law, Paul Ramsey was "the contemporary Protestant moralist who learned most profoundly from the Catholics."[23]

Ramsey was also a "genuinely biblical theologian."[24] Beginning from a robust confidence in the authority of the Protestant Christian tradition in which he worked, Ramsey appropriated and adapted natural law theory in a novel way, grafting it on to his own understanding of covenant. His early work had derived an ethic of love from the biblical notion of covenant as a living relationship.[25] "Covenant means . . . unclaiming love."[26] To live in covenant is to live in principled practices beyond legalism.[27]

Reflecting on the arguments against legalism in Paul's letter to the Galatians and those against libertinism in Paul's first letter to the Corinthians, Ramsey articulates how, on a Christian account, the faithful are to conduct themselves in the absence of codified norms.

> In place of rules for conduct . . . comes not irregularity but self-regulation, and not merely the self-regulation of free, autonomous individuals but the self-regulation of persons unconditionally bound to their neighbors by "faith working through love. . . ." What should be done or not done in a particular instance, what is good or bad, right or wrong, what is better or worse than something else, what are "degrees of value"—these things in Christian ethics are not known in advance or derived from some preconceived code, they are derived *backward* by Christian love by what it apprehends to be the needs of others.[28]

Faith working through love is responsive not to what the situation requires but to the neighbor's *need*. Such need must be discerned neighbor by neighbor, but not situation by idiosyncratic situation. Faith working through love is a practice, "a prolongation of the incarnation . . . among those in need."[29] It is discovering that one is freely loved and therefore bound—called—also to love.

Whereas situation ethics is predicated on the uniqueness of situations requiring a decision and the novelty of each loving response, Ramsey emphasized "the similarities among situations . . . the likeness of one person who bears a human countenance with every other person and his needs and claims."[30] And, important for Ramsey, one discerns what response the neighbor's need calls for "not only by asking which singular action is the most loving, but also asking which *principles* of action or *rules of practice* will prove to be most love-embodying or love-fulfilling."[31] Love as covenant-fidelity was to become the central tenet of Ramsey's medical ethics, and the articulation of such love-embodying principles of action as respect for persons the methodological pivot point.

MORAL INTERPRETATION

Over the course of the decade following the publication of Ramsey's seminal work, *The Patient as Person* (1970), the search for methodological clarity became urgent as the new bioethics came into being. With only slight exaggeration, it can be said that this search came to a successful conclusion in 1979 with the publication of Tom L. Beauchamp and James F. Childress's *Principles of Biomedical Ethics*, which promised to "bring some order and coherence to the discussion of [biomedical] problems."[32] Other claimants to the title of ruling methodology appeared (modern casuists were formidable contenders), but it was principlism that carried the day.[33] With the subsequent popularization of principlism and its corollary, the valorization of the principle of autonomy, bioethics became preoccupied with ethical reasoning—"procedures and standards for deliberation and justification."[34] Even Ramsey's principled theological approach to moral inquiry seemed assimilable to philosophical principlism. But the collapsing of Ramsey's robust covenantal notion of "awesome respect"[35] for persons into the then reigning principle of respect for individual autonomy came at the cost of neglecting existential elements of moral life—virtues and vices and the search for meaning and understanding.

Prior to principlism's heyday, Ramsey had written, "Ethos determines what is felt and done more than ethical reasoning does; indeed, ethos is another word for accepted practice."[36] And much earlier, he wrote: "The relationship of doctor to patient is primarily a moral, personal one. . . . Perhaps we should say that diagnosis and cure are processes which go on *between* doctor and patient."[37]

The ethos of medical practice and research was (and is) morally dense. It must be interpreted. And moral interpretation requires the participation of the interpreter. He or she must enter the ethos, engage it, and get a feel for it before saying how things seem to him or her as participant-observer. Some such sense of the need for "reasonable and compassionate moral reflection"[38] must have drawn Ramsey to Georgetown University Medical School in the late 1960s. There he observed what transpired between doctors and patients, reflected with physicians about the moral dimensions of their practice, and rendered his interpretation of what it means "to be attentive to the patient as person."[39] This he did as a Christian ethicist who held that "covenant-fidelity is the inner meaning and purpose of our creation as human beings."[40] From the fact that Ramsey placed this avowal of his moral identity and his professional angle of vision on the first page of the preface to *The Patient as Person*, one can safely surmise that he considered it important for readers to know where he was coming from. But contrary to what the cultured despisers of religion might be inclined to infer from this authorial act, Ramsey did not then proselytize. Instead, he interpreted. He was "content to extract and extend the moral wisdom which he finds already operative . . . among . . . conscientious professionals . . . , and less concerned therefore to supplement, correct, or 'transform' it on the basis of Christian insights."[41] Discerning, illuminating, articulating, and extending the moral wisdom latent in practices is a good working definition of problematic theology.[42]

But is this approach to moral inquiry not characteristic in broad outline of the methods and aims of many cultural historians and anthropologists, literary theorists, philosophers who see things pragmatically or phenomenologically—indeed, of any number of humanists of an interpretive bent? Of course it is.[43] What, then, is the theological angle? In one of two epigrams that announce his last book, *Ethics at the Edges of Life*, Ramsey reproduced an entry from Kierkegaard's journals in which the author regretfully ponders the prospect of the dissipation of "a simple and profoundly passionate admiration and wonder of things which is the motive power of ethics."[44] Each of us who is engaged in moral inquiry and interpretation in the province of medicine is motivated by some passion or other, some sympathy, some admiration, some vision of the way things could be and often latently are. Such passions and visions, although not idiosyncratic, are nonetheless distinctive. Each of us comes from somewhere, and yet we all stand inside the hermeneutic circle.[45] Therefore, it behooves us as scholars and commentators, teachers and caregivers, to reveal to our readers and listeners, students and patients, where we are coming from and how things look from where we stand just now. This, I presume, is why Paul Ramsey identified for his readers his way of seeing the ideas and issues he was about to take up in *The*

Patient as Person as that of a Christian ethicist and then went on to say what he understood that vocation to entail.[46] It is also why each of us owes it to our conversation partners to be as forthcoming as we can about the formative forces and motive power that animate us and call us to our vocation.

THE MORAL WORK OF MEDICAL ETHICS

Thirty years ago John Cobb described Christian theology as culturally marginal, and Alasdair MacIntyre considered it morally ineffectual. The available options according to Cobb were to "accept and live the death of God" or to batten down the hatches and retreat from the world into enclaves of faith. For MacIntyre, theologians who wished to engage in moral debates could continue to use God-language, which was becoming less and less intelligible, or, in a bid to be heard, they could drop theistic language and join the secular conversation but have nothing to say that was not being said by other people of good will and sound mind. Many theologians who went to work on medical ethics 25 or 30 years ago, myself included, made MacIntyre's second move. Jonsen notes: "With few exceptions, the theologians and the philosophers who were partners in the early medical ethics merged into one—the bioethicist."[47] Lumping was more important in those days than splitting, and getting a hearing took priority over pushing the distinctiveness of one's perspective.

As soon as principlism became something of a party line in bioethics, however, that early move had to be reconsidered. Moreover, as a sophisticated understanding of the embeddedness of moral knowledge and intellectual work evolved throughout the humanities, the question of where each of us stands in the hermeneutic circle required individual answers.

When I migrated from undergraduate teaching in religious studies (a gradual transition in my case) and began to work full-time in the medical humanities, I did not think of myself as having let theology slip away. Nor do I think that way now, although for nearly 25 years[48] I have not been a practicing theologian but an ethnic Christian—accepting and living the death of God, doing moral and intellectual work in medicine alongside others similarly engaged with a vast variety of passions and visions motivating them, some theological, most not. This is our late modern circumstance, and I do not find it desperate. I do not think we live in a world of moral strangers,[49] and I think the significance of the fragmentedness of moral knowledge has been overblown. Moral wisdom resides now as always in practices; however, medical practice today is under siege, pushed by social change and pulled by cultural forces, with the result that the moral wisdom in the practice is obscured. The work of medical humanists, problematic theologians among them, is to discern that wisdom, draw it out, focus it, illuminate it, and extend it so that medical and other healthcare practitioners can reconnect with their moral purposes.

As ethnic Christian and problematic theologian, I construe those purposes in a covenantal context as "a prolongation of the incarnation . . . among those in need."[50] Covenant connotes a fundamental fidelity that runs deeper than contractual relations, reaches beyond the spoken and the spelled out, and does not depend on procedural norms. It is an ethos. In covenant, one receives others as one receives a gift—in trust— and one passes the gift on in response to need, with due regard for the recipient, and without calculation. This is the context within which I, as a practitioner of problematic theology, view the moral work of medical ethics. And I go about asking my fellow moral inquirers how they see it, and what calls them to focus on the human scene.

ACKNOWLEDGMENT

Dedicated to William Hamilton—radical theologian, mentor, friend— and to the memory of Ronald Gregor Smith, Doktorvater—ethnic Christians both.

NOTES

1. W. Hamilton, "The Death of God Theologies Today," in *Radical Theology and the Death of God*, ed. T.J.J. Altizer and W. Hamilton (Indianapolis, Ind.: Bobbs-Merrill, 1966), 36-7. On the 20th anniversary of Bonhoeffer's execution, Hamilton wrote of Bonhoeffer, "He is forcing us to shift our center of attention from theology, apologetics, criticism of culture, the problem of communication, and even hermeneutics, to the shape and quality of our lives. He has enabled us to note, in Protestantism, perhaps he has even brought about, the end of theological confidence, and the beginning of a time of confusion between theology and ethics. The communication of the Christian in our world is likely to be, at least for a time, essentially ethical and nonverbal." W. Hamilton, "Dietrich Bonhoeffer," in *Radical Theology and the Death of God*, (reprinted from *Nation*, 19 April 1965), 118.

2. W.F. May, "Why Theology and Religious Studies Need Each Other," *Journal of the American Academy of Religion* 52 (December 1984): 751. May is a

practitioner *par excellence* of problematic theology. See, W.F. May, *The Physician's Covenant* (Philadelphia: Westminster Press, 1983); W.F. May, *The Patient's Ordeal* (Indianapolis, Ind.: Indiana University Press, 1991); W.F. May, *Testing the Medical Covenant* (Grand Rapids, Mich.: Eerdmans, 1996).

3. According to Cobb, "It was they and not the remnants of nineteenth century liberalism who gave effective leadership to resistance against Hitler." See J.B. Cobb Jr., "From Crisis Theology to the Post-Modern World," in *The Meaning of the Death of God: Protestant, Jewish, and Catholic Scholars Explore Atheistic Theology*, ed. B. Murchland (New York: Vintage Books, 1967), 139.

4. It is no coincidence that it was from Karl Barth, dialectical theologian *par excellence*, that Paul Ramsey took his theological bearings in *The Patient as Person* (New Haven, Conn.: Yale University Press, 1970): xii. Ramsey wrote: "I hold with Karl Barth that covenant-fidelity is the inner meaning and purpose of our creation as human beings. . . ."

5. See note 3 above, p. 140.

6. Ibid.

7. Ibid.

8. A. MacIntyre, "The Debate about God: Victorian Relevance and Contemporary Irrelevance," in *The Religious Significance of Atheism*, ed. A. MacIntyre and P. Ricoeur (New York: Columbia University Press, 1969); 25.

9. MacIntyre brought this analysis to bear on medical ethics in "Can Medicine Dispense with a Theological Perspective on Human Nature?" in *Knowledge, Value and Belief*, ed. H.T. Engelhardt Jr. and D. Callahan (Garrison, New York: Hastings Center, 1977), 25-43. Ibid.

10. MacIntyre, "The Debate about God," see note 8 above, p. 29.

11. Ibid., 26; This, as MacIntyre remarks elsewhere, is particularly true of liberal Protestantism, which "was so anxious to address the secular world in that world's own categories that it obliterated stage-by-stage all that was distinctive in Christianity, making it increasingly banal, uninteresting and vacuous." Roman Catholic theologians come in for a different kind of criticism. They "all too often give the impression of being only mildly interested in either God or the world; what they are passionately interested in are other Roman Catholic theologians." See A. MacIntyre, "Theology, Ethics, and the Ethics of Medicine and Health Care: Comments on Papers by Novak, Mouw, Roach, Cahill, and Hartt," *Journal of Medicine and Philosophy* 4, no. 4 (1979): 440.

12. MacIntyre, "Theology, Ethics," see note 11 above, p. 442. See also "A Rejoinder to a Rejoinder," where MacIntyre challenges Paul Ramsey thus: "Let Ramsey provide one decisive position on a question disputed in contemporary medical ethics; let him provide one belief about the Lord of heaven and earth; and then let him show us how the former is derived from the latter. Until he has done this, what he is asserting will remain quite unclear." A. MacIntyre, "A Rejoinder to a Rejoinder," in H.T. Engelhardt, Jr. and D. Callahan, *Knowledge, Value, and Belief*, see note 9 above, p. 76. MacIntyre says that what Ramsey

asserts is "that the Jewish people and the Christian community in all ages are standing 'meta ethical' communities of discourse about substantive moral matters; they propose to shape and fashion how that discourse should proceed. There is no theological statement that is not at the same time an ethical claim, no ethical statement that does not indicate its theological reason." See A. MacIntyre, "Kant's Moral Theology or a Religious Ethics?" in *Knowledge, Value, and Belief*, p. 60.

13. MacIntyre, "Theology, Ethics," see note 11 above, p. 441.

14. A. MacIntyre, *After Virtue* (South Bend, Ind.: Notre Dame University Press, 1981).

15. See, for example, F.S. Carney, "The Virtue-Obligation Controversy," *Journal of Religious Ethics* 1, no. 1 (1973): 5-19.

16. J. Fletcher, *Situation Ethics: The New Morality* (Philadelphia: Westminster Press, 1966), reissued in 1997 with an introduction by J.F. Childress. Fletcher's 1954 book, *Morals and Medicine* (Boston: Beacon Press), although similar in outlook and approach, generated no such stir. See also H. Cox, ed., *The Situation Ethics Debate* (Philadelphia: Westminster Press, 1968).

17. Fletcher, *Situation Ethics*, see note 16 above, p. 36.

18. Fletcher called his method "neocasuistry" but, as Albert R. Jonsen has observed, "for the casuist, the situation is framed by cases that approach it, illuminate it, and challenge it," whereas for the situationist no such context exists. See A.R. Jonsen, "Casuistry, Situationism and Laxism," in *Joseph Fletcher: Memoir of an Ex-Radical*, ed. K. Vaux (Louisville, Ky.: Westminster/John Knox Press, 1993), 23.

19. Wilford O. Cross noted: "The tendency of situationism to treat love as a sort of intellectual-emotional substance in itself and give it verbs of action, saying love does such and such, creates manifold confusion of thought." See W.O. Cross, "The Moral Revolution: An Analysis, Critique, and Appreciation," in *The Situation Ethics Debate*, see note 16 above, p. 157.

20. Fletcher, *Situation Ethics*, see note 16 above, pp. 60-1, 90.

21. As Mary Faith Marshall has observed, "Without knowing what love means in a given situation, one is hard pressed to determine how to realize it." See M.F. Marshall, "Fletcher the Matchmaker; or Pragmatism meets Utilitarianism," in *Joseph Fletcher: Memoir of An Ex-Radical*, see note 18 above, p. 42.

22. P. Ramsey, *War and the Christian Conscience* (Durham, N.C.: Duke University Press, 1961), 6. On exceptionless rules, see especially P. Ramsey, "Two Concepts of General Rules in Christian Ethics," *Ethics* 76, no. 3 (April, 1966): 192-207; P. Ramsey, *Deeds and Rules in Christian Ethics* (New York: Scribners, 1967); P. Ramsey, "The Case of the Curious Exception," in *Norm and Context in Christian Ethics*, ed. G. Outka and P. Ramsey (New York: Scribners, 1968), 56-135. In this last-cited article, Ramsey clarifies his use of the term *rule* as follows: "Heretofore, when treating the methods and the options for adducing or elaborating the full contents of a normative ethics upon the

basis of the ultimate norm in Christian ethics (*agape*, or whatever is a more adequate or fruitful name for our basic Christian perspective upon the moral life), I have used the word 'rule' as shorthand for 'principle,' 'orders,' 'ordinances,' 'ideal,' 'direction,' 'directives,' 'guidance,' the 'structure' of *agape* or of *koinonia* life, the 'style' of the Christian life, the 'anatomy' or 'pattern' of Christian responsibility—as well as for 'rules' strictly so called" (p. 73).

23. J.M. Gustafson, *Protestant and Roman Catholic Ethics* (Chicago: University of Chicago Press, 1978), 151. For a demurrer see C.E. Curran, *Politics, Medicine, and Christian Ethics: A Dialogue with Paul Ramsey* (Philadelphia: Fortress Press, 1973).

24. MacIntyre, "Theology, Ethics," see note 11 above, p. 441.

25. "In the Bible God appears as a covenant-making, covenant-restoring and covenant-fulfilling God; Israel, a people of the covenant and a covenant-breaking people. In both these respects, Christians conceive themselves to be heirs of the covenant." P. Ramsey, *Basic Christian Ethics* (Chicago: University of Chicago Press, 1950), 367.

26. Ibid., 388.

27. Judith Shklar defines *legalism* as "the ethical attitude that holds moral conduct to be a matter of rule following, and moral relationships to consist of duties and rights determined by rules." J. Shklar, *Legalism* (Cambridge, Mass.: Harvard University Press, 1964), 1. See John Ladd's "Legalism and Medical Ethics," in *Contemporary Issues in Biomedical Ethics*, ed. J.W. Davis, B. Hoffmaster, and S. Shorten (Clifton, N.J.: Humana Press, 1978), 1-35.

28. See note 25 above, pp. 78-79.

29. Ibid., 151.

30. P. Ramsey, "The Biblical Norm of Righteousness," *Interpretation* 24, no. 4 (1970): 422.

31. Ibid. I have tried to show that Ramsey was a "principled casuist" in "Paul Ramsey, Principled Protestant Casuist," *Medical Humanities Review* 2, no. 1 (1988): 24-35.

32. T.L. Beauchamp and J.F. Childress, *Principles of Biomedical Ethics* (New York: Oxford University Press, 1979), vii.

33. "Almost from its birth, bioethics was an ethics of principles, formulated as 'action-guides' and little else. . . . This confined scope gave the early bioethics the appearance of a set of rules and procedures and truncated its growth in certain directions, particularly in the realms of moral character and virtue." A.R. Jonsen, *The Birth of Bioethics* (New York: Oxford University Press, 1998), 333. Beauchamp and Childress have continued to refine their method with the publication of each subsequent edition of their book (1983, 1989, 1994). A considerable literature critiquing and defending methodological principlism has evolved which, to review, would digress from the aims of this article. See especially S. Toulmin, "The Tyranny of Principles," *Hastings Center Report* (December 1981): 31-9; *A Matter of Principles? Ferment in U.S. Bioethics*, ed. E.R.

DuBose, R. Hamel, and L.J. O'Connell (Valley Forge, Pa.: Trinity Press International, 1994); R.B. Davis, "The Principlism Debate: A Critical Overview," *Journal of Medicine and Philosophy* 20 (1995): 85-105; "Theories and Methods in Bioethics" (special issue), *Kennedy Institute of Ethics Journal* 5, no. 3 (September 1995). For a detailed account of principlism's rise to methodological hegemony, see A. Jonsen's *The Birth of Bioethics*, especially chapter 10, "Bioethics as a Discipline," 325-51.

34. See note 32 above, p. vii.

35. See note 34 above, p. xiii.

36. P. Ramsey, "Ethical Dimensions of Experimental Research on Children," in *Research on Children: Medical Imperatives, Ethical Quandaries, and Legal Constraints*, ed. J. Van Eys (Baltimore: University Park Press, 1978), 58.

37. P. Ramsey, "Freedom and Responsibility in Medical and Sex Ethics: A Protestant View," *New York University Law Review* 31 (November 1956): 1191-2.

38. See note 4 above, p. 18.

39. Ibid., p. xi.

40. Ibid., p. xi-xii.

41. P.F. Camenisch, "Paul Ramsey's Task: Some Methodological Clarification and Questions," in *Love and Society: Essays in the Ethics of Paul Ramsey*, ed. J.T. Johnson and D.H. Smith (Missoula, Mont.: Scholars Press, 1974), 67-89.

42. *Problematic* theology is decidedly not to be mistaken for *quandary* ethics. For a criticism of the latter, see R.A. Carson, "Interpretive Bioethics: The Way of Discernment," *Theoretical Medicine* 11 (1990): 51-9.

43. The recent scholarly attention to virtue ethics and narrative ethics indicates a broadening of methodological scope in the field. I have spelled out my understanding of "medical ethics as reflective practice" without reference to any particular discipline in a chapter bearing that title in *Philosophy of Medicine and Bioethics*, ed. R.A. Carson and C.R. Burns (Dordrecht, The Netherlands: Kluwer Academic Publishers, 1997): 149-57.

44. P. Ramsey, *Ethics of the Edges of Life* (New Haven, Conn.: Yale University Press, 1978), vii.

45. Every narrative has a moral, including bioethical narratives, as Tod Chambers has persuasively shown in "Retrodiction and the Histories of Bioethics," *Medical Humanities Review* 12, no. 1 (Spring 1998): 9-22. See also R.A. Carson, "The Moral of the Story," in *Stories and Their Limits*, ed. H.L. Nelson (New York: Routledge, 1997), 232-7.

46. Taking a different tack in his study of the ordeals that patients suffer, William F. May makes explicit in a postscript to *The Patient's Ordeal* the central notion of "Jesus's solidarity with those whose stricken identity has been the subject of this book." See note 2 above, pp. 200-6.

47. Jonsen, *The Birth of Bioethics*, see note 33 above, p. 58. Jonsen notes elsewhere that "theological ethicists let their theology slip away as they forged into the ethical complexities posed by technology and the life sciences." A.R.

Jonsen, "The Ethicist as Improvisationist," in *Christian Ethics: Problems and Prospects*, ed. L.S. Cahill and J.F. Childress (Cleveland, Ohio: Pilgrim, 1996), 218.

48. R.A. Carson, "The Motifs of *Kenosis* and *Imitatio* in the Work of Dietrich Bonhoeffer, with an Excursus on the *Communicatio Idiomatium*," *Journal of the American Academy of Religion* 43, no. 3 (September 1975): 542-53.

49. That we live in a world of moral strangers is uncritically assumed in much of the bioethics literature. For an early and influential articulation of this assumption, see H.T. Engelhardt Jr., "Bioethics in Pluralist Societies," *Perspectives in Biology and Medicine* 26, no. 1 (Autumn 1982): 64-78.

50. See note 29 above.

4

Religion, Morality, and Public Policy: The Controversy about Human Cloning

James F. Childress

INTRODUCTION

Although theologians had central roles in the emergence of modern bioethics, religious discourse became marginalized within bioethics before being partially restored. Bioethicists now commonly attend to religious beliefs and practices, particularly in settings where clinicians need to consider their patients' religious beliefs in order to determine how to respect them as persons, or where they need to consider the implications of their own religious beliefs.

On the one hand, questions arise about when if ever it is justifiable to override the religiously based decisions of Jehovah's Witnesses, Christian Scientists, faith healers, or others. There is clearly a need for greater familiarity with particular religious traditions when philosophers confuse, for example, Jehovah's Witnesses and Christian Scientists, whose fundamental beliefs and practices differ so much.[1] However, as Dena S. Davis reminds us, it is not sufficient to study religious traditions' official or dominant beliefs and practices, because individuals who identify with those traditions may have quite different conceptions.[2] Even religious "heretics" have a right to respect in the context of medical care. To take one example, it would be a mistake for a physician in the Indian Health Service to withhold information about the risks of a medical procedure from a particular Navajo patient on the grounds that, according to traditional Navajo beliefs, negative medical information can actually cause medical problems because language creates reality, rather than merely reflecting it.[3] A particular Navajo may, however, have rejected that traditional position.

On the other hand, clinicians may consider how their own religious traditions bear on their actions—for example, does the clinician's particular religious tradition permit participation in abortion and, if so, under what conditions? Such reflections have long been part of traditional medical ethics, as articulated within particular religious communities, while the effort to learn about patients' religious traditions expresses a modern concern to respect patients as persons within a pluralistic society.

Still another question arises about religion and bioethics, and that is the question addressed in this chapter: What is the proper role for religious convictions in the formulation of bioethical public policy in a liberal, pluralistic democracy? This question arises in at least two contexts. It may arise when adherents to a particular religious tradition claim exemption from some legally mandated conduct, such as providing conventional medical care for a child. For example, it arises when Jehovah's Witness parents refuse a blood transfusion on behalf of their child when that transfusion appears to be necessary to save their child's life. It may also arise when there is religious objection, for example, by some Native Americans and Orthodox Jews, to the application of the legal standard of "brain death."[4] The question about the proper role of religious convictions in bioethical public policy may also arise in debates about the moral content and direction of public policy, apart from any claims for exemption from legal duties or legal standards. To address what role religious convictions should play in debates about bioethical public policies, this chapter focuses on the controversy about human cloning that erupted upon the announcement in February 1997 of the birth of a cloned sheep, "Dolly," several months earlier.

In response to the announcement, President William Clinton declared a ban on the use of federal funds for research to clone humans, called for a voluntary moratorium in the private arena, and asked the National Bioethics Advisory Commission (NBAC), which had been appointed in late 1996 to deal with issues in genetics and in research involving human subjects, to prepare a report and recommend appropriate public policies within 90 days. The debate about appropriate public policies toward human cloning, both within the NBAC and in the society at large, affords one way to examine how religious convictions may legitimately contribute to the formation of public policy in a liberal, pluralistic democracy, which involves reasoning and giving reasons to other citizens in a deliberative forum.[5] Instead of addressing constitutional issues, which obviously set the background for such debates, this discussion considers only the social ethics or public morality of speaking in and listening to religious voices in public reasoning and justification.

THE NATIONAL BIOETHICS
ADVISORY COMMISSION

Even though these reflections draw on my participation in the NBAC, I do not profess to speak for the commission. Others inside and outside the commission may have quite different interpretations, as some of the commission's critics certainly do.[6]

NBAC's June 1997 report, *Cloning Human Beings*, recommended continuing the moratorium that President Clinton had imposed on the use of federal funds for research related to cloning humans to create children, continuing his call for a voluntary moratorium in the private arena, and passing federal legislation to prohibit somatic cell nuclear transfer to create children. NBAC rested its recommendations to a great extent on the following argument: "At this time it is morally unacceptable for anyone . . . to attempt to create a child using somatic cell nuclear transfer cloning . . . because current scientific information indicates that this technique is not safe to use in humans at this time."[7] Why? Dolly was the only birth out of 277 attempts, even though 28 other fusions developed to the blastocyst stage, and there are at least theoretical reasons to worry about the effects of the mutations accumulated by the aging somatic cells that are used in cloning. For instance, there are questions about whether such mutations will lead to cancer and other diseases.[8] (The phrases "human cloning" or "cloning humans" are used here to refer to somatic cell nuclear transfer cloning to create children, unless otherwise indicated.)

Some critics charge that NBAC, a "bioethics" commission, copped out because it based its recommendations largely on a *scientific* argument about safety rather than on an *ethical* argument. That charge is misdirected; it reflects an inadequate understanding of ethics. More accurately, NBAC, in light of the available scientific evidence, reached a *moral* conclusion, based at least in part on the ethical obligation not to harm or impose serious risks of harm on potential children. Safety is a fundamental ethical consideration. It is not merely a scientific consideration, even though it obviously rests on scientific evidence. Any procedure that creates a substantial risk of harm to children is morally problematic.

There is no reason to believe that safety problems are permanently insurmountable in cloning mammals, or that this ethical barrier will long endure. Hence, it is crucial to consider other important ethical issues that arise from the prospect of human cloning, such as the probable effect on the family. These issues require careful, thoughtful, and imaginative reflection over time so that society will be ready to respond appropriately to human cloning if and when the technique appears to be safe.

For these reasons, NBAC recommended a sunset clause in federal legislation, review by "an appropriate oversight body" prior to the expiration of the sunset period, and "widespread and continuing [public] deliberation"—in short, a national dialogue—on the whole range of ethical and social issues so that society can formulate appropriate long-term policies toward human cloning. It also attempted to identify, at least in a preliminary way, some of these issues and to start to construct a framework for addressing them. However, it did not attempt to resolve—nor is it likely that it could have resolved—the other ethical and social issues that emerge once the safety problems associated with cloning are resolved.[9]

THE ROLE OF RELIGIOUS CONVICTIONS IN THE DEBATE ABOUT PUBLIC POLICIES TOWARD HUMAN CLONING

When President Clinton asked NBAC to consider the cloning of human beings, he commented that "any discovery that touches upon human creation is not simply a matter of scientific inquiry, it is a matter of *morality* and *spirituality* as well."[10] Shortly thereafter the commission set up two days of hearings, with particular attention to scientific, ethical, and religious perspectives.

Why religious perspectives? Some were surprised that NBAC solicited religious perspectives along with the customary philosophical perspectives. However, attention to religious perspectives is not unprecedented in debates about public policies for new technologies. For instance, in the early 1980s the report of President's Commission's for the Study of Ethical Problems in Biomedical and Behavioral Research, *Splicing Life*, included religious perspectives in its discussion of genetic engineering.[11] In particular, it focused on "playing God," which often has a secular as well as specifically religious significance. (President Clinton also invoked that language, which seems to focus on unwarranted human claims of unlimited power and unlimited accountability.)

NBAC recognized that public policy in the United States cannot be based on purely religious considerations—that its own reasons for its recommendations could not and should not be religious. But, for several reasons, NBAC still believed that it was important to examine religious perspectives, along with philosophical perspectives, on human cloning, in its process of analyzing and assessing moral arguments. In two places in its report NBAC listed several reasons, in slightly different language, for its attention to religious perspectives. Religious traditions "influence and shape the moral views of many U.S. citizens and religious teachings over the centuries have provided an important source of ideas and inspiration." "Policy makers should understand and show respect for diverse moral ideas regarding the acceptability of cloning of human beings in this new manner." Often religious ideas "can be stated forcefully in terms understandable and persuasive to all persons, irrespective of specific religious beliefs." NBAC wanted to determine whether "various religious traditions, despite their distinctive sources of authority and argumentation, reach similar conclusions about this type of human cloning" since a convergence among them, as well as among secular traditions, would be instructive for public policy. "All voices should be welcome to the conversation." And a range of moral views should be considered in determining the feasibility and costs of different policies that might be affected by vigorous moral opposition.[12]

This chapter develops in a more systematic way some of these reasons, along with several others that did not appear in the report or in the commission's discussion. It challenges some conceptions of "public reason" in a liberal, pluralistic democracy that seem or even seek to exclude religious convictions from public decisions and justifications.

EMOTION AND
IMAGINATIVE DELIBERATION

When Dolly made human cloning a realistic prospect, passionate outcries were heard everywhere—"repugnant," "offensive," and "revolting." Even Ian Wilmut, Dolly's creator, found the prospect of cloning a human "offensive." NBAC, according to one analysis, needed to understand "why people reacted with such passion"—their "gut reactions," in Chairman Harold Shapiro's words—and so they "started with religion."[13] That oversimplifies why religious perspectives were important to the commission, even though some religious spokespersons had certainly responded passionately in condemning human cloning, and their responses clearly played some role in the rush to propose legislation in Congress and elsewhere.

Religious perspectives not only help *explain* passionate responses. In public discourse, they may also *instruct* or *inform* emotions and passions. Harvard law professor Martha Minow gives an instructive example. A trial court judge approved a couple's petition to become the legal guardians of a child with Down's syndrome when the biological parents refused to authorize medical treatments that were considered necessary to save the child's life. Judge Fernandez granted their petition, against the biological parents' objections, and in a footnote cited "the Holy Bible, 1 Kings 3:26," which tells the story of King Solomon's threat to cut a child in two when he could not determine which of the two women who claimed be the mother actually was the mother. This biblical story instructed Judge Fernandez's emotions, as the judge noted, and it offered a way for him to reflect on his own anguish as a decision maker in a most difficult case.[14]

The biblical story or stories of creation in Genesis may have functioned in a similar way for some commissioners, even if they were, in Max Weber's terms, "religiously unmusical," and even though religious thinkers used these biblical passages to reach quite different conclusions. Of particular importance in the discussion of the possibility of human cloning is Genesis 1: 27-28 (New Revised Standard Version): "So God created humankind in his image, in the image of God he created them; male and female he created them. And God blessed them, and God said to them, 'Be fruitful and multiply, and fill the earth and subdue it; and have dominion over the fish of the sea and over the birds of the air and over every living thing that moves upon the earth.' "

Such stories, whether they are religious or secular, may also be important in public imagination, as part of public reasoning closely connected with the emotions. A strictly rationalistic model of public reasoning neglects the important role of imagination and reimagination in public policy, just as it neglects the role of the emotions. As a result such a model usually demands that religious views, when offered, be restated or translated into common, secular language. NBAC, or at least some of its commissioners, did ask religious thinkers if they could restate their views in secular terms. And some commissioners "later complained that whenever they asked religious people [in the hearings] to translate their feelings into terms that were more accessible to nonbelievers, they received hate mail accusing them of demeaning spiritual faith."[15] However, a strictly rationalistic model that requires translation of religious language for public reasoning is inadequate. As Martha Minow reminds us, it forces religious people to make constant efforts "to check their religious language and conceptions at the door." This parallels what some towns in the Old West might have required—visitors had to check their guns at the door of meeting places, such as bars. Minow continues, "That seems to be how lots of people talk about excluding religion from public discourse."[16]

But religion is not the only "gun" in town; there are other "comprehensive views" as John Rawls calls them. Furthermore, religious views are not always "weapons." Rather than functioning only as conversation stoppers, they may be quite relevant to the conversation inside the meeting hall, especially if the task is to imagine or reimagine, as is certainly the case when the topic is a dramatically new technology, such as cloning humans.

One NBAC member (Laurie Flynn) reported that she "had been especially moved by [theologian Gilbert] Meilaender's description of children as a gift."[17] Meilaender's description came in the context of the biblical story of creation and his distinction between children as gifts and children as products. It also came in the context of his distinction, drawing on the Nicene creed, between "begetting" and "making."[18] These were heady religious concepts for public discourse about human cloning. As I remember our conversation, Meilaender had asked me, when I called on behalf of NBAC to invite him to testify, whether his *theological* approach would be appropriate, and I assured him that it would. Then individual commissioners asked for translation into secular language, with one commissioner wondering whether it was necessary to use religious categories to express "principled" views, such as the distinction between "making" babies and "begetting" them.[19]

If public reasoning includes imagination, and not only rational deduction from shared secular premises, then even religious stories and theological concepts may enable us to imagine and reimagine in ways that are fruitful for public policy. What does human cloning mean? What are its potential negative and positive effects? Rather than excluding religious views, we should consider them on their own terms to see what we might learn from them. They may yield insights.[20] And they may do so through imagination and reimagination, enabling us to see the technology for cloning humans from different perspectives. This revisioning may be important for public policy, even if in the end policy makers or advisors reject the positions that the religious stories and concepts support or shape and justify a policy on secular grounds. Such revisioning may occur even when the religious positions diverge, as they did in many respects in testimony before NBAC.

One argument for the possible positive role of biblical stories and other religious categories in public imagination focuses on the place of the Bible in American culture. John Coleman suggests that "biblical religion" often provides a "powerful and pervasive symbolic resource" for public ethics in the United States. He notes that major contributors to public life, such as Abraham Lincoln, Reinhold Niebuhr, and Martin Luther King Jr., all appealed to biblical religion, not as revelation, but rather an important source of "insights and symbols [that] convey a deeper human wisdom. . . . Biblical imagery . . . lies at the heart of the American self-understanding. It is neither parochial nor extrinsic."[21] From this standpoint, then, appeals to a biblical story may sometimes be less parochial than some secular appeals.[22] Similar points may hold for concepts and norms that may have originated in specific religious traditions.[23]

Many of us on the commission wanted to hear religious positions in their own terms—in part because they might help us imagine and reimagine—and yet we also wanted to learn whether there might be secular equivalents. Such an inquiry does not impose an unfair burden on religious thinkers and traditions.[24] Listening fairly and attentively to religious positions in their own integrity does not preclude also seeking translation or, if translation is too strong, seeking to determine whether there might be an overlapping consensus.

OVERLAPPING CONSENSUS

Religious communities and traditions often present moral positions and arguments that are not merely or exclusively religious in nature. Their conclusions may rest on premises that are not religious, or not specifically religious, even when they fit within a larger religious framework. For instance, a judgment about human cloning may appeal to "nature," "basic human values," or "family values"—all categories that are not reducible to particular faith commitments and that may be accessible to citizens of different or no faith commitments. Some may serve as "middle axioms," which religious communities may share with nonreligious ones.

A good example appears in the *prima facie* or presumptive moral requirement not to harm others. Even if, in particular traditions, this moral principle is connected to specific theological convictions, its meaning and significance are not necessarily limited to those connections. And this principle provides a moral basis for holding that human cloning is wrong and should be seriously restricted or even prohibited—at least for now—because of the potential harm to children so created. To be sure, particular religious traditions will develop fuller conceptions of this principle, including the nature and significance of various harms.

An overlapping consensus also appears in the conclusion many reached that it is unethical, at least at this time, to engage in somatic cell nuclear transfer cloning to create children. Lisa Cahill argues against Christian ethicists who hold that we can identify only scattered moral fragments of past traditions in our society, in part by pointing "to the *fact* of intercultural and interreligious understanding and social cooperation—however halting, partial, and ambivalent." This fact challenges the claim that "universal human experiences, values, and virtues are simply illusory." One of Cahill's examples is "the recommendation this year of the National Bioethics Advisory Commission to provisionally ban human cloning, reached after fairly inclusive hearings and debates by an interdisciplinary committee formed from various religious and political traditions."[25]

To determine whether there is a *de facto* consensus about public policy toward human cloning, one might think that it is enough merely to count "religious heads"—that is, to find out what religious people, as well as nonreligious people, think. Surveys would perhaps be sufficient for this purpose. However, for purposes of public policy, it is also important to understand the reasons for any overlapping consensus. On the one hand, knowing the reasons might enable policy makers to gauge the intensity and depth of views on human cloning. This might be important as part of a cost-benefit analysis of different possible public policies (for instance, predictable serious and sustained opposition might count as a major cost). On the other hand, the reasons that religious and other thinkers support a particular policy could point in quite different directions under different circumstances (for example, if human cloning proves to be safe for the children so created), and that is important to understand as well.

Even though some religious thinkers, especially those within the Roman Catholic tradition, focus on universal principles or values, a more historicist interpretation of the overlapping consensus is also possible. Sometimes a consensus may emerge because important social-cultural norms are historical deposits of religious traditions. In the secularization debate a number of years ago, sociologist Talcott Parsons among others offered a positive interpretation of secularization as the institutionalization of religious norms in the wider social-cultural context. Originating within particular religious traditions, these norms, such as equality, had become secular—that is, they had become embedded in the society and culture.[26] Whatever their historical origins, they may now operate on their own tracks, to use one of Max Weber's metaphors, as part of the "background culture" and the public political culture.

MORAL REASONING ABOUT PUBLIC POLICY
IN A PARTICULAR POLITICAL CONTEXT

It was not always easy for the commission to determine and keep in clear view its primary target. That target can be described as proposing and justifying a prohibitive, a restrictive, or a permissive public policy with regard to somatic cell nuclear transfer cloning to create a child. In doing public ethics, it is necessary to explicate the premises and presumptions of moral discourse in a particular society. Commissioners need to ask which acts and policies are justifiable within the society's evolving moral framework, not merely which they themselves view as morally justifiable. For several commissioners, the premises and presumptions of a liberal, pluralistic, democratic society placed the burden of proof on those who argued for restrictive or prohibitive legislation directed against human cloning. For them, that burden of proof was met by the safety argument or by the concerns about other ethical issues or by both in combination whether as equal or as primary and secondary arguments.

Another point about context is also crucial. Many liberal political theorists who debate the role of religion in public policy focus on the nature of liberal, pluralistic democracy as such, but too many factors about a particular liberal, pluralistic democracy are relevant to permit such a high level of generalization. Hence, the debate about the appropriateness of religious convictions must occur within a particular liberal, pluralistic democracy, such as the United States, with its own specific history, traditions, institutions, and practices.[27]

Within this specific context, the following additional points are also important. First, arguments for and against a significant role for religious convictions in public policy appeal to two different fears, which may be more or less plausible depending on the particular liberal, pluralistic democracy at a particular time. On the one hand, opponents often fear religion's divisiveness. John Rawls begins his book on political liberalism with the story of religious conflict in the West, and we know full well religion's role in conflicts around the world.[28] Many who argue for a reduced role, or no role at all, for religious convictions in public policy share this fear, and it is not unreasonable. On the other hand, many who argue for an increased role for religious convictions find the "public square" in the United States too empty, and believe that religious contributions could enhance the moral quality of our deliberative process.

The appropriateness of appeals to religious convictions may depend on particular institutions and roles within the democracy. For instance, many liberal theorists take the courts as the paradigmatic institution in a democracy that should not make decisions on religious grounds or give religious justifications for their decisions. Theorists' views vary more widely when they consider legislators, executives, and citizens. NBAC consists of citizens, appointed by the president, to advise the White House Office of Science and Technology Policy; President Clinton specifically asked for advice on policies toward cloning humans, which he then used to propose federal legislation. The kind of information gathering, analysis, and reasoning that NBAC pursued could, in principle, be much more open to religious perspectives than would be appropriate for some other institutions and roles within our democracy.

There is an appropriate role for religious perspectives in the *process* of formulating public policies, as NBAC attempted to do in an advisory capacity, even if it is necessary to limit their role in the *content and justification* of those policies. The process of reaching a decision—or, in NBAC's case, a recommendation—should attend to the widest possible range of positions and reasons for those positions, but the outcome in substance and public justification needs to involve a sufficient or adequate secular—that is, nonreligious—reason.[29] This is especially true when the policy involves coercive measures, as so many do; for example, NBAC proposed a temporally limited ban on cloning humans, and the legislation that the White House subsequently proposed included criminal sanctions.

Even the strongest critics of the place of religious convictions in public reasoning about public policies, particularly ones that potentially involve coercion, tend to recognize a legitimate place for religious convictions in the "background culture," which according to Rawls includes "nonpublic reasons . . . the many reasons of civil society" and which obviously shape how a new technology such as cloning may be viewed.[30] However, it may be very difficult to draw a hard and fast line between background culture and public political debate, particularly on new technologies such as human cloning. Since the background culture tends to spill over into the public debate about appropriate policies, it is better simply to welcome all arguments and assess their worth in public.

PUBLIC SCRUTINY OF
RELIGIOUS-MORAL REASONS

One version of this last argument for inviting religious contributions to debates about public policy also rests on specific features of the background culture and political life in the United States. This argument holds that, since religious convictions inevitably play a role in citizens' proposals for public policies, at least in the United States, those reasons need to be brought into public view so that they can be subjected to appropriate testing too.

By contrast, Richard Rorty suggests that it is appropriate to make religion private and keep it away from the public square, even to the extent of "making it seem bad taste to bring religion into discussions of public policy."[31] Against this argument, Michael Perry contends that we need to "public-ize" religion, not privatize it: "We should welcome religiously based moral arguments into the public square (where we can then test them), not try to keep them out."[32] Perry's argument proceeds this way: Given the fact—and he takes it as a fact based on opinion surveys and other data—that so many Americans are religious, it is inevitable that some legislators and some citizens will rely on religious arguments in making political choices. "Because of the role that religiously based moral arguments inevitably play in the political process, then, it is important that such arguments, no less than secular moral arguments, be presented in, so that they can be tested in, public political debate."[33] Perry is not very clear about how this testing might proceed, since he seems to suggest at one point that it occurs, at least ideally, "by competing scripture- or tradition-based religious arguments," but that surely is too limited for public political debate.

When religious convictions are brought into the public square they are subject to—and should be subjected to—close public scrutiny, just as any other positions should be. For instance, some of them may be mutually contradictory. The fact that a position is religiously based gives it no special claim or privilege in public political debate. Just as a position should not be excluded or rejected merely because it is religious, so it should not gain any special advantage just because it is religious. The model of "religious and moral engagement" (in Michael Sandel's language) that appears appropriate, as a form of mutual respect, in a deliberative democracy entails inclusion but also scrutiny.[34]

The fundamental concern about religious convictions and arguments in public political debate, Perry argues, is not that they are brought to bear, but rather *how* they are brought to bear. For example, they may be asserted dogmatically. And concerns about how fundamental convictions are brought to bear extend to secular convictions no less than to religious convictions.[35] This point is often neglected.

To take one example of this neglect, R.C. Lewontin, in criticizing NBAC for "inviting" religious discussants to the table, fails to see that religious as well as secular arguments, including philosophical ones, may display the same flaws and deficiencies in this regard.[36] He claims that theologians attempt to "abolish hard ethical problems" and avoid "painful tensions." (I will ignore his phrase "internal contradictions," which he includes along with "painful tensions," because both philosophers and theologians try to avoid "internal contradictions" in order to develop defensible positions.) Many theologians as well as many philosophers, in testimony to NBAC and in other contexts, do recognize these painful tensions. Neither group as a whole fails to appreciate the moral conflicts involved in cloning humans, in various scenarios, or in different public policies toward cloning humans, even if different thinkers resolve them differently. And NBAC's own reflections benefited greatly from both theological and philosophical perspectives and considerations. In contrast to Lewontin's interpretation, those religious reflections not only appear in the chapter entitled "Religious Perspectives," but also are interwoven into the chapter entitled "Ethical Considerations," along with philosophical reflections.[37]

Scholars within religious traditions had already engaged in sustained moral analysis and assessment of the prospect of human cloning, beginning as early as the late 1960s and early 1970s. In response to scientifically premature proposals for human cloning, Protestant ethicist Paul Ramsey responded negatively, worrying about its dehumanization. Joseph Fletcher, who by then thought mainly within a secular framework, responded positively by viewing human cloning, along with other reproductive technologies, as more human than "normal" sexual reproduction; according to Fletcher we are most human when we create and use technologies, rather than simply yielding to "nature."[38] They and others mined resources in different religious and philosophical traditions to arrive at their judgments and recommendations. In some ways, then, some religiously based thinking was at least as far along, and may have had more to build on, than some philosophical reflection for analyses and assessments of human cloning.

For such reasons, it was appropriate and even important for NBAC to invite testimony from several religious thinkers. The commission heard from scholars in Jewish, Protestant, Roman Catholic, and Islamic traditions, and it contracted with Professor Courtney Campbell of Oregon State University for a paper on these and other religious perspectives (including Eastern Orthodox, Buddhist, Hindu, and Native American perspectives).[39] In addition, public testimony often reflected religious perspectives. Furthermore, as follow-up to NBAC's report, Senator William Frist organized a hearing before the U.S. Senate Labor and Human Resources Subcommittee on Public Health and Safety entitled "Ethics and Theology: A Continuation of the National Discussion on Human Cloning."[40]

SELECTED RELIGIOUS POSITIONS IN THE DEBATE ABOUT PUBLIC POLICY TOWARD HUMAN CLONING

RELIGIOUS ARGUMENTS

Presenters of religious perspectives identified several relevant ethical concerns about cloning humans, as did presenters of philosophical perspectives. They did not always agree about the significance of those concerns, perhaps in part because some problems would not erupt unless human cloning became a widespread practice (and asexual reproduction does not seem likely to replace sexual reproduction!). Their concerns included physical harm to children so created (the safety issue), psychosocial harm to children, wrongs to children and others through objectification and commodification, harms to the family, and injustice in the allocation of resources.

There is disagreement among particular religious traditions, and in the society at large, about whether, in light of these different ethical concerns, any conceivable acts of human cloning could ever be justified if the technique were safe for the children so created. On the one hand, some thinkers, especially those in the Roman Catholic tradition, hold that cloning humans is wrong in and of itself (that is, intrinsically wrong), and that it would thus be wrong under any conceivable circumstances. Any use would violate human dignity, the natural law, the natural order, or some other fundamental principle or value. The emotional response to this violation would appropriately take the form of revulsion.[41] On the other hand, many hold that human cloning would be wrong in some, perhaps most, circumstances but not in others that could be imagined. Although there are numerous variations, many Protestant and Jewish thinkers, along with many secular thinkers, take this second position and worry about inappropriate uses or abuses of human cloning rather than about every single use. Some who take this second position view human cloning as a morally neutral technology, as Rabbi Elliot Dorff does; others, such as Protestant ethicist Nancy Duff, view it as morally problematic but not intrinsically wrong.[42]

Several possible scenarios are considered—cloning because of problems of infertility, cloning to provide a compatible source of biological material (such as bone marrow) for treatment for leukemia, and cloning a dying child. Many who hold that human cloning could be justified under some circumstances would not view all these scenarios as ethically acceptable. In any event, virtually all religious and secular positions that accept some possible cases of human cloning presuppose that the procedure is sufficiently safe for the child created by cloning and that the child's rights and interests will be adequately protected. Otherwise, human cloning even for legitimate purposes would be morally unjustifiable.

On one point a strong consensus, perhaps approximating unanimity, exists among Jewish, Roman Catholic, and Protestant thinkers. A child created through somatic cell nuclear transfer cloning would still be created in the image of God. This point is important because some commentators on religious views on cloning overlook it. One distinguished political scientist even suggested that religious thinkers would obviously oppose cloning because the children would be "soulless."[43]

Such a misunderstanding may result from the claim, made by some religious traditions and thinkers, that cloning would *violate* the dignity of the child created this way. However, at the same time, they also contend, as one Roman Catholic thinker emphasizes, that it would not *diminish* that child's dignity.[44] In different language, Rabbi Dorff emphasizes that cloning would create "a new person, an integrated body and mind, with unique experiences," however difficult it may be for such persons to "establish their own identity and for their creators to acknowledge and respect it."[45] And Rabbi Bryon Sherwin notes that none of the Jewish sources "suggest that the clone would not have his or her own unique individual human identity."[46] (These comments reflect two views of the violation of human dignity. On the one hand, human dignity involves being brought into being through sexual intercourse of a married couple; on the other hand, it involves independent identity and respect for that identity.)[47]

Religious thinkers who reject all human cloning as immoral tend to favor a permanent legislative ban. By contrast, those who believe that human cloning could sometimes be ethically justified may argue for a ban (usually temporary), or regulation, or permission, depending on the circumstances. At this time, in view of the great uncertainty about the safety of human cloning, a temporary ban or strict regulation seems plausible to many. Nevertheless, concerns quite properly arise about the range and scope of any ban or regulation as well as about its potential effectiveness.

CONSERVATIVE AND LIBERAL POSITIONS—CULTURE WARS?

Sociologist James Hunter has observed that conservatives (orthodox) in a particular religious tradition may share more with conservatives in other religious traditions than with liberals in their own tradition; the same point also applies to liberals (progressives).[48] It is quite striking, however, that this pattern does not uniformly hold with respect to human cloning.

Organizers of a conference for the conservative Center for Jewish and Christian Values, held in Washington, D.C., and sponsored by conservatives in Congress, were visibly uncomfortable when their expected united front of Protestant, Catholic, and Jewish views against human cloning turned out to be somewhat divided. The organizers, who had expected to present strongly the main religious arguments against human cloning and against any policies that would permit it, were mildly startled when Rabbi Bryon Sherwin, a conservative rabbi, indicated that Orthodox and Conservative Jewish thinkers, on the basis of their legal tradition, find it difficult to condemn human cloning *per se*, and that much Jewish opposition to human cloning, particularly in Reform Judaism, reflects categories outside Jewish law. "In my view," Sherwin argued, "Jewish theological, ethical and legal tradition can endorse the propriety of cloning human beings, albeit with certain restrictions."[49]

Religious and secular thinkers alike insist, in what is clearly an overlapping consensus about the moral minimum, that it is morally obligatory not to inflict serious harm on children created through human cloning. One such harm is physical. Cloning would be wrong at least for now, according to many religious thinkers, because cloners could not be sure that they would not be doing unacceptable physical harm to children. This is also the position NBAC took, based on broad societal moral norms, in holding that safety is a fundamental ethical issue (although not the only one) and that, at least for the time being, human cloning to create a child should not be undertaken and should be prohibited through legislation. Such prohibitive legislation would also provide a window of opportunity for the society to determine whether safe human cloning would have unacceptable moral costs and should be severely restricted or even banned.

Consensus on these arguments meant, however, that NBAC did not have to try to resolve the larger debate about the probable effects of acts and especially of widespread practices of human cloning on social values that are not reducible to harms or wrongs to individuals. Under a temporary prohibition, there would be time for society to address the other ethical concerns. One such major concern is human cloning's potential effect on the family, especially if cloning were to become a widespread practice rather than an occasional, isolated act. Among the risks, which some commissioners considered speculative, are threats to fundamental responsibilities within the family, including intergenerational relationships. Certainly questions arise about how to understand relationships—for example, between the source of the cloned tissue and the child created (delayed identical twin)—but our language about family also identifies different responsibilities.

NBAC sought to engender and sustain in its own meetings and in its report serious national moral discourse about human cloning and about public policies toward human cloning. Hence, it listened to and attempted to understand as fully as possible various religious and philosophical positions. And it called for a similar national process over time. It is not clear what to expect from a period of sustained "moral and religious engagement." Unfortunately it appears that this engagement may occur without the deliberative space created by a temporary ban.

ACKNOWLEDGMENTS

The author is indebted to several institutions and individuals, particularly members of the National Bioethics Advisory Commission. An earlier version of this chapter was presented as the 1997 Sorensen Lecture at Yale University Divinity School; a portion was given as testimony at a hearing before the U.S. Senate Subcommittee on Public Health and Safety of the Committee on Labor and Human Resources; and some of the materials appeared in "The Challenges of Public Ethics," in the

Hastings Center Report 27, no. 5 (September-October 1997): 27-9. The author is grateful for helpful discussions at Yale University Divinity School, as well as with the Hastings Center working group on religion and biotechnology. Discussions with Courtney Campbell have also been very valuable.

NOTES

1. For confusion of Jehovah's Witnesses with Christian Scientists, see G. Dworkin, "Paternalism," in *Morality and the Law*, ed. R. Wasserstrom (Belmont, Calif.: Wadsworth, 1971); M. Bayles, "Paternalism," *Principles of Legislation* (Detroit, Mich.: Wayne State University Press, 1978).

2. D.S. Davis, "It Ain't Necessarily So: Clinicians, Bioethics, and Religious Studies," *The Journal of Clinical Ethics* 5, no. 4 (Winter 1994): 315-9.

3. J.A. Carese and L.A. Rhodes, "Western Bioethics on the Navajo Reservation: Benefit or Harm?" *Journal of the American Medical Association* 274 (13 September 1995): 826-9.

4. For a discussion of a New Jersey statute that exempts certain religiously based objections to the brain-death standard, see R. Olick, "Brain Death, Religious Freedom, and Public Policy," *Kennedy Institute of Ethics Journal* 1 (1991): 275-88.

5. For a helpful depiction of "deliberative democracy," especially in relation to bioethical issues, see A. Gutmann and D. Thompson, "Deliberating about Bioethics," *Hastings Center Report* 27, no. 3 (May-June 1997): 38-41.

6. For a critical review of the NBAC Report, see R.C. Lewontin, "The Confusion over Cloning," *New York Review of Books* (23 October 1997).

7. *Cloning Human Beings: Report and Recommendations of the National Bioethics Advisory Commission* (Rockville, Md.: NBAC, June 1997): iii.

8. Ibid., 22-4.

9. Subsequent discussions among individual commissioners suggest that there is some disagreement about whether the recommended temporally limited ban rested equally on safety and the other ethical concerns, or it rested primarily on safety with the ban presenting further opportunity to address other ethical concerns. Individual commissioners may have had different reasons for supporting the ban, and there is some textual evidence for both of these reasons.

10. See note 7 above, p. 12.

11. President's Commission for the Study of Ethical Problems in Biomedical and Behavioral Research, *Splicing Life* (Washington, D.C.: U.S. Government Printing Office, November 1982).

12. See note 7 above, pp. 7-8, 39-40.

13. S. Cohen, "A House Divided," *Washington Post Magazine,* 12 October 1997, 15.

14. M. Minow, "Political Liberalism: Religion and Public Reason" (a sym-

posium), *Religion and Values in Public Life* 3, no. 4 (Summer 1995): 4-5.

15. See note 13 above, p. 15.

16. This paragraph and the next one are greatly influenced by Martha Minow's comments and language. See note 14 above, pp. 4-5, 11.

17. See note 13 above, p. 16.

18. G. Meilaender, "Remarks on Human Cloning to the National Bioethics Advisory Commission," 13 March 1997, reprinted in *BioLaw* 2, no. 6 (June 1997): S114-18.

19. See note 13 above, p. 15.

20. As Meilaender puts it, the theological language he used seeks "to uncover what is universal and human." See note 18 above, S114.

21. J.A. Coleman, quoted in M.J. Perry, *Religion in Politics: Constitutional and Moral Perspectives* (New York: Oxford University Press, 1997), 48.

22. Of course, proponents of religious positions may decry the loss of the distinctiveness of religious positions in public debate when stories function as part of the background culture, but it is outside the scope of this chapter to explore such intrareligious concerns. Nevertheless, even if the Bible is not as significant in the background culture in the United States as Coleman supposes, biblical stories may by their difference or oddness still stimulate the imagination, just as any good story might. For an argument that a certain kind of literary imagination can also be part of public rationality, see M.C. Nussbaum, *Poetic Justice: The Literary Imagination and Public Life* (Boston: Beacon Press, 1995).

23. For instance, one of the major shifts in public policy toward the allocation of organs for transplantation occurred when the national Task Force on Organ Transplantation held that donated organs belong not to the procurement teams and transplant surgeons who remove them from the cadaver but rather to the public, to the community at large, and that procurement teams and transplant surgeons only hold those organs in trust, as stewards, for the community. This fundamental shift in perspective occurred in part through language influenced by biblical accounts of stewardship. See U.S. Department of Health and Human Services, Report of Task Force on Organ Transplantation, *Organ Transplantation: Issues and Recommendations* (Washington, D.C.: U.S. Department of Health and Human Services, 1986).

24. Contrast this with the discussion in C. Campbell, "Prophecy and Policy," *Hastings Center Report* 27, no. 5 (September-October 1997): 15-7.

25. L.S. Cahill, "Beyond MacIntyre," *Religion & Values in Public Life* 5 (1997): 7.

26. T. Parsons, "Christianity and Modern Industrial Society," in *Secularization and the Protestant Prospect,* ed. J.F. Childress and D.B. Harned (Philadelphia: Westminster, 1970), 43-70.

27. See K. Greenawalt, *Private Consciences and Public Reasons* (New York: Oxford University Press, 1995).

28. J. Rawls, *Political Liberalism* (New York: Columbia University Press, 1993).

29. R. Audi, "Liberal Democracy and the Place of Religion in Politics," in *Religion in the Public Square: The Place of Religious Convictions in Political Debate*, R. Audi and N. Wolterstorff (Lanham, Md.: Rowman & Littlefield, 1997), 24-33. The principles of (adequate) secular rationale and (adequate) secular motivation are part of Audi's conception of civic virtue.

30. See note 28 above, p. 220, note 42.

31. R. Rorty, "Religion as Conversation-Stopper," *Common Knowledge* 1 (1994): 3, quoted in M.J. Perry, *Religion in Politics: Constitutional and Moral Perspectives* (New York: Oxford University Press, 1997), 49.

32. Perry, see note 32 above, p. 49. Emphasis added. Elsewhere Perry writes that it is "important that religious arguments be presented—principally, so that they can be tested—in public political debate" (p. 6).

33. Ibid., 45.

34. See M. Sandel's comments in "Political Liberalism" (note 14 above), especially p. 3. He argues for an expansive conception of public reason, "a public reason of moral and religious engagement," which expresses the idea "that mutual respect among citizens means *addressing* our fellow citizens, not just talking at them or appealing to reasons that can't possibly engage them in moral argument."

35. Perry, see note 31 above, p. 49.

36. See note 6 above.

37. This observation also serves in part to rebut Courtney Campbell's objection that "in the NBAC hearings, the contributions of religious perspectives were deemed politically important and ethically insignificant." See note 24 above, p. 17.

38. P. Ramsey, *The Fabricated Man: The Ethics of Genetic Control* (New Haven, Conn.: Yale University Press, 1970); J. Fletcher, *The Ethics of Genetic Control* (Garden City, N.Y.: Anchor, 1974).

39. C. Campbell, "Religious Perspectives on Human Cloning," *Cloning Human Beings: Report and Recommendations of the National Bioethics Advisory Commission*, vol. 2: Commissioned Papers (Rockville, Md.: NBAC, June 1997).

40. "Ethics and Theology: A Continuation of the National Discussion on Human Cloning," Hearing before the Subcommittee on Public Health and Safety of the Committee on Labor and Human Resources, U.S. Senate, 105th Congress, First Session, 17 June 1997.

41. See, for example, L.S. Cahill, "Hearings on Cloning: Religion-Based Perspectives," and A.S. Moraczewski, "Cloning and the Church," testimony before NBAC, 13 March 1997, both reprinted in *BioLaw* 2, no. 6 (June 1997): S100-05. For an emphasis on repugnance and revulsion, see L. Kass, "The Wisdom of Repugnance: Why We Should Ban the Cloning of Humans," *New Republic*, 2 June 1997, pp. 17-26.

42. N.J. Duff, "Theological Reflections on Human Cloning," Testimony before NBAC, 13 March 1997; Rabbi E. Dorff, "Human Cloning: A Jewish Perspective," both reprinted in *BioLaw* 2, no. 6 (June 1997): S106-13, 118-25.

43. Nevertheless, in discussion at NBAC and at the Hastings Center, Gilbert Meilaender thought that the status of the child created by cloning at least merited more reflection.

44. A.S. Moraczewski, see note 41 above.

45. Dorff, see note 42 above.

46. B.L. Sherwin, "Religious Perpsectives on Cloning," (paper presented at a conference on Religious Studies in Cloning at the U.S. Capitol, Washington, D.C., 24 June 1997), 6.

47. The NBAC report rightly avoided all uses of the term *clone* or related terms to refer to the children created by this process, on the grounds, as one commissioner put it, that we should not create a new social category that could create mischief, provide the basis for discrimination, and so forth. It does appear in some writings, including some that condemn cloning. For example, L. Kass (see note 42 above) refers to the "clonant" (p. 20).

48. See J.D. Hunter, *Culture Wars: The Struggle to Define America* (New York: Basic Books, 1991), 96. "The theologically orthodox of each faith and the theologically progressive of each faith divided consistently along the anticipated lines on a wide range of issues," such as sexual morality, family issues, and capitalism.

49. See note 46 above, p. 2.

5

Relativizing the Absolute: Belief and Bioethics in the Foxholes of Technology

Dolores L. Christie

INTRODUCTION

" 'Beware of the dog.' There are doubtless many people around who believe that an analogous sign is in place when a theologian is present to discuss the ethical dimensions of biomedicine. Theologians just might bite. Or worse, they may not."[1] In his discussion of the connections between a particular theological stance—Roman Catholicism—and its effect and influence on bioethics, Richard McCormick expresses the difficulty that many people have with the intersection of believers, theologians, and scholars of religions with the bioethical project. Are they dangerous, as he suggests some believe? Or are they, like many dogs, merely harmless or even useless? McCormick's musings point to the question that prompted this book. In this chapter I shall offer my own musings on the subject.

Professionally I wear two hats. I hold an academic appointment in a department of religious studies in a frankly religiously oriented college. In that small department, my teaching load includes the usual utilitarian and eclectic array of entry-level religion and theology courses. Although a number of my students do not share the religious affiliation of the institution, many of the courses offered consciously espouse and promote those beliefs, albeit in an academic rather than a proselytizing context. My other hat is that of philosopher, as I teach one bioethics course each semester in the department of philosophy. To complicate the issue, I profess to believe in God and am academically trained as a theologian. This network of identities has prompted some thinking on how religion and bioethics connect.

This chapter examines the results of that internal conversation. First, it looks at the development of bioethics as a field, its preferred methodologies, and their limits. Second, it examines the scope of religion and of bioethics. Third, it presents three distinct modes of intersection between bioethics and religion and their potential contributions. Finally, the chapter concludes that a religious perspective, properly understood, may function effectively and profitably to enrich bioethics.

NONRELIGIOUS MODELS

INTRODUCTION

The rich soil in which bioethics was planted some 30 years ago with seeds from a variety of disciplines was not particularly adverse to religion. The first edition of *The Encyclopedia of Bioethics*, for example, contained a number of articles that linked the concerns of bioethics with the principles and professions that some mainline American religions hold.[2] Yet while many early authors in bioethics were themselves religious people and indeed wrote professionally from a religious bias, the mainstream of bioethical dialogue has not reflected a serious conversation with religion. Although bioethics has been and continues to be an interdisciplinary field, the contributions of religion have been marginalized at best and ridiculed at worst. For example, although articles on Roman Catholic and Jewish perspectives on abortion appear in the original *Encyclopedia* and explorations of various religious perspectives on bioethical issues have continued to appear in the literature, such work has proved to be somewhat peripheral to the main development of the field. Mark Siegler speaks of the "secularization of American bioethics," which he perceives as a shift away from what are the important values and beliefs of the parties involved.[3] Religion has been the eccentric shirttail relative, begrudgingly present at family celebrations but without a serious function in the conversation at the dinner table. The favored paradigm for bioethics has become that of philosophy. Its moral methodology, which tends to systematize procedure and method rather than define content and values, has emerged as dominant.

PRINCIPLE-BASED BIOETHICS

The influence of the Enlightenment can be seen in the basic development of the philosophical model, at least in the United States. Two paths have emerged: the first is principle-based ethics, the second is the philosophical methodology of deontology and teleology. Beauchamp and Childress, whose book is still considered a standard for teaching bioethics, use the foundational values of medicine and render them normative for moral action in the form of bioethical principles.[4]

Beauchamp and Childress offer a "framework for moral judgment and decision making" in light of scientific, technological, and social developments in contemporary society.[5] They are not concerned with the development of definitive standards for the good, but with "action guides"[6]—engines that drive the process of solving a moral dilemma. Their appeal to content—what comprises rightness and wrongness—seems somewhat slippery. It derives from popular consensus, what they call "common morality."[7] Although the fabric of their methodology is reinforced by the use of deduction, induction, and attainment of a coherency, the nature and relevance of introducing threads of value is never seriously addressed. What is the basis in the good for the rules that precede and ground the process? Beauchamp and Childress themselves admit the limitations of deduction and induction, noting that the answers at which decision makers arrive with regard to a particular question (the example they use for a deductive method is abortion) may find their ground "less on moral rules and principles than on beliefs about the nature and development of the fetus."[8] They remark that moving from the particular to the general in the inductive process leaves haziness about the role of particular experience and individual judgment."[9] Methodology alone, however complete and elaborate, does not justify answers to concrete moral dilemmas.

The solution to the deficiencies of deduction and induction offered by Beauchamp and Childress is a Rawlsian "reflective equilibrium," which provides a *prima facie* judgment about the rightness of a particular action, based on a common agreement of what is the good. Liberation theologians and others have questioned reliance on the good as defined by popular consensus. They have demonstrated that the strong voice and abundant power of the dominant culture sometimes mask the continuation of real evils as part of the normative structure.[10]

One does not need to travel too far afoot to see illustrations of this assertion. There are the Tuskegee studies, which for many years exploited men who were poor and without status. Although today we would have a totally different perspective on those studies, at the time the culture did not even question whether to tell the truth to a group of poor and powerless individuals. In a more contemporary example, we can lift up the denial of informed choice of medication to pregnant women with acquired immunodeficiency syndrome (AIDS) in third-world countries.[11] Although this discussion does not mean to imply that Beauchamp and Childress would support exploitative research or that using their method likely results in bad decisions, these extreme examples illustrate the potential folly of trusting "common wisdom" to define what is the good. Ungrounded decision making may open to the exploitation of those with faint voice and little power. Perhaps my viewpoint is prejudiced by a religious perspective, but I am reluctant to book passage on the good ship "Common Consensus." In the final analysis, Beauchamp and Childress offer an attractive package, a house of cards marvelous in its balance and logic, but inadequate as a complete method for moral decision making. It is vulnerable to a shift in the wind of common morality, which could disturb its fulcrum or topple it altogether.

ETHICS OF DUTY AND CONSEQUENCE

Philosophy offers bioethics the formula of duty and consequences worked out by C.D. Broad in the 1930s[12] and brought to the modern reader in the work of William Frankena.[13] Like a principle-based approach, the methodology of duty and consequences must use content, but it too has no formula for ascertaining precisely what content or values should take precedence over others. Deontological formulas presuppose but do not define certain values that are preserved in expressions of duty. Consequentialists draw, often unreflectively, on values to sort possible choices in a. case, or they employ paradigmatic events (rule consequentialism: if these conditions are present, following this rule will achieve good consequences) to arrive at the good and therefore the right answer to a dilemma. Ultimately the manipulation of the duties and the consequences, acts or rules, is done on the basis of a corpus of beliefs that the decision maker holds, but may not bring to consciousness. As Richard McCormick has observed, "Discursive reflection does not *discover* the right and good, but only *analyzes* it."[14] The content of the right and the good, which takes the form of rules, taboos, values, and so forth, is the subject of this analysis. That the necessary "right" or "good" content remains largely undefined may explain why persons using the same methodology can arrive at different answers to the same dilemmas, and persons claiming different methodologies ("It is my duty" meets "I gotta do what works") sometimes arrive at the identical answer to a moral problem. This can be seen time and time again in the classroom, where the methodology a student uses eventually is less important than the particular belief system that he or she holds.[15]

CONTEMPORARY VOICES IN ETHICS

It may be this lack of attention to content in the methodology described above that has precipitated the growing suspicion that a strictly philosophical approach to bioethics is insufficient to address the complexity of contemporary issues. To address this perceived inadequacy, attempts have been made to admit other voices to the bioethical conversation. The profession has added new tools.[16] For example, it has become increasingly common to speak of virtue ethics, a "new" way of dealing with the appropriation of values in both the deed and the doer. The spotlight has widened to explore the character and moral reality of the doer, in contrast to an approach that focuses substantially on the nature of the action itself.[17] The contention is that how I am, my moral dispositions and attitudes, has an influence on the character of what I do. The moral adjudication of actions cannot be determined solely by their content; it must include their motivation. Common sense suggests that morally right actions are more apt to be performed by those of morally upstanding character.

Beauchamp and Childress acknowledge a deficiency in an actor-neutral approach and try to address it in their text. They outline the moral character that is desirable for the medical professional, situating its source in the professional relationship or in the codal models peculiar to the profession. They note the evolution of these codes into the contemporary form that eliminates nearly all vestiges of reference to virtue.[18] Often those who speak of virtue ethics speak of them in a frankly religious mode. The recent work of Pellegrino and Thomasma,[19] for example, underlines the importance of religious commitment, with its emphasis on attitude and virtue, to the bioethical project.

In addition to the virtues approach, there is a growing body of literature on the so-called feminine ethics of care (beginning with the work of Carol Gilligan) and on feminist ethics, which uses a political or liberation methodology as well as a gender-sensitive perspective to address the serious issues in the field.[20] Feminine ethics emphasizes a particular value in the process of decision making, that of care, placing importance on the context of the decision and calling into question any fixed or arbitrary solutions.[21] This approach is a strong challenge to the dispassionate and objective model that has characterized medicine for a long time. Feminist ethics examines the political and power issues that are embedded not only in individual moral decision making, but in the very structures that dictate where money goes, how attitudes are formed, and so forth.[22]

Recently, we have witnessed the reanimation of case-based ethics, with the emphasis on model cases to help solve current dilemmas.[23] By attending to the particular case, those who use this method have tried to fill the lacunae in a purely principle-based or philosophical approach. Modern casuistry has the advantage of addressing the particulars of a dilemma without neglecting the paradigms or principles that may apply to it. However, this method does not possess the tools to mediate diverse perspectives on the good. If I believe that autonomy is the most important value, another person's passionate appeal to society's good and to slippery-slope arguments against my anticipated suicide will not change my resolve to kill myself. If a physician is convinced that a transplant is the only response to a patient's medical situation, the patient's wish to remain home and to die in a shorter time but without surgery and immunosuppressing drugs will not even get a hearing. This is especially apt to occur if the patient is limited in the ability to express his or her preferences or is perceived to be unable to understand the merits of the suggested treatment. Historically, casuistry underwent significant development within the Christian tradition, which proved to be the strength of the method. Ultimately, however, connections with religion may have been the genesis of its decline in the late 19th century and early 20th century, when philosophical ethics became dominant.[24]

THE SCOPE OF RELIGION

Does religion and its study have anything to add to the mix? The very word itself tends to be thrown around as if everyone had a common understanding of its meaning. Religion is difficult to define, since it evokes a cluster of meanings both among believers and among those who reject its claims. In general, however, religion claims to offer explanations that satisfy the human quest for meaning. It professes to answer such questions as "What can I know?" "What should I do?" and especially, "What may I hope?"[25] Religion and its claims exist, at least in part, in an extratemporal context, gathering human experiences and attempting to explain them in light of a supreme being or transcendent idea, critiquing culture and its manifestations through the filter of the resultant belief system, and offering solutions to the situations of life that seem insoluble by scientific knowledge or action alone. All human cultures have some religious dimension—beliefs, rituals, and behavior patterns. Rudolf Otto's "holy,"[26] Mircea Eliade's "sacred,"[27] and Paul Tillich's "ultimate concern"[28] all address an idea of a being or direction that is not delimited by a positivistic view of the world. Some religions name and define the holy or the sacred in a frankly personal fashion; others do not. A tentative definition of religion can be constructed: religion is a system of beliefs professed by individuals and within a community that struggles with ultimate questions, offers a set of answers to those questions, and prescribes behavior consistent with that construct.

WHAT RELIGION OFFERS

Religion proposes to offer many advantages to the individual. First, it may provide an identity, an articulation of *who* the believer is. Religious persons are never merely individuals, standing alone with only a singular goal. Their identity is caught up in the existence of others—both the significant other (the god or supreme being) and the "others" who share the community of belief. This notion of the believer's essential connectedness to community is exemplified in the work of such Christian thinkers as Janssens, Häring, and Hauerwas.

Embedded in religious language are answers to questions of identity; anthropology; and concepts about self, others, the world, and the divinity. My religious anthropology may tell me I am good—an *imago dei*—and that I should trust my judgments about reality. There is a self-confidence created by such a stance that will serve believers well in their life projects.

Starting with a different anthropology, religion may tell me that I am a sinner and untrustworthy, and therefore dependent on another, an authority figure, to tell me what to do. It may even name that moral mentor for me. The authority may be called physician, family, elder of the church, or divine voice. Transfer of responsibility for decision making to another may provide security to believers; they will be relieved of the awesome task of making decisions for dilemmas that confound them.

Second, religion offers the believer a *what*—a particular and concrete story that defines origins, identity, and destinations in the form of religious myth. Religious myths not only tell believers who they are and what they are worth, they articulate religious answers to dilemmas that seem inadequately addressed by a scientific methodology. Religion offers a perspective on such difficult questions as the meaning of life and death and the place of suffering in human existence. Such answers, be they the promise of an afterlife or the hope of returning to a new life with better prospects, provide believers a corpus of meaning. They articulate not only what is to be believed, but why. At the bedside of a dying child, the pain of medical hopelessness may be relieved more effectively by the language of heaven than with words that define in exquisite detail the type of cancer that is sapping a nascent life. For the religious person, whether the belief is true or false is less at issue than whether that belief works to provide consolation and comfort in the face of life's illogical conundrums.

Religious tradition may affirm the goodness of the material world and its connectedness to humanity, or it may eschew that connection on the basis of a dualistic understanding of the material world. Attitudes toward medical treatment, sustaining of life, or how to treat the body will be informed by such beliefs. Religious story may affirm God's jurisdiction over the world. In that sense it relativizes the need to find complete and definite solutions to all the problems that living presents; it puts into a larger frame the questions that press urgently on the bioethical agenda. This can be problematic.

Third, religion articulates a *where*—a location that situates the believer in relationship to the sacred. The suggestion of transcendence, something beyond the human being, relativizes the dogma and conclusions of science—and even of bioethics. If I am not my own genesis, my attitude toward my own reality is modified. In a religious worldview, the value of human life is not completely defined within the frame of bodily function—a biological commodity to be preserved, disposed of as I wish, or even bartered for another good. A religious perspective may not view the individual as "a collection of cells and organs and their functions . . . a diseased organ or a system of organs"—what Häring calls "sacralization of the physiological aspect of human nature."[29] Such questions about identity and the meaning of human life are currently being raised in bioethics, but are not adequately answered. Contemporary issues that illustrate this lacuna of answers include human cloning and patenting human genetic material.[30]

In a religious worldview, death as the "final frontier" of science, as noted in Daniel Callahan's work, can give way without regret. Not only does this have implications for decisions about who is ultimately in charge at the bedside and what must be done, it has the potential to effect change in the more global issues of macro-management of funds for healthcare.

If perfecting human technology, fending off death, and minute tinkering with human life to achieve its ideal form are no longer the only and ultimate goals of human existence, those who allocate funds for medical purposes can relax a bit. It may not be necessary to do all things for all people. Keeping multiple Helga Wanglies alive indefinitely is not the only reasonable goal. Religion has the potential to suggest the basis for alternatives. This discussion is not advocating a nihilistic approach to medicine, but it is suggesting an alternative vantage point.

Fourth, religion functions to give the believer a certain attitude or set of attitudes—a *how*. The discussion above mentioned the attitude of relativization of some of the values that science, and likewise medicine and bioethics, tend to hold sacred. In addition, if one were to examine the stories and beliefs of any specific religious tradition, one would uncover certain traits of character that the "religious" person embodies. Note that there is no attempt here to claim that such attitudes are unique to the religious person. However, because of the specification through religious narrative, the reinforcement of the community, and the conscious espousal and practice by the individual believer, these attitudes are highlighted in religion in a systematic manner often wanting in other arenas. Such values as compassion, hope, generosity, and patience are exemplary but not exhaustive.

Finally, religion offers the believer a community—a *with whom*. The word *religion* comes from the Latin, *religio*, meaning to bind. Religion as a serious endeavor requires the personal investment of the individual in a set of beliefs. It often includes the commitment to and participation in a community of believers who preserve, teach, and pass on what is believed to the next generation. Such commitment generally exhibits a pledge to certain behaviors that are shaped by the content of the beliefs and the practice of the community. The individual "binds" himself or herself to certain ideas, people, and actions. The prescribed actions—morality—are generally the outgrowth of what the religious group believes to be important and of value. For example, the Christian Scientist who is in pain may call in a "practitioner"—a type of minister and member of the community who prays with the believer in times of trial and pain.

Community is an extension and reinforcement of the individual person's identity to an identification with others. Other members may be viewed as like ourselves, deserving of respect and consideration. Individual decisions must therefore include a concern for the well-being of the others who are like ourselves.[31] Should the rich, 75-year-old businessman consent to be placed on a list for liver transplant—even attempt to use his financial resources to manipulate his rank on that list—when there are younger persons in triage for the same list? Can the goals of the individual be realized at the expense of the needs of the many? An orientation toward the common good, the well-being of all members of the community, which religion invokes, will change the conclusions and character of decision making.

There is a concreteness to all aspects of religion—a clear *who, what, where, how,* and *with whom* that evolve from the historical and ongoing religious experience of the group but are appropriated in a unique fashion by the individual.[32] Religion does not function as an entity disconnected from persons or from contexts, however. Religion is enfleshed, peculiar to this concrete believer, rendering the attempt to define religious claims and boundaries complicated. Religion can mean a variety of things to different people, and a particular canon or code can be appropriated selectively by an individual believer even from within a clear and established religious tradition. The woman who embraces Christian Science but consents to pain medication immediately after an elective surgery and the avowed Roman Catholic who uses birth control pills exemplify this selective diversity. In the end, persons choose to live their lives based on a self-selected set of values, based in their own personally composed story, and acted out in the moral choices of their lives. Jonathan Z. Smith observes: "While students of religion may employ the generic term 'religion,' they know full well that there is no one who lives such a 'religion.' "[33] That this is true must be taken into account in exploring the connections between the study of religion and bioethics.

Likewise, religions' claims to truth do not rest solely on their ability to be proven through scientific means, although that does not mean they are necessarily unscientific or illogical. It is the nature of religious claims to be in a different category of truth from the truths of science or philosophy, as Tillich demonstrated.[34] It is precisely this issue that sometimes causes religious assertions to be dismissed as irrelevant in bioethics, whose methodology intersects with the patently scientific field of medicine.

THE TASKS OF BIOETHICS

In contrast to religion, bioethics has its own set of tasks. First, bioethicists wish to contribute to the solution of concrete dilemmas. The function especially of the clinical bioethicist is to add expertise, both scientific and methodological, to the concrete decision-making projects of patients, family, and medical personnel. A bioethicist is sufficiently knowledgeable about medicine to understand the procedure or treatment under consideration and to apply the peculiar expertise of method to a moral dilemma. The bioethicist's value as a professional is enhanced if he or she understands the psychology of human interaction, the place of emotions and power issues in decision making. The function of the ethicist is not to make decisions, it is to facilitate the decisions of the proper decision maker—in most cases the patient or the patient's appointed surrogate (at least in North America). Whatever the bioethicist brings in terms of his or her own belief system may be added to the mix of discussion; it may not override that of the person whose decision it is to make.

Second, the bioethicist is concerned with breaking open the many aspects of an issue, bringing to bear methodologies and values that may shed light and understanding. He or she may use scholarly leisure to think about the complexity of an issue, to try to uncover all its aspects. Naturally, the bioethicist brings a particular point of view, nourished by his or her own experiences, training, and system of beliefs. The literature is filled with articles that explore issues from a variety of viewpoints.

Third, the bioethicist has an influence and authority that extends to policy making. Not only is there need to resolve whether a concrete Sarah should have an abortion or a real-life Tom should have life support removed, there is concern about specific policies on abortion or futile treatment for particular hospitals or nursing homes. Such policies must take into consideration a multiplicity of values and concerns as well as the interests of all the people who will be affected. The power of bioethicists to influence decision making at this macro level may extend to questions of allocation of funds, government policy, and even law. It is an awesome power. What, if anything, does religion offer to this important task? Since I can reflect only on my own experience, the answer proposed here represents that perspective. How do I function as a believer, whose canoe finds itself afloat in the choppy river, "Bioethics"? As a theologian, do I have something to offer the field? What do I teach the students who enroll in my classes in religious studies? Is this different from what I teach in bioethics, in the department of philosophy?

THREE MODELS OF INTERSECTION
BETWEEN RELIGION AND BIOETHICS

Three models that exemplify ways in which religion may intersect with bioethics are examined below. Each model—believer, theologian, and scholar of religion—is an example of the "practice" of religion.

THE BELIEVER

The believer may play the role of patient or of bioethicist. Either enters the bioethics stage with a set of values and perceptions about life that may be different from those of other professionals, caregivers, and so forth. This is a good thing. Personal religious belief may function as a stabilizing force in the kinds of crises medical decisions sometimes bring. A potential transplant recipient testified that "her husband, daughter, and her religion [constituted] her support system."[35] For believers religious belief offers the adherent strength, consolation, and sometimes explanations for what is happening to them. Religion may offer hope to those who medically seem to have no hope. There is a growing body of literature that attempts to address so-called alternatives to traditional medical practice, some of which have a basis in religion. Faced with a serious life-or-death medical decision, the believer often relies on religion as a rudder in a frightening sea. Bioethicists who are also believers will understand this element in a particular case, either because of familiarity with the patient's belief system or at least by analogy from their own belief systems. Although this is not a unique function for the bioethicist—in fact, it is more pertinent to work of the hospital chaplain or religious minister—it is an added dimension to the role.

On the other hand, religion may navigate the believer to the shores of a decision that is problematic—a situation where the tenets and especially the practice of religion seem to interfere with the person's ability to choose a medically efficacious procedure or path. Religious belief seems sometimes to function as an impediment to good decisions. Because religion is by its very nature not totally dependent on factual or scientific data to substantiate its claims,[36] religion's conclusions may appear to clash with those of science. Medicine, and perhaps by extension bioethics, grounds its conclusions in scientific method; what one can demonstrate through data gathering and empirical observation is what one will believe. This approach is positivistic, of course, finding truth only where proof of that truth is available. Because many of the same issues and the same people are involved in medicine and in bioethics, there is bound to be a carryover of assumptions and method. "What is the *right* answer?" has been asked many times in ethics committee meetings, as if some datum will emerge to support a definitive solution to a sticky question. Many unresolved areas in bioethics appear to await scientific solutions. For example, if it can be determined once and for all when death actually occurs, somehow that will resolve the moral issues connected with organ retrieval; if a certain percentage of women develop breast cancer before the age of 40, the determination of whether a particular woman should have her breast removed prophylactically will be answered. The problem is one of mixing unlike categories, expecting facts to solve moral dilemmas. Although such data are important, even essential, to the decision-making process, facts alone do not provide answers to moral problems.

Some religious claims seem to rest so completely and preemptorily on nonscientific bases that very little common ground can be found between them and other discourse. Often it is precisely these forms of religious thought that are lifted up as mainstream and normative—straw men, as it were, to be batted down. They are presented as clear and definitive evidence that religion has little to say in a sophisticated contemporary dialogue. The result is that all forms of religious thought may be dismissed as irrelevant to a serious bioethical conversation; religion and its study are then rejected as quaint relics from a premodern culture. As Stephen Post notes in his discussion of the attitude of psychiatry toward religion: "Reductive interpretations of religious phenomena inevitably lead to insensitivity and lack of empathy toward those persons who manifest particular beliefs and behaviors of a religious nature."[37]

While Post goes on to argue the efficacy of taking seriously religion in all its manifestations, there are some instances of belief that cannot contribute much to an effective interdisciplinary dialogue. Because they often are lifted up as representative examples of all religion, they contribute to the marginalization of religious discourse from the area of bioethics. Such instances need to be named and examined, if only to set them apart from the premise that religion and bioethics have a place of common discourse. It is important, however, not to confuse the strongly held beliefs of an individual, which ought to function in a preemptive manner in decision making *for that individual*, and those beliefs as serious data in a partnered dialogue with other positions. Bioethicists would do well to examine their own belief systems to ascertain where they fit in this spectrum.

Stumbling Blocks

Stumbling blocks to the dialogue between religion and bioethics take many forms. Some affect only the individual; others affect the larger community. This is true especially of those beliefs that claim a preemptory grounding in religion, but that may embody values that are seen by nonbelievers as unacceptable even for those who hold them. These beliefs all have a common root. They are based in a kind of supernatural absolutism[38]—what is moral is a function of God's approval or disapproval—or in religious positivism, which may profess no interest in the logic of empirical evidence or the conclusions of the collective experience of the culture.

The first type of supernatural absolutism encompasses a religious perspective and a consequent mode of action that may seem morally suspect to the majority of onlookers. This is not particularly problematic, however, if the only ones affected by the belief are the believers themselves. The Christian Scientist who refuses treatment or the Jehovah's Witness who does not consent to a lifesaving transfusion of blood may bring consternation to the surrounding medical personnel, nurses, and consulting ethicists, but the actions the believer takes affect only herself. It may be difficult for others to stand by in such cases, especially in light of medicine's commitment to cure and to care. It is important to distinguish the proper moral jurisdiction and moral agent—in this case the patient—from that of the professional. It is not the professional who, as moral agent, "kills" a patient by nonintervention; it is rather the choice of the proper moral agent, the patient, to forgo treatment for religious reasons, invoking values that override those of medicine. In neither case is there need for the unwilling, active[39] participation of another or for the extension of a financial or care burden on the medical system. Neither Christian Scientist nor Jehovah's Witness patients expect those who do not share their beliefs to do what they do, although the devout might judge nonbelievers to be in danger of losing what some religions prize—the possibility of eternal life. Although the example of such strong religious belief has much to edify, it provides little occasion for dialogue. It provides the occasion for respect, however, and for clear definitions of decision-making boundaries.

Those who depend solely on arbitrary divine control to give them direction for medical decisions may pose a problem to the implementation of good medical care. Courtney Campbell has delineated two extreme positions in this regard.[40] On the one hand, religion can provide an attitude of fatalism, committing the believer to await God's pleasure in the medical arena. "Since it is God's will that determines whether my child will live or die, there is nothing medicine can offer. I need just to pray and to wait for God's action." This approach leaves little room for discussion, acting as a trump card[44] to short-circuit medical intervention, even in the face of its compelling logic. In the emergency room or at the bedside, medicine is not sympathetic to this position. The other pole is characterized by the espousal of vitalism,[42] says Campbell, which dictates that all forms of medical intervention be used. "I have no say in deciding when this person should die; that is God's decision. Therefore I must continue to do everything I know how to do to save him." Such an attitude prompts the sometimes desperate continuation of treatment when there is no likelihood that the patient will return to health. In an age of cost-containment and growing recognition that some interventions are indeed futile, medicine and society are less and less comfortable with such a stance.

It is consistent with the values of a liberal society to react toward such positions with an attitude of laissez-faire, even in the face of large cost and considerable discomfort.[43] The compassionate may offer kindly, if reluctant, support. A seemingly arbitrary religious stance often preempts other options, cutting off exploration of alternate solutions to the medical and moral dilemma. In fact, for the patient there is no dilemma. The action that must be taken is seen as required by divine command, with no other evidence or reason needed to support it. Such a position is often not accepted by others, however, and persons who embrace such a point of view are generally marginalized in the bioethical conversation.

A second stumbling block to discussion between religion and bioethics concerns actions or attitudes that affect not only adult believers but others under their care, usually minor children or in some cases the unborn. While the data are mixed, there is consistency in legal precedent to deny jurisdiction to parents of already born children, if parents or guardians wish medically harmful things to be done. Intervening actions in the case of pregnancy have been less criticized, since the moral status of the conceptus—at least in this culture—is determined by the woman in whose body the conceptus resides.[44] Although some have tried to make the case for forced treatment of addicted pregnant women and others have suggested the dual-patient status of the mother-fetus dyad,[45] little consensus is evident. When the reasons for withholding accepted medical intervention are religious, however, the pressure to override the woman's choices may be greater. For example, the Hmong woman who, for religious reasons, refuses Cesarean section for her unborn child may be looked upon as an uneducated individual whose beliefs need not be respected. She is not immediately seen as a free moral agent in a liberal society, who may do what she wants with the fetus she carries. There is little consideration for her position or hurry to discuss common ground. There is, in fact, discomfort with such a position; it is viewed as an unreasonable stance in the face of sound medical advice.

Sometimes practices supported by religious belief do not seem to be benign, even for the believer, when viewed from outside the faith context. What should be the bioethicist's attitude toward a claimed religious reason to circumcise and infibulate young girls, for example? Circumcision for male Jews is performed in a cosmopolitan culture generally without question. Although some justify male circumcision for reasons of health, the practice can be accepted on religious grounds alone. No attempt is made to interfere with the cutting of the male foreskin, even though the "patient" has not reached the age of consent and does not appear particularly happy about the surgery. Anthropologists, feminists, and even the talking heads on the evening news have begun to join bioethicists in raising questions about the genital alteration of girls. Is it essentially different from that of boys? If so, why is it different? Do not both these actions, the circumcision of boys and of girls, find their justification in religious and cultural tradition? It is necessary to explore the issue in greater depth before an answer becomes clear. That exploration must venture into the realm of values, basic religious beliefs, and choices. To raise these questions, however, is at least to open the door to dialogue with seemingly irrefutable positions. These are questions that cannot be answered without an avenue for dialogue between the fields of religion and bioethics. A potential facilitator for this dialogue is described below.

THE THEOLOGIAN

The function of the professional theologian is different from that of the believer. While in a sense all believers do theology, and some would argue that theologians ought to be believers, there is an expertise proper to the field of theology. The theologian begins with the premise that a particular religious tradition is valid, or at least defensible—as does the believer. However, the theologian's professional task goes further.

There are two vital tasks for the theologian to perform in intersection with bioethics. First, he or she functions as a prophet. This function is external to the community of belief; its primary focus is communication with those who do not share the particular belief system. The theologian is a bridge builder with the awesome responsibility to articulate clearly and effectively to the greater community the particular perspectives that his or her religion espouses. The theologian can point to and interpret the importance of what McCormick calls "the fullness of our own reality"[46] that religion articulates. In a sense, theologians must speak a second language that translates clearly the message and moral response of their communities of faith to others. If professionals who understand the particular religious story and its moral implications cannot or will not do this, who will?

Theologians can help expose the grand stories that represent the enduring religious traditions of human history. I have seen the effectiveness of such activity in the religious studies classroom. In presenting a course called "End-of-Life Issues and Catholic Teaching," I have become convinced that a clear position of advocacy is a better vehicle for understanding than the relativistic presentation of all views as having equal value, as one might advocate in philosophy. For example, students could see in the frankly theological exposition what the Catholic Church teaches on suicide, evaluate the reasons offered to support that position, and judge for themselves—in dialogue between their (personal, lived experience) story and the story told by the church. Forming one's viewpoint on these serious questions over against the clear articulation of moral norms from a strong religious tradition is easier than forming it in the relativistic context of philosophy. The viewpoints that students form may not and need not agree with official church teaching or theological opinion, but the latter offer a clear position for students to embrace or to reject.

Sometimes the prophet's job is to preach what is politically distasteful but religiously sound. The theologian can do this both for believers—who may need clarification of what the tradition teaches—and for the greater community, articulating clearly and unashamedly what is found in the narrative and norms of the particular religion. In any case, the job of the prophet is to interpret and to articulate as well and clearly as possible the reality that is perceived.

Second, the person who does theology has an obligation to reflect on the nature and conclusions of his or her particular tradition in light of contemporary reality and experience. To do so is to achieve a corrective balance to monolithic and unbending positions that may result from too narrow adherence to religious formulations inherited from the past. This function is, in a sense, an internal one. The ongoing struggle of mainstream Catholic theologians today to read "the signs of the times" in light of their unique tradition is an example of such work. New situations call for new answers—a historical worldview demanding that ongoing reflection on the conclusions of the past precipitate fresh (although not necessarily or completely different) conclusions about the present. We can point to the change in attitude among Catholic thinkers toward the moral acceptance of kidney transplants. Violation or mutilation of the body, including removal of a healthy kidney from a healthy body, was in the past viewed as an immoral action. Given time and reflection from a new perspective, however, this opinion of the church has given way to acceptance of kidney transplants from live donors.

Contemporary issues in biomedical technology desperately need the input that theologians can offer. What does a particular religious stance about human dignity and integrity or a belief in afterlife or divine stewardship have to say about Dolly the sheep and what she represents—the potential to clone human beings? Although there seems to be an uneasy expectation that persons of faith would find cloning immoral, religious voices have only begun to speak out on this issue. And the chorus is mixed in its opinions. The religious "solutions" to such questions are not foregone conclusions; they demand careful thought and dialogue.

There is a call for theologians to reflect on issues surrounding the patenting of genes. Mark Hanson has raised questions about dignity and meaning, the disparity of values held in the marketplace and in places of worship, and the need to think more completely about the meaning of "ownership" of the code of humanness. He notes that "we experience our world largely as we construct it."[47] It is important that the "engineers" of theology put on the necessary hardhats to influence the building as it goes up. Facile conclusions are insufficient for such important technological advances.

Ultimately it is a matter of professional integrity for theologians to reflect on their traditions and bring that reflection to bear on contemporary issues. They must constantly ask difficult questions. Is the tradition that we defend (and likely espouse) still valid for today? If not, is there a possibility to update or to apply this belief to the sticky contemporary issues without damaging or destroying the core of the tradition? Is discontinuity between yesterday's dogma and today's dilemma a matter of content or merely a matter of language in need of translation? What has our tradition to offer for the difficult questions that contemporary bioethics faces? If theologians can keep on task, they will have a great deal to offer bioethics. They are the ones who connect the time-tested insights of a particular religious tradition and the novel dilemmas of contemporary bioethics. As Delwin Brown put it: "The academic theologian attempts to understand a community's religious beliefs in their context . . . and what these beliefs actually do in the context. The academic theologian asks how these beliefs can be evaluated in relation to various normative horizons, of adjacent communities [that is, the bioethics community]. . . . Finally, the academic theologian explores the various alternatives to the beliefs in question, whether they are options implicit in the tradition itself or possible adaptations from the outside."[48]

THE RELIGIOUS SCHOLAR

Finally let us examine the possible contributions of the scholar of religion to the bioethics debate. Even within the field, religious scholars are divided on what the profession means or how it properly functions.[49] It is generally accepted, however, that the scholar of religion "starts by accepting the beliefs as true or meaningful in the eyes of the believer and then proceeds to wherever the subsequent discussion might lead."[50] The expertise of the religious scholar is distinct from that of the theologian. There are at least two contributions such scholars can make to bioethics. First, they bring a methodology. The study of religion is one that includes sociological analysis of the history and the development, and the doctrines and codes of religion. In a sense, scholars of religion bring to bioethics the skills of scientific professionals at a table of scientific professionals. They bring what Smart calls an "informed empathy."[51] They are capable not only of translating the meat and morality of a particular religious tradition but also of "[taking] account of beliefs, motivations, and so forth of human beings."[52]

Story tells us where we come from. If I tell someone my story, I will identify myself with a particular history or event—the founding account of my story of meaning. If I tell the religious part of my story, not only will the tale include what I believe—my religious identity (content)—but it will reveal the sources of that identity (context). What I am religiously, perhaps a Reform Jew, is a function of a long-ago event—the Passover and Exodus from Egypt. That is where I come from. As noted above, even the most philosophical methodology needs content, and for each person the story is the basis for that content. Scholars of religion are skilled in listening to and articulating the stories that give meaning to people's lives. At the bedside, both the patient who needs to decide and the medical personnel who stand by with cure and care have stories that influence the manner in which they manipulate the data through the methodologies of bioethics. Since it is these stories that ultimately give significance to the individual small and large actions that people perform, they are important elements in the decision-making process. These stories are religious. Someone needs to represent them to those whose perspective is not religious.

Religion offers a concrete corpus of normative material that may be helpful as a starting point, and perhaps offers possibilities for an end point in bioethical dilemmas. It is not accidental that norms from different religious traditions often draw on similar pools of values. Throughout history, human communities have collected such bodies of wisdom that, while neither foolproof nor unadaptable to new situations, may serve as a helpful resource in the formation of policy and law and as an aid in making individual decisions. In the final analysis, however, religious scholars need to bring a particular perspective to the bioethics debate—the critical eye of one who "exposes the mechanism whereby [religious] truths and norms are constructed in the first place, demonstrating the contingency of seemingly necessary conditions and the historical nature of ahistorical claims."[53] In doing so, such scholars will contribute a great deal to a field that must weave satisfactory private decisions into adequate public policy with strands from a multiplicity of religions and other cultures.

SOME FINAL THOUGHTS

Although I have argued that all three practitioners of religion—believer, theologian, and scholar of religion—have something to offer bioethics, all can shape their contributions better. First, believers can reflect more fully on their own belief systems to clarify with serious reflection what is believed and why and prepare to articulate this to the bioethics community. Believers must, however, be willing to give ground in the face of the common good. This may require compromise in areas that are not central to particular beliefs as well as recognition of the need to use healthcare dollars prudently and justly. Believers must recognize the discomfort that others feel when confronted with positions that seem contrary to good medical practice and try to respond with understanding. This advice can be applied not only to believer-patients but to believer-bioethicists.

Second, theologians should be more proactive and less apologetic in the transmission of their traditions. The gathered wisdom of religious traditions has much to say to contemporary society—and, by extension, to the field of bioethics—both in the making of individual decisions and in the construction of public policy. Theologians will succeed in contributing only if they are really ready to enter into dialogue. The theologian who spends professional energy talking only to those within the tradition will impoverish the bioethics project. According to Pellegrino and Thomasma: "If religious influence is denied, insights about the deeper meaning of illness and healing in a community of healers may be missed."[54] If this is true, it is imperative that theologians articulate clearly and reflectively the insights they represent. Essential qualities include confidence that what they say is important, a clear "second language" to communicate insights, humility to listen and to reassess in the face of the valid insights of others, and the courage to enter into an arena that often does not take them seriously. McCormick observes: "To claim that such distinct outlooks and onlooks (theology) have nothing to do with bioethics is either to separate faith from one's view of the world (which is to trivialize faith by reducing it dualistically to an utterly otherworldly thing), or to separate one's view of the world from bioethics (which is to trivialize bioethics by isolating it from the very person it purports to serve)."[55]

Third, scholars of religion must enter into the field more aggressively, articulating and owning the unique gifts they bring. Their training and their nonpartisan stance will not only help the understanding and appreciation of religious diversity in medical decision making, but also add methodology and insight at the macro level for policy making. Perhaps it is the religious scholars who can fashion "some ordering principles that cannot be trumped"[56] to bolster the inadequate contributions of philosophical ethics.

Does religion really have a serious role to play in bioethics? This chapter began with a canine metaphor. I have always liked dogs, especially big ones. My own experience with them, like my experience with religion, is that they are neither fearful nor useless. Dogs bring comfort and companionship, they offer a loud and relatively inexpensive security system, they provide the occasion to chat with neighbors on daily walks, and they remind us that we are responsible for sentient beings other than ourselves. Maybe I feel this way because I have been around dogs all my life. Much the same could be said about believers, theologians, and religious scholars. Perhaps we need to invite these not-so-hairy animals more seriously into the bioethics house. They might surprise us, barking in the face of danger, consoling us with undeserved affection, and perhaps imposing a few demands that we would rather not face. After awhile, it will be hard to see how we ever managed without them.

NOTES

1. R.A. McCormick, "Theology and Bioethics," *Hastings Center Report* 19, no. 2 (March-April 1989): 5.

2. W.T. Reich, ed., *The Encyclopedia of Bioethics* (New York: Free Press, 1978).

3. M. Siegler, "The Secularization of Medical Ethics," *Update: Center for*

Christian Bioethics 7, no. 2 (June 1991): 2.

4. T.L. Beauchamp and J.F. Childress, *Principles of Biomedical Ethics*, 4th ed. (New York: Oxford University Press, 1994). In the preface to the latest edition the authors note the changes and additions to this standard text. They suggest that, in spite of the additions, "some readers may prefer to read the chapters devoted to various principles" before they explore other facets of the book (p. vii.).

5. Ibid., p. 3.

6. Ibid., p. 4.

7. Ibid., p. 5.

8. Ibid., p. 16.

9. Ibid., p. 19.

10. The underlying thesis of liberation theology is that powerful structures and narrative support enduring systematic oppression of less powerful, often voiceless groups; people of color or of less economic means are kept in bondage, financial or actual, by the dominant White culture, who could justify their behavior by interpreting biblical texts to say that this was God's will. See G. Gutierrez, *A Theology of Liberation*, trans. C. Inda and J. Eagleson (Maryknoll, New York:: Orbis Books, 1973). Women have been considered to have a "permanent status of inferiority because of sex." See L.M. Russell, *Human Liberation in a Feminist Perspective—A Theology* (Philadelphia: Westminster Press, 1974), 29. These structures and their supporting narratives function to enshrine in the culture certain things as "values," which in reality are systemwide evils. "Evils" can masquerade under the rubric of "goods" by popular consensus. Therefore, it is necessary to be wary of defining "value" by such a method.

11. The examples of Tuskegee and of the withholding of azidothymidine (AZT) from third-world, pregnant women are both controversial. Some would argue that standards for research evolve over time and/or cannot be universally established for cultures different from our own. See "Research on AIDS in Poor Nations Raises an Outcry," *New York Times*, 18 September 1997, sec. 1, A1, A18. Nevertheless, both examples illustrate instances where individuals without power have been sacrificed to values accepted by the dominant culture by common consensus.

12. C.D. Broad, *Five Types of Ethical Theory* (London: Routledge and Kegan Paul, 1930).

13. W.K. Frankena, *Ethics* (Englewood Cliffs, N.J.: Prentice Hall, 1963).

14. R.A. McCormick, "Does Religious Faith Add to Ethical Perception?" in *Introduction to Christian Ethics*, ed. R.P. Hamel and K.R. Himes (New York: Paulist Press, 1989), 141.

15. Such conclusions may or may not be congruent with what might be termed a "favored methodology" of a particular religious tradition. It is my experience that either such a methodology does not exist, or that students have not internalized it at their particular stage of development. Carl Elliott explores the enigma of the breach between ethical theory and personal choices in "Where

Ethics Comes from and What to Do about It," *Hastings Center Report* 22, no. 4 (July-August 1992): 28-35. He notes, "Ordinary people pay little attention to theories when they make their moral decisions."

16. For a thorough discussion of this development, see E.D. Pellegrino, "The Metamorphosis of Medical Ethics: A 30-Year Retrospective," *Journal of the American Medical Association* 269, no. 9 (3 March 1993): 1158-62.

17. Focus on the action itself promotes an illusion of certainty which, I believe, is most compatible with medicine itself. Medicine tends to be a discipline of science, which traditionally has claimed an objective purity, free from the bias of the personal or emotionally particular. In many of the issues upon which bioethics had focused (such as turning off machines), the search for a sure and scientifically based answer is more harmonious to science and its bias than a "messy" solution, which brings in the values, hidden agendas, and emotions of the parties involved.

18. See note 4 above, p. 464.

19. E.D. Pellegrino and D.C. Thomasma, *Helping and Healing: Religious Commitment in Health Care* (Washington, D.C.: Georgetown University Press, 1997).

20. Only about 10 percent of the editorial board of the first edition of the *Encyclopedia of Bioethics* were women. The field has changed considerably since that time.

21. Although the emphasis on care *per se* arises from Carol Gilligan's work, *In a Different Voice* (Cambridge, Mass.: Harvard University Press, 1982), the elements of a contextualized approach to ethics is not new with her. See, for example, C.E. Curran, *Themes in Fundamental Moral Theology* (Notre Dame, Ind.: University of Notre Dame Press, 1977), 67.

22. See, for example, B.H. Andolsen, "Elements of a Feminist Approach to Bioethics," in *Feminist Ethics and the Catholic Moral Tradition*, vol. 9, ed. C.E. Curran, M.A. Farley, and R.A. McCormick (New York: Paulist Press, 1996), 341-82.

23. A.R. Jonsen and S. Toulmin, *The Abuse of Casuistry: A History of Moral Reasoning* (Berkeley, Calif.: University of California Press, 1988).

24. Ibid.

25. R. Viladesau and M. Massa, *Foundations of Theological Study: A Sourcebook* (New York: Paulist Press, 1991), 94.

26. R. Otto, *The Idea of the Holy* (New York: Oxford University Press, 1958).

27. M. Eliade, *The Sacred and the Profane*, trans. W.R. Trask (New York: Harcourt Brace Jovanovich, 1959).

28. P. Tillich, *Dynamics of Faith* (New York: Harper and Row, 1957).

29. R.P. Hamel, "On Bernard Häring: Construing Medical Ethics Theologically," in *Theological Voices in Medical Ethics*, ed. A. Verhey and S.E. Lammers (Grand Rapids, Mich.: William B. Eerdmans, 1993), 223-4.

30. M.J. Hanson, "Religious Voices in Biotechnology: The Case of Gene

Patenting" (special supplement), *Hastings Center Report* 27, no. 6 (November-December 1997): 1-21. Hanson affirms that the issue of biotechnology needs the input of religious thinking, but that there is much work to be done in the dialogue. So far, religious "answers" have been vague or inadequate.

31. Louis Janssens uses the Flemish word, *evennaste*, to describe this relationship. The word recalls the English, "bosom buddy," connoting a close identification of the self of another with one's own self. See D.L. Christie, *Adequately Considered: An American Perspective on Louis Janssens' Personalist Morals* (Louvain, Belgium: Peeters Press, 1990), 41.

32. This section draws loosely on the work of James Smurl.

33. J.Z. Smith, "Are Theological and Religious Studies Compatible?" *Council of Societies for the Study of Religion Bulletin* 26, no. 3 (September 1997): 61.

34 Ibid., p. 30-5.

35. This comment, taken from a typed summary of the psychosocial evaluation for a candidate for transplant in Ohio, is representative of the kinds of things people mention when faced with difficult and especially life-threatening medical procedures. I perceive it to be a variation on the theme: there are no atheists in foxholes.

36. Divinity cannot be titrated and precipitated in a test tube, although belief in God is not in itself illogical. For an extended discussion of the distinction between faith and science, see Tillich, *Dynamics of Faith*, chap. 5, note 28 above.

37. S.G. Post, *Inquiries in Bioethics* (Washington, D.C.: Georgetown University Press, 1993), 56.

38. R.M. Veatch, "Does Ethics Have an Empirical Basis?" *Hastings Center Report* 1, no. 1 (1973): 57.

39. Not everyone is willing to distinguish between active intervention and allowing something to happen (often termed "passive"). See, for example, J. Rachels, "Active and Passive Euthanasia," *New England Journal of Medicine* 292, no. 2 (9 January 1975): 78-80. This article has seen multiple reprints, attesting to the ongoing controversy over this distinction.

40. C. Campbell, "Religious Ethics and Assisted Suicide in a Pluralistic Society," *Kennedy Institute of Ethics* 2, no. 3 (1992): 253-7.

41. I believe this term was first used by Russell B. Connors, Jr. and Martin Smith.

42. See note 40 above, p. 257.

43. Some challenge to this position can be noted, however. Examples include laws that provide for forced blood transfusions for minor children of Jehovah's Witnesses and cost-cutting measures initiated in the face of managed care. I foresee increasing pressures to stop futile treatment, even for those who espouse a vitalist position.

44. Recent discussion in the courts and in the media with regard to suicide and assisted suicide has tended to favor the opposite view.

45. See T.H. Murray, "Moral Obligations to the Not-Yet Born: The Fetus as Patient," in *Biomedical Ethics*, 3rd ed., ed. T.A. Mappes and J.S. Zembaty (New York: McGraw-Hill, 1991), 463-72.

46. See note 1 above, p. 7.

47. Ibid., p. 15.

48. D. Brown, "Academic Theology and Religious Studies," *Council of Societies for the Study of Religion Bulletin* 26, no. 3 (September 1997): 65.

49. See an extended discussion on this topic in *Council of Societies for the Study of Religion Bulletin* 26, no. 3 (September 1997).

50. This idea is borrowed from Schubert Ogden. See A. Sharma, "On the Distinction Between Religious Studies and Theological Studies," *Council of Societies for the Study of Religions Bulletin* 26, no. 3 (September 1997): 51.

51. N. Smart, "Religious Studies and Theology," *Council of Societies for the Study of Religions Bulletin* 26, no. 3 (September 1997): 67.

52. Ibid.

53. R.T. McCutcheon, "A Default of Critical Intelligence? The Scholar of Religion as Public Intellectual," *Journal of the American Academy of Religion* 65, no. 2 (Summer 1997): 453.

54. Ibid., p. 6.

55. See note 1 above, p. 10.

56. See note 19 above, p. 73.

6

Whose Religion? Which Moral Theology? Reconsidering the Possibility of a Christian Bioethics in Order to Gauge the Place of Religious Studies in Bioethics

H. Tristram Engelhardt, Jr.

GAUGING THE PLACE OF
RELIGIOUS STUDIES IN BIOETHICS

Why should religious studies play any role in bioethics? Where could it fit? After all, philosophical bioethics analyzes issues, clarifies arguments, and assesses justifications for claims. What more could one want? What more would one need and why? No full answer can be given regarding the appropriate role of religious studies in bioethics without examining the place of religion itself in bioethics. One knows the role that philosophy plays in bioethics as the guardian of sound, rational argument and the careful explication of concepts. One must then determine the role of religion to assess the plausibility of the role of religious studies. The role of religious studies in bioethics depends crucially on the role, experience, and meaning of religion in bioethics.

A judgment regarding the role of religion in bioethics involves assessing the place of the theological issues that shape the religious phenomena to which religious studies could direct their energies on behalf of bioethics. The focus of this essay is on theological issues that frame the meaning of moral theology and the significance of its contribution to the ethics of bioethics. This focus on the phenomenon of religious bioethics is restricted to Western Christian bioethics and the conceptual issues it raises for a study of the role of religion in bioethics. It is Western

Christianity that determined much of the moral and metaphysical assumptions of the culture within which modern medicine and the biomedical sciences have developed and within which the contemporary phenomenon of bioethics originally took shape.

It is far from clear what contribution, if any, religious concerns in bioethics can make to the understanding of the various problems confronting contemporary medicine. First, one associates religion with the prescientific past. The challenges of contemporary medicine are predominantly those rooted in recent scientific developments and in new forms of technology. The past, out of which most religions draw their traditions, is prescientific and pretechnological in most of the senses of science and technology that make contemporary medicine especially problematic. In turning to religious roots for bioethics, it may then appear that one is turning to the past. Second, religious bioethics as the focus of religious concerns in bioethics speaks with many voices. Science and technology appear to speak with only one voice. That is, contemporary science and technology appear to share a common understanding of knowledge and reality, while the various traditions of religious bioethics are separated by their different and competing views of true knowledge and the deep meaning of reality. If one focuses more narrowly on the phenomenon of religious bioethics, the problem becomes even more difficult. Religious bioethics, because of its ties to the past and because of the diversity of the moral positions it compasses, would seem to offer greater confusion rather than more clarity. Finally, ours is an age of faith in science and technology, not an age of faith in divine powers and transcendent truths. The contemporary loss of faith in traditional notions of the divine is so significant that many who would speak in the name of religious ethics have also lost faith in the religions whose morality they interpret.[1] The result is that a religious bioethics is in many circumstances not theological in the strong sense of being oriented toward a transcendental, personal God.

In the face of a crisis of belief, providing a religious bioethics commits one to reexamining the very nature of religious morality. A religious bioethics may be religious in the sense of identifying a particular culture, narrative, or way of understanding values that was once anchored in a transcendent faith. The significance or force of such a religious bioethics is not derived from a grounding in God or a true revelation, but rather in the richness of the tradition on which it draws, the poetic power of the narrative it possesses, or the perceptiveness of its particular cultural insights into the human condition. A turn to religious bioethics for a focus for religious studies must then be examined with care. One must determine whether the invocation of religion is meant to offer a transcendent truth and a connection with noumenal meaning, or whether the appeal to religion is instead an invocation of a special humanism with a particular sensitivity for concerns with questions of ultimate significance. In the latter case, the *studia divinitatis* are transformed into the *studia humanitatis*, thus domesticating the religious by moving from the noumenal to the worldly. Although questions regarding the transcendent are entertained, answers are given in terms of an analysis of immanent experience and through discursive argument.

This essay assesses the possibility of a religious bioethics in the strong sense of a theological bioethics—a bioethics grounded in the revelation of a transcendent God. Such an assessment involves determining the moral and epistemological consequences of such a deep grounding, as well as why such a project should command our interest. Taking such a project seriously leads to understanding why philosophical bioethics is not able to give a full and complete account of the moral issues raised by healthcare. Indeed, the case will be made that it is philosophical bioethics that is most disabled by the challenges of postmodernity—the recognition not only of the absence of a canonical, universal, moral narrative, but also of philosophical reason's inability to establish foundationally one among the many competing moral narratives as canonical. Content always appears to be secured by begging the question or engaging in a circular argument. The project of a religious bioethics thus encounters a choice between ever more universal moral norms that are at the same time ever more impoverished in content, or moral norms that maintain content at the price of being parochial. Universality involves a loss of content, despite ecumenical desires to the contrary. Content involves particularity. Moreover, content divides. It separates communities whose content-rich moral claims differ from those of other communities. A study of the possibility of religious bioethics offers an insight into the possible future roles of religion in healthcare ethics.

THE HUMAN CONDITION AND THE QUEST FOR RELIGIOUS ANSWERS

There is nothing like facing death, experiencing severe disability, or enduring significant suffering to wake such questions as "What is the meaning of life?" "Why did this happen to me?" and "Is there any ultimate significance to my suffering?" The concern to find deep meaning in the major passages of life, from reproduction and birth to suffering and death, appears to be part of human nature. However, as Kant, Hume, and others have told us, we find ourselves confined within a sphere of immanent experience, such that a breakthrough to the transcendent is impossible. Yearnings and questions that appear to point to the transcendent are reconstructed so as only to have immanent significance. Still, in the heart there is a gnawing sense of the transcendent. Following Leibniz, it would have been simpler had there been nothing: the difference between nothing and something is infinite. It requires an infinite explanation, so that a sufficient explanation is at the very least an all-powerful, self-conscious God. Although discursive reasoning finds itself embedded in the sphere of the finite, the human heart still sees through to the presence of a transcendent meaning. If such a meaning is available, then an ethic can be articulated that can place the passages of human life, which medicine addresses, within a context of ultimate meaning. The experiences of reproduction, birth, disability, suffering, and death could then be appreciated through a narrative into which one finds oneself told, not one among many narratives into which one might decide to tell one's experiences.

The allure of a religious account that would be more than a cultural account is that it would provide not just one among many other accounts of healthcare values. It would place the personal experience of our suffering in terms that are more than individual or even communal. A theological account could unite the justification, motivation, and genesis of morality in the ultimate source of all being.[2] If morality has its source in an infinite and all-knowing God, morality will be given not only a ground for its claims, but an ultimate assurance of its appropriate enforcement. The source of morality would be found not in a particular tradition or even in human reason, but in the ground of all being itself. In such an account, there need be no ultimate tension between the right and the good. The narrative within which one should come to understand reproduction, birth, suffering, and death, and the appropriate interventions of medicine could be anchored in an ultimate account of sin and salvation.

The provision of such an account of human experience has been the traditional role of most religions. This has also been the role played by most religious reflections on biomedical issues for well over 2,000 years—to place human choice in terms of the will of God and an ultimate account of sin and salvation. The difficulty for a contemporary religious bioethics is not only that religion appears prescientific and that the religions are plural, but also that many leading religionists no longer have faith in their own religion or are at least uncomfortable with its claim of providing ultimate meaning. This loss of faith in Faith has in great measure been tied to a traditional Western Christian assumption that reason can prove the existence of God and justify the general lineaments of moral theology. When this promise could not be kept, Western Christianity was itself brought into question. A faith in reason led to a crisis in belief.[3] Yet the response has in general been to fortify the alliance with secular moral rationality.

Such a reorientation toward the secular seemed necessary, because traditional religion was culturally marginalized. As Peter Berger observed: "Probably for the first time in history, the religious legitimations of the world have lost their plausibility not only for a few intellectuals and other marginal individuals, but for broad masses of entire societies. This opened up an acute crisis not only for the nomization of the large social institutions but for that of individual biographies. In other words, there has arisen a problem of 'meaningfulness' not only for such institutions as the state or the economy but for the ordinary confines of everyday life."[4] Berger's conclusions bear on the role of religion in general. They disclose a fundamental problem for religious bioethics in almost all of the industrialized countries of the world. The very project of providing a religious grounding of the content of ethics has been brought into question. What can religion add to the ethics or ethos of healthcare?

The moral theologies of most of the mainline Christian religions entered into a period of foundational crisis, just as they were offered the opportunity to give moral guidance. They were not able to provide an ethics or ethos for the new medical science and its technologies. Rather than being able to offer guidance, most Christian religions attempted to guide themselves through a crisis of identity and grounding. It was no longer clear to many what the tradition could teach them concerning the moral content of ethics. Their moral traditions had been brought into question. It was also unclear as to how they could provide a special grounding for their moral claims. The metaphysical assumptions within which they had framed their arguments had been called into question not only by others, but by themselves as well.

As the Roman Catholic moral theologian Edward Schillebeeckx noted: "The Christian revelation, in the form in which it has been handed down to us, clearly no longer provides any valid answer to the questions about God asked by a majority of people today. Neither would it appear to make any contribution to modern man's meaningful understanding

of himself in this world and in human history. It is at once evident that
more and more of these people are becoming increasingly displeased and
dissatisfied with the traditional Christian answers to their questions."[5]
The result was a remarkable change in the character of much Christian
moral theology.

With respect to its impact on Roman Catholic moral theology, Richard McCormick made the following observation in 1973: "The Second Vatican Council, after speaking of the renewal of theological disciplines through livelier contact with the mystery of Christ and the history of salvation, remarked simply: 'special attention needs to be given
to the development of moral theology.' During the past six or seven
years moral theology has experienced this special attention so unremit-
tingly, some would say, that the Christianity has been crushed right out
of it."[6] A new moral theology emerged whose claims were much closer
to those of secular morality.

Jeffrey Stout's study of these changes in the character and standing
of moral theology with an accent on reformed moral theology reveals a
similar problem. His account of the de-Christianization of Protestant
Christian theology begins with a variation on the theme of choice between universality and content, between the general language of secular
morality and a particular moral language grounded in belief.

Academic theology seems to have lost its voice, its ability to command attention as a distinctive contributor to public discourse in
our culture. Can theology speak persuasively to an educated public
without sacrificing its own integrity as a recognizable mode of utter-
ance? This dilemma is by now a familiar one, much remarked upon
by theologians themselves. To gain a hearing in our culture, theology has often assumed a voice not its own and found itself merely
repeating the bromides of secular intellectuals in transparently figu-
rative speech. Theologians with something distinctive to say are apt
to be talking to themselves—or, at best, to a few other theologians of
similar breeding. Can a theologian speak faithfully for a religious
tradition, articulating its ethical and political implications, without
withdrawing to the margins of public discourse, essentially unheard?[7]

Either choice has significant costs. Because the general culture of the
West is no longer shaped by traditional Christian moral beliefs, for a
Christian bioethics to speak to many in this culture it must cease to be
Christian in a traditional sense and instead assume the language and argu-
ment of secular thought. On the other hand, if it remains true to the

moral content of its tradition, Christian bioethics will appear sectarian, parochial, and anachronistic.

Stout's fine-grained analysis of Christian theologians' distancing themselves from traditional Christian belief (such as, belief in the Resurrection and immortality) takes as a major example the theological work of James Gustafson. The austere theocentrist morality that Gustafson develops out of the Christian past is substantively disconnected from the traditional content of Christian morality. As Stout keenly notes, the result of such religious austerity is "a momentum that seems bound to carry us . . . to atheism."[8] In such circumstances, the difference between religious and secular moral accounts regarding bioethical issues becomes vanishingly small—indeed, only a difference of vocabulary and cultural resonance. In such circumstances, the articulation of a religious bioethics has at best a limited cultural significance: it can provide moral guidance for those patients who happen to possess a particular religious cultural background and who wish to understand their illness and encounter with medicine in terms of a moral language taken from this background. But the substance of the morality is brought into accord with the claims of secular morality. The moral core of a religious bioethics then runs the risk of collapsing into a secular bioethics.

The trend to reduce moral theology, which might have given a special basis for religious bioethics, to a special variety of secular moral reflection has been fortified by developments in Roman Catholic moral theology that have denied a substantive difference between moral theology and secular moral thought. In such accounts, moral theology and secular moral thought become materially equivalent. The Roman Catholic moral theologian Joseph Fuchs advocated this position in the following observation:

> Christians and non-Christians face the same moral questions, and . . . both must seek their solution in genuinely human reflection and according to the same norms; e.g., whether adultery and premarital intercourse are morally right or can be so, whether the wealthy nations of the world must help the poor nations and to what extent, whether birth control is justified and should be provided, and what types of birth control are worthy of the dignity of the human person. Such questions are questions for all of humanity. If, therefore, our church and other human communities do not always reach the same conclusions, this is not due to the fact that there exists a different morality for Christians from that for non-Christians.[9]

In such circumstances, one is invited to believe that all Roman Catholic bioethical commitments can be derived from rational arguments.[10]

When the assumption that one can by reason secure all that one once believed by faith becomes implausible, then as long as one remains committed to the central role of reason in justifying morality, it becomes necessary to abandon that moral theological content that cannot be justified in general secular terms. Moral obligations that cannot be justified by reason cannot be required by faith. Father Charles Curran, a critic of Roman Catholic views regarding contraception and other matters, supports the material equivalence of moral theology and secular morality with a force that suggests the appropriateness of rationally reassessing the claims of moral theology.

> Obviously a personal acknowledgment of Jesus as Lord affects at least the consciousness of the individual and his thematic reflection on his consciousness, but the Christian and the explicitly non-Christian can and do arrive at the same ethical conclusions and can and do share the same general ethical attitudes, dispositions, and goals. Thus, explicit Christians do not have a monopoly on such proximate ethical attitudes, goals, and dispositions as self-sacrificing love, freedom, hope, concern for the neighbor in need, or even the realization that one finds life only in losing it. The explicitly Christian consciousness does affect the judgment of Christians and the way in which they make ethical judgments, but non-Christians can and do arrive at the same ethical conclusions and also embrace and treasure even the loftiest of proximate motives, virtues, and goals that Christians in the past have claimed only for themselves. This is the precise sense in which I deny the existence of a distinctively Christian ethic; namely, non-Christians can and do arrive at the same ethical conclusions and prize the same proximate dispositions, goals, and attitudes as Christians.[11]

Fuchs and Curran, along with many others, make the point that morality is morality.[12] Therefore, there cannot be a special Christian morality. From this line of reasoning, it follows as well that there cannot be a particular religious bioethics, such as a Christian bioethics. All of this becomes plausible within a posttraditional religious-moral experience and understanding.

This view of religious ethics and therefore of religious bioethics has a number of attractions. First, insofar as philosophical reasoning can disclose substantive moral conclusions, the seeming plurality of religious perspectives can be overcome in a unity of philosophical moral conclusions. This hope is an expression of the Enlightenment aspiration to overcome religious divisions in a morality all can share despite the apparently divisive particularities of religious conviction. Such a unity would form the basis for secular moral authority and the moral unity of secular societies. Religion would not divide. Religious authority could even be recruited to support secular moral authority through supporting secular morality. Second, the material equivalence of moral theology and secular morality would have religious significance for ecumenical aspirations aimed at disclosing a fundamental unity transcending confessional boundaries. All religions should share and support the same moral vision.

As attractive as this circumstance might seem, it is inadequate to three sets of important phenomena. First, many of the existential questions provoked in the confrontation with suffering and death (What is the meaning of my suffering? Is this life all there is?) involve transcendental concerns that focus on answers that reach beyond the powers of immanent reason. If there are ultimate meanings to life, suffering, and death that transcend human discursive proof, then these could not be established by secular philosophical argument. Transcendent concerns regarding the meaning of reproduction, suffering, and death point beyond whatever success secular discursive reasoning might have in disclosing a fundamental moral unity binding all persons. Such concerns in involving a personal quest for meaning point toward a meaning that is more personal than discursive. Also, they reach beyond secular ethics. Given the infinite gulf between the finite and the infinite, the phenomenal and the noumenal, there would be no secure basis for holding that God as transcendent would require only obedience to that morality that human discursive reasoning could justify.

Second, there are obviously real religious bioethical differences. Religions have substantive views and disagreements regarding the morality of contraception; third-party assisted reproduction; abortion; special selfless, supererogatory charitable undertakings such as those supported by celibate orders of brothers and nuns; the allowability of physician-assisted suicide; and the moral propriety of euthanasia. Actual religious traditions have real differences, which would be denied through the claim that differences are due only to errors in reasoning. The moralities at stake are substantively different, at least until sound argument corrects them. If moralities can be distinguished in terms of different foundational moral premises, rules of moral evidence, rules of moral inference, as well as views as to who may be in moral authority to settle moral controversies, then different religions with different views of revelation and different ecclesiologies will have substantively different moralities, which even sound rational argument could not unite. The disagreement regarding basic premises and rules of evidence and inference would be enough to ensure the discursive irresolvability of the differences that separate the various moralities.[13]

Finally, the problem of plurality is precisely the problem that postmodernity lays at the feet of secular philosophy: secular moral philosophy had aspired to providing a universal moral narrative that could encompass everyone without dependence on the particularities of any one culture or claims of religious revelation. Were this possible, moral content could have been derived from the nowhere of universal reason. It should therefore be acceptable to all. Postmodernity is not just the sociological condition of being beset with the pluralism of a moral babble. It is the recognition that secular moral philosophical reason cannot discover a way out of this pluralism. The difficulty lies in the circumstance that the acquisition of guiding moral content requires a foundational choice among different rankings of moral values and among different orderings of fundamental moral principles. Such choices presuppose a background moral or value sense to ground and guide them. To establish any particular morality, one must already presuppose the authority of particular moral intuitions, a particular theory of the good, a particular understanding of moral rationality. As with Hegel's critique of Kant, all moral content comes to be recognized as contingent.[14] Within the immanence of secular moral thought, one can forward a particular moral view only by begging the question or engaging in a circular argument. Postmodernity has its roots in secular philosophy's inability to discover a canonical moral content to justify that content.[15]

Given the inability of secular moral rationality to establish a canonical moral content, religious bioethics may attempt to forgo normative claims in favor of an invitation to experience a deeper appreciation of the human values at stake in biomedical interventions. If one regards religious bioethics as a special genre of the humanities, one directed to the sensitive appreciation of the fine grain of particular cultural understandings and framings of the human narrative, one does not escape the problems facing secular bioethics. Or rather, one escapes by no longer offering a normative bioethics. Religious studies and religious bioethics would then not be able to provide the normative guidance many still seek. Instead, one would offer accounts of alternative moral narratives and of the geographies of various religious moral understandings.

In such circumstances, one articulates maps that disclose differences, harmonies, and insights. But one does not possess a privileged position from which to indicate how to use such maps. One cannot authoritatively say what differences to avoid, what harmonies to endorse, or what insights to affirm. One may appreciate the beauty of the differences and the affinities that provide certain unities. But in such circumstances, one has ceded the aspiration to a normative ethical account in favor of an aesthetic account. The normatively good and the morally right will have given way to an aesthetic of the holy. The attempt to domesticate religious bioethics either reduces the field to secular bioethics clothed in a special jargon, or it recasts the field in the image and likeness of a humanistic sociology and anthropology. In the first case, the normativity of religious bioethics is at root secular. In the second case, if there is normativity, it is aesthetic rather than moral.

BEYOND SECULAR MORALITY AND THE AESTHETIC OF THE HOLY: TOWARDS A RELIGIOUS BIOETHICS WITH TRANSCENDENT CLAIMS

If a religious bioethics should wish to be more than a secular moral account using a special language, or a humane appreciation of the depth of religious moral narratives as they address medicine's role in reproduction, cure, caring, and the accompaniment of death, then religious bioethics will need to find a radically different anchor for its meaning and purpose. If a religious bioethics is to break out of the hermeneutic circle within which secular moral thought can have content only by begging the question, then it will need to ground itself in a radical claim of a normative revelation. If it is to provide more than cartographies of religious narratives as these are experienced in healthcare, then it will need to find resources to provide normative guidance. In short, in order to avoid the problems of secular morality and to provide more than an insightful humanistic anthropological geography of alternative religious experiences, religious bioethics will need to be religious in a traditional sense.

Such an understanding of religious bioethics involves epistemic and normative claims that will set it apart from secular moral bioethics. First, this involves claims to nondiscursive but compelling knowledge: religious revelation that warrants moral claims. Second, religious bioethics must recognize that, since its normativity will not be deducible from general rational reflection, it will have a particularity. Religious bioethics will not be materially equivalent to secular bioethics. If it is to respond to the profound religious questions that people pose when confronted with disability, suffering, and death, religious bioethics must step beyond the confines of secular morality. Such a step requires taking seriously the moral differences that religion contributes.

The differences go against the tastes of the age. The moral content offered by traditional moral theological reflection stands in contrast to many secular moral assumptions, as illustrated by the "culture wars" that have developed around the issues of abortion, physician-assisted suicide, and euthanasia. The very language of a traditional religious bioethics goes against the grain of much of the surrounding culture; the root assumptions of moral reflection in our societies are no longer religious, but secular. As T.S. Eliot observed in 1937 in the shadow of the moral catastrophes of National Socialism and Soviet Russia:

> We must remember also that the choice between Christianity and secularism is not simply presented to the innocent mind, *anima semplicetta*, as to an impartial judge capable of choosing the best when the causes have both been fully pleaded. The whole tendency of education (in the widest sense—the influences playing on the common mind in the forms of 'enlightenment') has been for a very long time to form minds more and more adapted to secularism, less and less equipped to apprehend the doctrine of revelation and its consequences. Even in works of Christian apologetic, the assumption is sometimes that of the secular mind.[16]

A religious bioethics that takes itself seriously will also need to take seriously the peculiarity and integrity of its experience.

To develop a plausible account of a religious bioethics, one may very well need to abandon many of the core assumptions of Western Christian moral theological reflection. Such a project would likely return Christian bioethical reflection to the moral concerns it possessed prior to its Westernization.[17] Such a shift would involve a change in epistemology and a commitment to a knowing from the heart or a mystical apprehension of the truth. One can appreciate the contrast in these epistemological assumptions by comparing the moral reasoning of John Paul II, Pope of Rome, and that of the church of Shenouda III, Pope of Alexandria. John Paul regards the current moral disarray of the West as due to a loss of faith in human reason. "Once the idea of a universal truth about the good, knowable by human reason, is lost, inevitably the notion of conscience also changes."[18] The church of Pope Shenouda (the 116th successor to St. Mark) recognizes that "it is most faulty to think that philosophical terms and expressions could confine theological meanings which are purely divine."[19] Instead of a philosophical grounding of moral theology, a grounding is sought in a mystical apprehension that has sustained the Christian experience since the first centuries. As Abba Gregorios emphasizes:

> There are many mysteries in our religion which we accept with deep acquiescence just because they are revealed by God. We believe in them contrary to the evidence of our senses and to our reason if we may use the word, just because they are proved to be from God. As we believe in God and in His omnipotence, so we believe in the mysteries of our religion without any need to ask why and how. A philosophical mind cannot agree to this mystical faith. But a philosophical mind is not in fact a true religious mind. It rather believes in its own capacities and measures. Religion to a philosophical mind is a science that could be treated on the same level as any other branch of human knowledge. A philosophical mind applies to religion the scientific method. Here analysis, classification, philology and so on enter into religion, in order to make it more reasonable and acceptable to a philosophical mind. Also in this kind of dealing with our religion we cannot understand the spirit of our religion. Where reason interferes, mystical experience disappears. We have to use our minds up to a certain point, but beyond that we should leave our minds to the guidance of a mystical experience.[20]

Such an orientation would involve a de-Westernization of Christian religious bioethics—a substantial change, indeed. Yet, such a return to the roots of Christian tradition and its epistemological and metaphysical assumptions may likely afford the only opportunity for sustaining a Christian religious bioethics that will neither collapse into the concerns of secular moral thought (and its irresolvable difficulties with postmodernity), nor reduce Christian religious bioethics to one of the secular medical humanities.

Religious bioethics reconsidered in this light would offer a response to the philosophical problems of postmodernity. It would need to invoke a theological basis for identifying the correct ordering of moral values and principles, an ordering needed to affirm the appropriate content-full morality. Since it is clear that discursive philosophical reasoning cannot make a principled selection among different orderings without begging the question, a way out of this problem can only be secured if Truth can in some way affirmatively break in and settle the matters at issue. This has been one of the traditional roles ascribed to God in the theologies of revealed religions. In such circumstances, moral theology and the bioethics it could sustain would retain their character and integrity over against secular morality, while also providing normative moral force. Such a moral theology would need to take seriously the experience of God as definitive of the content of morality. The knowing of the heart open to God would offer what discursive knowing could not secure.

Because the God to be known would enter into human experience from outside that experience, that God would transcend human categories for being. A moral theology in response to the encounter with such a God would affirm a metaphysics that could only be articulated in an apophatic theology grounded in a mystical epistemology. Such a grounding of moral theology and of religious bioethics would return Christian reflections to a framework of exploration that had already been well established by the time of St. Isaac the Syrian (seventh century). Such an undertaking would recast the very project of Christian bioethics.[21] As we rethink the possibilities for religious bioethics at the end of the second millennium, we are returned to the project of moral theology as it was understood in the first millennium. This reorientation will redefine the role of religious studies in the field of bioethics by bringing us to reconsider the very role of religion in the moral life.

NOTES

1. Of those worldwide who claim a religious affiliation and by implication would have an interest in a religious bioethics, most belong to one of the religions directed to the God of Abraham. The crisis of religious belief has not been a prominent feature of Islamic religious experience in the last few decades, as has been the case with Western Christianity. Since Western Christianity is associated with the contemporary flourishing of medicine, science, and technology, the focus of this essay is on the difficulties faced by Christian bioethics and their possible remedies.

2. In secular moral accounts, there is always the possibility of a tension between what is useful for one's self and what is demanded by moral rationality. For example, for the utilitarian, the greatest good for the greatest number may conflict with the pursuit of some of the most important goods of particular individuals. A Kantian deontologist may know that to tell a particular lie will incur blameworthiness, yet that telling the truth will most likely have disastrous personal consequences. It is for this reason among others that Immanuel Kant argued in his *Second Critique* that we must act as if God exists and as if we

are immortal, so that we can then rationally act under the conviction that there will in the end be a proportion between one's realization of the good and one's conformity to right action.

3. M. Buckley, *At the Origins of Modern Atheism* (New Haven, Conn.: Yale University Press, 1987).

4. P.L. Berger, *The Social Reality of Religion* (London: Penguin, 1969), 130.

5. E. Schillebeeckx, "Silence and Speaking about God in a Secularized World," in *Christian Secularity*, ed. A. Schlitzer (Notre Dame, Ind.: University of Notre Dame Press, 1969), 156.

6. R. McCormick, *Notes on Moral Theology, 1965 through 1980* (Washington, D.C.: University Press of America, 1981), 423.

7. J. Stout, *Ethics after Babel* (Boston: Beacon Press), 163.

8. Ibid., 182.

9. J. Fuchs, "Is There a Christian Morality?" in *Readings in Moral Theology No. 2: The Distinctiveness of Christian Ethics*, ed. C. Curran and R. McCormick (New York: Paulist Press, 1980), 11.

10. The commitment to grounding most, if not all, moral theological claims in general secular reasoning lies deep in the history of Roman Catholic moral thought. One thus finds in a Roman Catholic medical ethics textbook from the 1950s the following claim regarding the moral claims advanced in that text. "All men, then, are called upon to obey the natural law. Hence it matters not whether one be a Roman Catholic, a Protestant, a Jew, a pagan, or a person who has no religious affiliations whatsoever; he is nevertheless obliged to become acquainted with and to observe the teachings of the law of nature. In the present volume all the obligations which are mentioned flow from the natural law, unless the contrary is evident from the context." See E. Healy, *Medical Ethics* (Chicago: Loyola University Press, 1956), 7. It is important also to underscore that Roman Catholic moral theological reflection had for a long time maintained a view that revelation provided content for morality not available to natural reason. One finds this position taken, for instance, in the 1914 edition of *The Catholic Encyclopedia*. "Moral theology, correctly understood, means the science of supernaturally revealed morals. . . . It is also plain that although this Supreme lawgiver can be known by natural reason, neither He nor His law can be sufficiently known without a revelation on His part. Hence it is that moral theology, the study of this Divine law is actually cultivated only by those who faithfully cling to a Divine Revelation, and by the sects which sever their connexion with the Church, only as long as they retain the belief in a supernatural Revelation through Jesus Christ." See C. Herberman et al., ed., *The Catholic Encyclopedia* (New York: Encyclopedia Press, 1914), 14: 604.

11. C.E. Curran, *Catholic Moral Theology in Dialogue* (Notre Dame, Ind.: University of Notre Dame Press, 1976), 20.

12. For a sample of some of the relevant literature bearing on the material equivalence of Christian moral theology and secular morality, see J.-M. Aubert, "La spécificité de la morale chrétienne selon saint Thomas," *Supplément* 92 (1970):

55-73; F. Böckle, "Was ist das Proprium einer christlichen Ethik?" *Heythrop Journal* 13 (1972): 27-43; J.F. Bresnahan, "Rahner's Christian Ethics," *America* 23 (1970): 351-4; J. Fuchs, "Gibt es eine spezifisch christliche Moral?" *Stimmen der Zeit* 185 (1970): 99-112; J. Macquarrie, *Three Issues in Ethics* (New York: Harper & Row, 1970); R. Simon, "Spécificité de l'éthique chrétienne," *Supplément* 92 (1970): 74-104.

13. The resolution of controversies with significant moral overlay is examined at greater length in H.T. Engelhardt, Jr. and A. Caplan, ed., *Scientific Controversies* (New York: Cambridge University Press, 1987).

14. See, for example, G.W.F. Hegel, *Elements of the Philosophy of Right*, ed. A. Wood, trans. H. Nisbet (New York: Cambridge University Press, 1991), sec. 134; and G.W.F. Hegel, *Encyclopedia: The Philosophy of Spirit*, ed. A.V. Miller, trans. J.N. Findley (New York: Oxford, 1979), sec. 508. See also H.T. Engelhardt, Jr., "Sittlichkeit and Post-Modernity: An Hegelian Reconsideration of the State," in *Hegel Reconsidered*, ed. H.T. Engelhardt Jr. and T. Pinkard (Dordrecht, The Netherlands: Kluwer, 1994), 211-24; A. MacIntyre, *A Short History of Ethics* (New York: Macmillan, 1973), 190-8; and A.W. Wood, "Does Hegel Have an Ethics?" *Monist* 74 (July 1991): 358-85.

15. I have explored these issues more fully in *The Foundations of Bioethics* (New York: Oxford University Press, 1996).

16. T.S. Eliot, *The Idea of a Christian Society* (London: Faber and Faber, 1982), 190.

17. In great measure, both Roman Catholic and Protestant theology developed out of a Germanic cultural context, which set aside many of the understandings that formed the basis of Christianity in the first centuries. For an account of the crucial shift in cultural consciousness that framed the characteristics of Western Christian thought, see J.S. Romanides, *Franks, Romans, Feudalism, and Doctrine* (Brookline, Mass.: Holy Cross Orthodox Press, 1981).

18. John Paul II, *Veritatis Splendor* (Vatican City: Libreria Editrice Vaticana, 1993), no. 31, 51-2.

19. A. Gregorios, quoted in I. Habib el Masri, *The Story of the Copts: The True Story of Christianity in Egypt* (Nairobi, Kenya: Coptic Bishopric for African Affairs, 1987), 2: 404.

20. Ibid., 405.

21. H.T. Engelhardt Jr., "Moral Content, Tradition, and Grace: Rethinking the Possibility of a Christian Bioethics," *Christian Bioethics* 1, no. 1 (1995): 29-47.

7

Bioethics and Religion: A Value-Added Discussion

Thomas A. Shannon

INTRODUCTION

Two sets of concerns inform this chapter. One is autobiographical and professional and the other is more disciplinary or content oriented. Both dimensions of this topic are critical for me and helped shape my own orientation to various topics in bioethics. Thus, the chapter begins with some reflections on how the field of bioethics was shaped and then moves into how a religious dimension will add to the debate.

THE DISCIPLINE OF BIOETHICS

When I received my doctoral degree from Boston University in 1972, the field of bioethics was in its initial phases. I took a course in bioethics offered through the Boston Theological Institute, the consortium of theology schools in the Boston area. Joseph Fletcher was one of the instructors, and Robert Veatch made a guest appearance. Other guest instructors from various divinity schools in the area gave presentations as well. In this course some attention was given to the religious dimension of the various problems we discussed, but philosophical and social analysis also played an important part of the discussion. I wrote a paper on the moral status of the fetus using the Thomistic theory of delayed animation further developed and applied to contemporary embryology by Joseph

Donceel. But in all of this the orientation was mainly philosophical rather than religious.

Yet in the development of bioethics there is a very long tradition of reflecting on these issues in religious categories and within religious communities. Many religions, such as the Catholic tradition, use a philosophical framework for such discussions, but the thrust of the analysis is informed by theological principles or faith-derived values. Topics such as humans created in the image of God, stewardship, human finitude, the value of community, and immortality inform these discussions in critical and profound ways. And this is reflected in the fact that many seminaries or divinity schools treated such topics in their curricula, mainly under the rubric of pastoral care, a course on the administration of the sacraments, or as part of the general curriculum in moral theology. Thus, questions of ordinary and extraordinary means of treatment would be treated under the fifth commandment: Do not kill. Abortion would be treated there also. Issues having to do with reproduction were treated in Catholic moral theology in the course on the sacrament of matrimony. Although divinity schools offered very few explicit courses that we would today identify as bioethics courses, many of the problems we discuss today have a long history of debate in moral theology. For example, the discussion of ordinary and extraordinary means goes back, in the Catholic tradition, to at least the 14th century.[1]

In the early days of bioethics, it should come as no surprise that many of the individuals teaching in this area came out of seminaries or divinity schools. The Catholic side had both Gerald Kelly and John Ford. Kelly wrote a medical ethics text as well as frequent articles addressing such topics. Richard McCormick, Warren Reich, and Charles Curran picked up where Kelly and Ford left off. Other Catholic theologians followed their lead: James J. Walter, Lisa S. Cahill, Richard Gula, and James Keenan. On the Protestant side were individuals such as Joseph Fletcher, at least in his time as an Episcopalian priest; Paul Ramsey; William F. May; Robert Veatch; James Childress; Stanley Hauerwas; and Karen Lebacqz. Although these individuals incorporated philosophical analysis into their courses and writings, they also were informed by their religious traditions or religious values. Particularly in the Catholic tradition, new topics and problems were incorporated into an existing framework that was then re-articulated in light of the new problems. Professionally trained philosophers generally were not part of these early discussions, although such individuals (Daniel Callahan in particular) were eventually to play a major role.

My strongest memory about this phase of the development of bioethics—this would be in the mid-1970s—is that many professionally trained philosophers were not interested in this field or such problems because the focus was practical problem solving rather than broad, theoretical philosophical analysis. The few philosophers who became engaged in the bioethics discussion were referred to as "applied philosophers," and that phrase was frequently pronounced with a certain level of condescension, if not outright disdain. At that time, analytic philosophy still was the dominant methodology in many graduate schools of philosophy, so there was little professional incentive to think about such practical and conceptually messy problems as whether to turn off a respirator. Thus, the interest in thinking about such problems came primarily from individuals trained in religious studies or theology and who grew up in a tradition that was open to practical problem solving. Although theology and religious studies had their theoretical and historical debates, they also had space—mainly in the disciplines of moral theology, pastoral studies, and pastoral counseling—for practical problem solving. In addition, Catholicism brought to the discussion its own practical history of case discussions both from the tradition of casuistry and the training of confessors. Many religious orders, for example, had the practice of holding weekly or monthly discussions of "cases of conscience," in which a case was presented and then the members of the community discussed various resolutions of it. Such was the fertile ground in which the field of bioethics developed.

What changed to bring in the philosophers and recast the nature of the field? One major element was the foundation of the Hastings Center by Daniel Callahan, a professionally trained philosopher—but with a strong Catholic heritage sharpened during his years as editor of *Commonweal*—and Willard Gaylin, a psychiatrist who remained agnostic on religious issues. The founding of the Hastings Center coincided with technological developments in medicine such as various forms of life support and organ transplantation, as well as the prolonged debate over the recombinant-DNA technology. The Hastings Center validated the public discussion of these questions and conducted a discussion of the many sides of these issues. Many of the individuals who formed the research teams developed by the Hastings Center were the individuals named above. But others were also brought in because, by definition, the Hastings Center was not an advocacy center. It was not to represent a point of view other than an informed, critical discussion that would be helpful in forming public policy. Thus, although many of the individuals spoke from a religious tradition, they had to recast that tradition when speaking to public policy issues. The focus was on a debate accessible to the larger community rather than one directed to a particular religious tradition. Thus, the focus of the Hastings Center changed how bioethical issues were presented and debated. Although religion and religious issues were not eliminated, the priority was the development of an analysis for use in public policy debate.

A second major change in the field of bioethics was the inclusion of professionally trained philosophers in the discussion. These individuals brought with them the methodology, terminology, and viewpoint of their own professional training. And their contributions added significantly to the analysis of various topics in bioethics. So one major reason for philosophers' inclusion was the contributions they could make from their particular perspectives. But another reason is a bit more cynical. The disdain in which some held the developing field of "applied philosophy" was overcome by the availability of grant money and jobs. As bioethics came more and more to the public's attention and the problems became issues of public policy, academics became more interested. Centers were established; professional journals were founded; grant money became available; and universities, colleges, and medical schools began offering courses. Suddenly applied philosophy looked pretty good, particularly when the job market at universities in the 1970s and early 1980s was tight and jobs in bioethics were available. Today the term *applied philosophy* has almost vanished, and the consideration of problems in a variety of professions—medicine, law, business, engineering, and journalism, to name a few—is regarded as routine and appropriate in graduate philosophy programs.

The point of these comments is not to express dismay at philosophy's entering the bioethics debate, but rather to note its late entry and its need first to validate in some fashion the consideration of practical problems as a legitimate part of the discipline. At one meeting, Al Jonsen described working in a medical school as "doing philosophy in the trenches." Another philosopher told of defining a philosopher as a "professional bull shit detector" during an interview at a medical school. Such descriptions accurately capture critical elements of the practice of bioethics, but they are a far cry from various metaethical considerations or discussions of the fine points of various methodologies. And while a philosopher who is not carefully trained in the fine points of his or her discipline will not get very far as a professional philosopher, neither will that person succeed at bioethics if he or she cannot translate these concepts and methods into a language and analysis to shed light on problems that desperately need such illumination. Thus, rather than seeing philosophy as wasted on such practical discussion, the revised version correctly sees the value that systematic discussion and analysis can bring to complex and value-laden discussions that are a routine, but often confused, part of daily decision making in the practice of medicine.

A third factor that brought philosophers to the fore was the increased recognition of the pluralistic nature of the bioethics debate. An additional dimension of this was the shift to a more procedural resolution of problems—deciding them on the basis of whose right it was to make the decision rather than evaluating the merits of a decision. Recognition of pluralism and procedural resolution helped decrease the role of religion in public policy debates because, rightly or wrongly, religion was seen as partisan and imposing solutions from a faith-based perspective that was not subscribed to by the citizens at large. Or, to paraphrase the argument of the time, to use the position of a particular religion on a specific topic as public policy was to impose its solution on people who were not members of that religion. In the vacuum that followed this debate, philosophy quite naturally stepped in and offered itself as a more neutral approach to considering the issues; at least philosophy could spell out the arguments and show what was at stake without necessarily committing itself to a particular conclusion. In short, religion was seen as advocacy, philosophy as analysis.

The consequences of the introduction of philosophy into the bioethics discussion were quite significant. One was the development of the "Georgetown mantra" of *autonomy, beneficence, maleficence,* and *justice.* Each of these four concepts is quite important, and their application to various problem in bioethics has been significant in illuminating and resolving many problems. The doctrine of informed consent, for example, would probably not have the significant place in the practice of modern medicine that it does had it not been for the development of a strong concept of autonomy.

Ironically, two of the major contributors to this "mantra"—Veatch and Childress—were trained in divinity schools. One might think that, given the academic backgrounds of these early bioethicists, their analysis of these core ideas might have turned out a little differently. Yet the context in which these core ideas were developed was significantly different than a religious context: the focus was the individual and his or her rights in a public policy context. That is, given the context of pluralism, the strategy of proceduralism for problem solving, the primacy of argument over advocacy, and the focus on rights rather than duties, these four concepts were used to think through the decisions of individuals. In informed consent, the issue was the primacy of patient choice, not medical judgment, family, or social obligations. With beneficence or maleficence, the primary issue was goods or harms to the patient, not necessarily social benefits or social harms. With justice, the main consideration was fairness to the individual, not to society. Now to be sure, there were and are many discussions that also included a social dimension; the distribution of scarce resources continues to be a major theme in many debates. But the critical point of departure, and frequently the sole controlling factor for these discussions, was the individual and his or her rights. Again I cannot emphasize enough the importance of that contribution to the various debates, but the problem is that such viewpoints came to be seen as the only ones or as the only normative ones.

Thus the role of family, community, religion, social needs, and medical judgment fell to the side of the road—if not off it completely. Many of the discussions in bioethics focused on the protection of the individual and the attainment of his or her rights as the main, if not sole, agenda. That such an agenda is skewed is now becoming obvious, socially, philosophically, and religiously. Part of this broader discussion is being driven by the shift in the practice of medicine from more or less private practice to some sort of health-maintenance organization (HMO) or other social institutionalization of the practice of medicine. Here social and systemic issues quickly come to the fore, and analysis of individual needs is inadequate. To be sure, individual needs continue to be critical, but other needs that are socially driven also must be incorporated into the debate.

We are also beginning to recognize the limits of the philosophy of individualism that has been so strong in U.S. culture. Although we will continue to celebrate the individual and recognize the strengths and contributions of our celebration of individual freedoms, we are also recognizing that *individual* and *community* are not mutually exclusive terms and that communities can contribute to individual well-being. We are also learning that resolving the needs of many individuals does not necessarily contribute to social well-being, in spite of almost two centuries of tutoring by Adam Smith and his invisible hand. That is, the social good is not necessarily served by each seeking his or her individual good; in fact harm can be caused to society in this way. An individual requesting and receiving a full range of services for a particular problem may not be socially harmful, but when everyone seeks the same level of treatment—whether appropriate or not—then society's resources can be strained.

Philosophy itself is turning to the direction of community as a critical resource in the resolution of problems, but we are only at the beginning of that journey.

Finally we are recognizing that, as it is important to treat individuals justly, there are also implications of justice for society in how we resolve such individual needs. The point is not to cast this discussion as a "win-lose" formula, but rather to note that the resolution of individual problems has social consequences, which are also subject to justice considerations. We all recognize the importance of an organ transplant for an individual dying of kidney or heart failure. But we also recognize that how one gets to a particular place on the waiting list is as much a matter of social justice as of individual justice. So, too, the perception of health-care is shifting from a private good owed in justice to the individual to a social good owed in justice to the community. The consequences of this shift will be significant in how healthcare services are provided, but this is a clear issue of social justice.

Thus, we are coming to recognize the limits of the philosophical concepts and methodologies we have relied on in the past. As valuable and critical as they have been and still are, they cannot resolve all problems nor can they fully analyze the changing shifts in the delivery of healthcare in this country. Additionally, the needs of the community are coming to the fore, and we are recognizing that social justice is as important as individual justice. Finally, we are seeing that the individual cannot stand totally alone but needs grounding in the resources that a community can provide.

Religion is one resource that we can use in this rethinking of fundamental bioethical problems as well as the new challenges facing us. I am not arguing for religion as *deus ex machina* but as a resource available to help extend our analysis and to ground our arguments.

RELIGION AND BIOETHICS: ADDING VALUE TO THE DEBATE

The point of departure for this section is two experiences I had where religion added a value to the discussion. One occurred several years ago when my wife and I (Catholics) were invited to a discussion group whose members (Jewish) had been meeting off and on for many years. I was invited to give a presentation on withdrawing life support. The discussion that followed was lively and very moving. Finally, one person asked how my religion had influenced my discussion. In my typical academic fashion I began by saying how the discussion of forgoing extraordinary treatment was a centuries-old part of Catholicism. "No, no!" he said. "You must believe in immortality; otherwise you could not speak as you do." And then the discussion got very interesting because many others declared that they too did not believe in immortality, which was why so many of their decisions to end treatment had been so difficult. To withdraw treatment was to say an ultimate farewell. And then we discussed how, even if one believed in immortality, such discussions were also difficult, but that while one dimension of one's relation was over, the belief in the possibility of another remained. As one of the prayers in the Catholic liturgy for the dead says: "Life is changed, not taken away."

If one had directly asked me independently of this discussion group if I believed in immortality or some form of personal postdeath survival, I would have said yes, but I probably would have qualified that whole topic in a variety of ways so that even I would be unsure of its meaning when finished. But in the context of this discussion, I learned how deeply such a belief was part of me and how that belief has conditioned my thinking about such decisions.

A second experience is more recent. Ray, a friend who was a priest and campus minister among many other incarnations, was diagnosed with a virulent brain tumor. He died seven weeks later. My wife and I were unable to attend the funeral, but my sister-in-law sent us a tape of the funeral, which more than 2,000 people attended. Two things stood out for me. One came from the homily that was preached by a colleague of Ray's who accompanied him in this last journey. Of particular interest was their discussion of how in some ways this illness was like the testing of Job—random, unfair, and unintelligible. Yet what came ringing through so clearly was the grace and graciousness with which Ray responded to this, a response born of a depth of spirituality that was supported and nourished by a loving and attentive community. The other element of religion came from a letter to Ray that was read during the homily. Ray pursued peace and justice with the same zeal that he brought to an even earlier incarnation as a Marine. The letter stated that the author simply could not get Ray out of his mind, that he had emblazoned a message in him about justice that he could not rid himself of. This was message that was so clearly much more than a discussion of "to each his or her own." The preferential option for the poor based on Hebrew and Christian scriptures does not put forth the image of justice as a scale, but rather a concern for the marginalized. And so a religious perspective transformed Ray and those he met.

The sections that follow in the physician-assisted suicide/euthanasia debate and on the provision of healthcare present two issues for which, like the examples above, religion can add value to the debate.

THE PHYSICIAN-ASSISTED
SUICIDE/EUTHANASIA DEBATE

Although it is probably impossible to argue one into a change of position on the topic of physician-assisted suicide and euthanasia, it is possible to suggest gaps or deficiencies in arguments. The trick is to be respectful of the arguments and beliefs of others, to avoid prosyletizing or appearing condescending, and at the same time to show how belief changes an argument or an attitude and can add different elements to the debate.

An important and influential text with which to begin is Daniel Callahan's *The Troubled Dream of Life*.[2] This book is one of the strongest arguments against physician-assisted suicide and euthanasia I have seen. But what is most interesting is that it argues the case on secular or philosophical grounds. While Callahan does not deny religious arguments or seek to remove religion from the debate, he does not see them as meaningful for him and he seeks arguments elsewhere. Essentially the argument is grounded in dying a death both reflective of and worthy of the life one has lived. What emerges from the argument is a kind of Camus-like stoicism in the face of the inevitable. One takes what comes and deals with it as best as one can, hoping for a community that supports one, and for personal resources to make one's dying bearable. Yet even in this, Callahan does not shut the door. "I watch and I wait," he says.[3]

An irony found in the book is that although Callahan rejects a religious element to his argument, primarily on personal grounds, the whole tenor of the book reflects a type of secularized Catholicism. The religious roots of the book are closer to the surface than he admits. To lead a life worthy of one's dying or to have one's death reflect one's life is one of the most traditional of Catholic perspectives on death. One is admonished by the tradition to live in a state of constant preparedness, for "one does not know the hour or place." And when one does know this, there is a whole theology of redemptive suffering derived from the tradition of the suffering servant in the books of Isaiah the prophet and from the life of Jesus. The teaching is not a refined sado-masochism, but a gesture of solidarity and service to the community, in terms of the inspiration of the personal example of the one dying and also of a change in how members of the community see themselves and their lives.

Additionally, Callahan's discussion of the value and significance of the distinction between ordinary and extraordinary means of treatment is surely informed by traditional Catholic teaching. Callahan sharpens this distinction in his usual perceptive style, but the teaching is of a piece with the Catholic tradition. So too his argument coheres with the Catholic tradition's teaching on the value of the community and seeking the common good of the community.

Would Callahan's argument be any different if he had not had an earlier exposure to a religious tradition? Perhaps not, for one can find other philosophical argument making many of the same points. But Callahan came to this argument with a mind-set that already had a fair amount of spade work done and with much ground prepared. The main line of the argument did not have to be rethought from scratch. Additionally his argument was pointed in certain directions—the relation of one's life and death and the role of community—by exposure to his religious tradition. Clearly Callahan went beyond this tradition, refined it, and added other elements to his argument. But a tradition was already present that added important dimensions to his argument.

The religious tradition can provide a needed critique of elements of the physician-assisted suicide/euthanasia debate. This debate is cast in a variety of ways—relief from unbearable pain, an end to incurable terminal disease, a resolution of the uncertainties of the inevitable progress of a disease. But a core feature of the debate, in the judgment of many, is autonomy—the right to control one's destiny. The life I live is mine and mine only, and I choose the circumstances under which I live or—in this debate—die. The mythology underlying this value is at the core of American life—rugged individualism, self-sufficiency, the need to "do it my way."

This element of the debate is central to all dimensions of the physician-assisted suicide/euthanasia debate. This is because of the central role autonomy has rightly played in bioethics almost since the inception of the field. Many of the philosophical and policy gains have in no small measure been due to the significance of autonomy. And we are now coming to realize how deeply autonomy fits into the core values and mythology of American life. Thus the stage was set for this next application of autonomy in the physician-assisted suicide/euthanasia debate. For surely the right to end one's life at the time and circumstances of one's choosing is but a logical application of the right to choose in general and the right to determine one's life circumstances in particular.

And this is a difficult argument to overcome. The major fights in bio-ethics ranging from abortion to the right to refuse unwanted treatment have all been based on autonomy; appeals to it are almost a philosophical knee-jerk reaction. When all else fails, autonomy is the ultimate trump.

But think of the image of autonomy and the mythology underlying it: the solitary individual, the one unknown to all others, the only one who can speak for one's self, the only one who can be trusted with one's self and one's deepest desires, the self-made person. The price of autonomy is quite high—an ultimate aloneness. For truly no one can know me or what is good for me or what I might want in particular circumstances. Only the autonomous self can know this.

What religion can offer here is a correction of autonomy—a reminder that there is a reality called community in which we are born, nourished, educated, sustained, and ultimately flourish. This is not a rejection of autonomy or a tyranny of the many over the one. Rather it is a recognition that at our deepest levels we are not self-made individuals. Everything we bring to our existence we have received from others—our existence, our language, our education, our food, our clothing, our shelter. As we mature, we assume many of these responsibilities for ourselves and begin to build on these resources and gifts from the community in which we live. We also find a degree of fulfillment in our relations with others whether in friendship or in other forms of committed relations. Here we find new dimensions of fulfillment and even self-discovery. But these new discoveries come as a gift of the relationship itself. We are much more with and a part of a community than the prevailing ideology of autonomy would suggest.

And it is here that I recall various stories of my friend Ray's last weeks. For while surely Ray had a deep devotion to self-reliance and a strong sense of initiative and individual responsibility, he also recognized that his life was not totally of his own making. He knew that although he had an agenda there was also a larger scheme in which he was not the only or even the main actor. He knew that receiving was also an act of service and that participating in community also meant receiving from that community. In many ways his self-reliance gave way to trust, his autonomy gave way to companionship in community, and his setting his own agenda gave way to altering his course to fit another.

In all this, religious commitment played a large role. Much of what he did and experienced between the time of his diagnosis and death would be meaningless to someone without such a commitment. Yet Ray's path to his dying reveals dimensions of both living and dying that are important parts of our larger social discussion of these issues, even though one might not be led by the same lights as Ray.

One element common to religion is the role of community and its importance in sustaining and nourishing its individual members. All religions hold some form of a theory of individual accountability, but they also join this to community resources of prayer, service, and ritual to aid members in their individual journeys. Additionally religions affirm the value and frequently the necessity of service both to the members of the religious community and to all members of society. This is expressed in the mandate to assist others, to give alms, or to engage in other forms of volunteer work in the community. While religions affirm the value of the individual and strong theories of personal accountability for one's life, they also recognize that communities offer resources to individuals to make such responsibility more possible—more possible precisely because one engages in this process with and for others. Thus, community is not only a locus in which one acts out major elements of one's religious commitments, it is also reality that sustains and nurtures us in our journey.

Two areas of application follow. First, even in the strongest forms of the physician-assisted suicide/euthanasia debate, autonomy fails at a critical level. That is, after all the rhetoric and ideology settles, the argument is that individuals really cannot do it by themselves. They have neither the resources nor access to them, and they are physically unable to do the act by themselves. The only means available are unaesthetic, particularly for survivors. Thus the debate is over physician-assisted suicide or euthanasia administered *by another*. At a very deep level this debate seems to be an appeal to a community for assistance in carrying out one's desires, and the limits and even failure of autonomy as the keystone of the argument are clearly revealed. At a critical juncture in the debate autonomy fails and the necessity of the community is implicitly invoked, although this is in no way acknowledged by the proponents of physician-assisted suicide and euthanasia.

Second, the notion of community invoked in the physician-assisted suicide/euthanasia argument is a strange one. The community or representative of the community is to serve the individual by helping that individual end his or her life rather than by assisting that person in living, the usual role of community. The image of the individual seeking assistance in dying is usually a person who is alone or certainly feels alone. In the literature on this debate, seldom does one find discussions of individuals who have resources other than themselves, even when these are available. Even in the Dutch film that shows a man being euthanized, his removal from the community is apparent. Certainly this man has community resources—an excellent healthcare system, a personal physician who makes house calls, a comfortable house and physical resources, and a loving wife. But the dominant image in the film is withdrawal. The husband does not touch his wife and vice versa, they do not speak of friends, and medical assistance is absent. At the end, the physician puts his arm around the wife and repeats over and over: "Isn't this beautiful? Isn't this better?" And the isolation of each is never stronger than in that moment.

And this is where other memories of my friend Ray return. Granted, Ray was a priest and a member of a religious community with a lot of built-in care and support, but he also had a number of other friends outside the religious community who drove him to radiation treatment, visited him, and provided various forms of service. And what is interesting is that Ray, a very take-charge kind of person with the Marine Corps overlay, accepted the service with grace and graciousness. And in being served himself in his illness, he also served others.

Many will argue that this death is the exception and that it idealizes pain and suffering. Some made the same arguments about the dying of Cardinal Bernardin. My friend Ray and Cardinal Bernardin had healthcare and personal resources not available to most. But that truth stands as a judgment on the physician-assisted suicide/euthanasia debate and the treatment of many of the dying. Our culture frequently isolates the dying, we tend to overtreat and undermedicate them, and we do not provide a space for their dying other than the most technologically advanced. Our culture is a death-denying culture. One almost has the feeling at times that dying is somehow un-American, an affront to our standard of living. Thus, when dying rears its ugly head—and we must never forget its head is ugly—we seek to get it done as quickly and painlessly as possible, efficiency and comfort being other critical American values.

Thus, at a critical moment the individual is alone. The presence of community will not remove the terror, eliminate pain and suffering, or remove the burden. But a community may ease these, relieve the aloneness, bring comfort, and most importantly assure the dying person that he or she is not abandoned. Community certainly does not solve all problems associated with dying, but a community does hold the patient in its midst and show that the patient is valued and not alone. Certainly this vision of community permits a variety of modes of dying, but the context in which they occur is radically different than in the traditional philosophical debate. Religion offers a critical change in perspective in the dying process, a perspective that will not eliminate the reality of death and its terrors but that offers many more options. To eliminate the role of a community—whether of immediate family, friends, or voluntary organizations to which one belongs—from the debate, regardless of how that debate is ultimately resolved, is to shortchange both the individual and the community.

THE PROVISION OF HEALTHCARE

This section is also inspired by my friend Ray and his passion for justice and his commitment to the poor—a message he communicated to others and one that some could not forget. This is a message we too need to hear in our rethinking of healthcare in the United States.

That we are undergoing a revolution in the provision of healthcare is apparent to anyone who has been to a physician lately or to anyone who has been without insurance. The general verdict thus far is that the changes are not good, and many are dissatisfied with the way HMOs provide services. The so-called drive-through deliveries that limited care to an overnight stay after normal childbirth was a focal point that sparked a major debate.

Some background features of this debate are important. First, there are two major ways of receiving health insurance. Most Americans obtain medical insurance as a benefit of employment. Employers bear a large share of the cost of medical insurance, although a greater share of these costs are being transferred to workers. Also if one is poor or elderly, insurance comes through government programs, and here too one's copayment is increasing and fewer benefits are available. Consequently, for most unemployed, the underemployed, and many of the nation's poor, there is no medical insurance. The same is frequently true for those who are determined to have a "medical predisposition" to a disease, which disqualifies them from many insurance programs.

Second, we have some rather strange beliefs about medical care in this country. We seem to think, for example, that quality medical care means as much as possible for as long as possible. We seem to think that medical resources are infinite and need not be paid for. And we seem to think that because we have insurance, we are entitled to as many tests and opinions as possible. Healthcare thus seems to be for many an infinite supply of increasingly high-tech interventions that are very expensive and require an increasingly sophisticated cadre of individuals to use them. Such a vision, even given some degree of exaggeration, is coming up against some realities that are very hard for Americans to accept. Resources are not infinite; a plethora of equipment does not necessarily mean quality care; prolonged use of various therapies or technologies is not necessarily in the patient's best interest; and payment for services is becoming complicated, to say the least.

These two situations are creating a very hostile atmosphere around the issue of the provision of healthcare. Traditionally healthcare was provided in a fee-for-service model in which many of the costs were underwritten by employment-derived insurance. Here the physician was essentially a small business person who contracted directly with the patient, who came to the physician. The predominant ethic was that the physician acted in the best interest of the patient; although fees were derived from such transactions, predominant weight in the equation was given to the physician's judgment. Because of this factor, costs escalated and began to go out of control. Thus, there was a shift to HMOs or other managed-care programs. Managed-care organizations used market forces to help solve the cost problem by developing incentive programs for physicians to be efficient in the care they provided (only tests or treatment actually needed and provided as cost-effectively as possible) or by developing capitation programs (specific allocations from various diseases or services with cost overruns taken from the operating budget of the HMO). Thus the *culture* of the provision of healthcare changed rapidly. The word *culture* is emphasized advisedly because, anecdotal reports to the contrary, Americans do not seem to be less healthy than before.

Nonetheless, some features remain that raise critical problems. First, many are still uninsured or have coverage that is inadequate. Second, coverage is still linked to employment. Third, the focus is still on high-tech interventions or rescue medicine rather than prevention. Fourth, many see the changes coming from the shift to an HMO model as radically unfair. These issues need serious and sustained discussion, and religion can bring at least two contributions to this discussion.

First, many religions, and here the discussion focuses on Roman Catholicism, have a concept of justice. The Bishops of the United States presented their understanding of justice in the 1986 pastoral letter "Economic Justice for All."[4] In the approach of the bishops, justice mandates specific responses to the individuals we meet within our daily lives. Here justice as participation and as the preferential option for the poor would focus on the needs of individuals and ensure their participation within the decision-making structure of society. Justice would ensure that individuals are not marginalized because of their income or social status. Justice would ensure that the poor or disenfranchised are not the one who receive less or inferior treatment because of their inability or reluctance to speak out.

The vision of justice offered by the bishops has five basic dimensions.

1. It is necessary to develop a cultural consensus that places economic rights in the same position of honor enjoyed by other social rights such as civil rights, the right of free speech, and the right to privacy. Here human dignity is protected by ensuring adequate participation in the resources of the community.
2. Justice is realized when individuals and groups actively participate in the life of the community. Justice seeks to give voice and choice and to diminish social, political, or economic marginalization as much as possible.
3. Justice is to be reciprocal. That is, justice is served not only when individuals' needs are fulfilled, but also when individuals are enabled to be active and productive within the community. Thus, justice demands contributions to the common good as well as contributions from it.
4. Justice does not focus on the production of goods and services only. It also must evaluate the sources of production, the means of production, and patterns of distribution.
5. With regard to distribution of resources, unequal distributions must be evaluated with particular attention to their impact on those whose basic human needs are unmet. Also unequal distributions based on characteristic such as race, sex or other, arbitrary standers cannot be justified.

What is critical in this orientation toward justice is its focus on both the dignity of the person and the construction of social structures that enable participation in as well as reception from society. Additionally, the vision of justice looks to the poor and mandates that their needs be met. In fact, the letter says that the increased economic participation of the marginalized takes precedence over the preservation of privileged concentrations of power and wealth.

One can ask how this type of preferential option for the poor shapes our attitude toward the provision of healthcare. One response is to recognize the breadth of the mandate. This was aptly summarized by Cardinal Bernardin when he said: "Our moral, political and economic responsibilities do not stop at the moment of birth! We must defend the *right to life* of the weakest among us; we must also be supportive of the *quality of life* of the powerless among us, . . . the sick, the disabled, the dying."[5]

What this discussion of justice brings to the table is an expanded understanding of justice, one that sees the inclusion of all members of the community so that they can both receive from the community and contribute to it. The provision of healthcare to all is one way in which quality participation within a community is ensured.

A second concept related to this discussion of justice is the common good. Considerations of the common good have largely fallen by the wayside in the last several decades in mainstream discussions of social and political ethics. In part this has been because, as Bellah phrases it: "American culture has focused relentlessly on the idea that individuals are self-interest maximizers and that private accumulation and private pleasures are the only measurable public goods."[6] Downplaying of the common good is also reflected in our reliance on cost-benefit analysis for social decision making. What is given priority here is social efficiency and a neglect of the social consequences that follow from such decisions. Finally we continue to hear the rhetoric that the government and our institutions are the enemy of the individual. Although the Reagan mantra of "Get Government off our backs" is not as frequently invoked as it was in the 1980s, the sentiment remains alive; it can be seen particularly in many of the critiques of the Clinton health proposal as well as in the rhetoric that drives the "reform" of welfare. What we seem to have forgotten is that "even autonomy depends on a particular kind of institutional structure and is not an escape from institutions altogether."[7] And we have further forgotten that autonomy is "only one virtue among others and that without such virtues as responsibility and care . . . autonomy itself becomes . . . an empty form without substance."[8]

In discussing the common good, a double nostalgia must be resisted and ultimately rejected. The American version is derivative from a vision of rural or small-town America as seen though the idealization of the early days of the founding of our Republic or the paintings of Norman Rockwell. Another version is papal and longs for the Middle Ages. According to Pius XI:

> At one period there existed a social order which, though by no means perfect in every respect, corresponded nevertheless in a certain measure to right reason according to the needs and conditions of the times. That this order has long since perished is not due to the fact

that it was incapable of development and adaptation to changing needs and circumstances, but rather to the wrongdoing of men. Men were hardened in excessive self-love and refused to extend that order, as was their duty, to the increasing numbers of the people; or else, deceived by the attractions of false liberty and other errors, they grew impatient of every restraint and endeavored to throw off all authority.[9]

To be sure there are virtues to be admired and emulated in both visions, but our world is largely industrialized and urban. Our problems, although similar to those of past generations, cannot rely on the solutions of our forbears because our times and social context are quite different.

In Roman Catholic social theory, from which I derive my perspective, the concept of the common good has a rich and varied history. In "Rerum Novarum," the 1891 encyclical by Leo XIII that began the tradition of Catholic social thought, Leo defined the common good as that for the sake of which civil society exists and "is concerned with the interests of all in general, and with the individual interests in their due place and proportion."[10] More specifically Pius IX, in "Quadragesimo Anno," stated that "Those goods should be sufficient to supply all needs and an honest livelihood, and to up lift men to that higher level of prosperity and culture which, provided it be used with prudence, is not only no hinderance but is of singular help to virtue."[11] Both of these conceptions of the common good are derived from the static and hierarchically structured society in which these popes lived. Additionally, as Dennis McCann notes, these writers assumed that the common good derived from such a society was "self-evidently substantive, objectively knowable, and indivisible."[12] Such a perspective is overly optimistic at best and epistemologically naïve at worst, but nonetheless such a concern for the good of society and all of its members stays at the heart of the encyclical tradition.

John XXIII began a shift from such a hierarchical and static vision of society and the common good by identifying the foundation of the common good as the human person who has rights and obligations flowing from his or her nature.[13] This vision moved the focus from the structure of society to the person and used the concept of rights to ensure the protection and enhancement of the individual in society and the concept of obligation to guarantee that the person actively participate in the development of society. Such thinking led John to a vision of the common good that did not stop at national boundaries but included "the entire human family."[14]

The Second Vatican Council, in its pastoral constitution, "The Church in the Modern World," continued this line of thought by recognizing that "the concrete demands of this common good are constantly changing as time goes on."[15] This important document recognizes that the common good is a dynamic concept and one that must be responsive to the changing needs of human society.

The American Catholic Bishops then used this perspective to develop a vision of social justice that "implies that persons have an obligation to be active and productive participants in the life of society and that society has a duty to enable them to participate in this way."[16] Here they follow Pius XI, who said: "It is of the very essence of social justice to demand from each individual all that is necessary for the common good."[17] Thus, the bishops envision justice as a means through which the person achieves the perfection of his or her self through contributing to the well-being of society. In the perspective of the bishops, then, the core of justice is the establishment of "minimum levels of participation in the life of the human community for all persons"[18] rather than establishing zones of privacy whereby individuals attempt to seek their private good independently of the community.

The American Catholic Bishops make the following affirmation: "The common bond of humanity that links all persons is the source of our belief that the country can attain a renewed public moral vision."[19] And finally, the bishops state: "The dignity of the human person, realized in community with others, is the criterion against which all aspects of economic life must be measured."[20]

This orientation presents a vision of justice and the common good that is not quite in the mainstream of America libertarian theory. The bishops recognize this and argue that the next phase of the American experiment needs to secure for this vision of social justice the same status as the other rights we correctly celebrate. The significant difference is that the bishops' vision orients the person to his or her role in the community whereas our traditional vision focuses on the autonomous individual.

This vision, based in a particular religious tradition, can make a valuable contribution to the public debate over healthcare and particularly the question of insurance. Although one can argue that this vision supports a variety of particular policies in the general healthcare debate, its more important function is to be a kind of searchlight that illumines aspects of the debate frequently ignored. That is, this perspective mandates that a key element of the provision of healthcare be the inclusion of those who are marginalized or in the greatest need of healthcare services. It argues that the well-being of society can be achieved only when those at the margins are brought into the mainstream and enabled to make their contributions to the common good of all. One key element in this strategy is to ensure that such individuals receive appropriate healthcare. Such policies not only respect and promote the dignity of all citizens but also guarantee a more just society in which the good of society prospers through the participation of the many in its goals.

The contribution of religion to this aspect of the debate is not to propose particular policies or strategies, but to make sure the debate addresses the needs and concerns of all, to ensure that the needs of the voiceless are given voice, and to ensure that the marginalized are protected and thus enabled to make their contribution to society. The role of religion here is to guarantee a broad social debate and the representation of the needs of all.

CONCLUSION

This essay has reviewed some historical aspects of the development of bioethics that suggest why religion has been put to the side of much of the bioethics debate: the use of philosophical analysis, the focus on analysis of issues rather than advocacy, and the pluralistic nature of the public policy debate. This marginalization of religion was not necessarily intentional or motivated by hostility to religion. Rather it began happening gradually, and then religious voices began to be perceived more as sectarian critiques rather than as contributions to the mainstream discussion. Such an understanding of religion as sectarian, at least in its politics if not its theology, was certainly helped by the blatantly partisan alignment of several religious organizations with the Republican agenda and their sponsorship of individuals for public office. The rise of the "Moral Majority" set the discussion of religion and public policy back several decades.

In bioethical discussions, religion should not necessarily or primarily focus on making public policy proposals—although religious bodies and individual members of religious organizations are certainly entitled to do this as members of our society. Rather, religion can identify aspects of the bioethics debate not highlighted by customary political or philosophical analysis, it can help ensure a wider agenda of public policy discussion, and it can argue for the inclusion of a broader constituency in the provision of healthcare.[21]

What religious traditions have to offer is a broader vision of both individuals and society, a more inclusive vision of justice, an inclusive vision of the common good, and a view of human dignity that argues that individuals should receive from the community as well as participate in its well-being. This contribution does not directly translate into a set of policy recommendations but it does serve as a lens with which we can sharpen our view of various debates and critique them when appropriate.

NOTES

1. D.A. Cronin, "The Moral Law in Regard to the Ordinary and Extraordinary Means of Conserving Life," in *Conserving Human Life* (Braintree, Mass.: Pope John XXIII Medical-Moral Center, 1989).

2. D. Callahan, *The Troubled Dream of Life* (New York: Simon and Schuster, 1993).

3. Ibid., 371.

4. This letter as well as other papal encyclicals can be found in D.J. O'Brien and T.A. Shannon, ed., *Catholic Social Thought: The Documentary Heritage* (New York: Orbis Books, 1992).

5. J. Bernardin, "The Consistent Ethic of Life and Health Care Systems," in *Consistent Ethic of Life* (Kansas City, Mo.: Sheed and Ward, 1988), 52. Italics in the original.

6. R. Bellah et al., *The Good Society* (New York: Alfred A. Knopf, 1991), 50.

7. Ibid., 12.

8. Ibid.

9. Pius XI, "*Quadragesimo Anno,*" see note 4 above, p. 64.

10. Leo XIII, "*Rerum Novarum,*" see note 4 above, p. 33.

11. Pius XI, "*Quadragesimo Anno,*" see note 4 above, p. 59.

12. D. McCann, "The Good to be Pursued in Common," in *The Common Good and U.S. Capitalism*, ed. O. Williams and J. Houck (Lanham, Md.: University Press, 1987), 164.

13. John XXIII, "*Pacem in Terris,*" see note 4 above, p. 132.

14. Ibid., 147.

15. Vatican II, "*Gaudium et Spes,*" see note 4 above, p. 220.

16. American Catholic Bishops, "Economic Justice for All," see note 4 above, p. 595.

17. Ibid., 595.

18. Ibid., 596.

19. Ibid., 584.

20. Ibid., 584.

21. Many of my ideas about the common good and the relation of religion to society have been shaped by M. Himes and K. Himes, *Fullness of Faith: The Public Significance of Theology* (New York: Paulist Press, 1993).

8

Bioethics and Religion:
Some Unscientific Footnotes

Stephen E. Lammers

INTRODUCTION

Bioethicists might well raise questions about the existence of collections like this one. "Why another collection of articles speaking about religion or religious studies and bioethics?" After all, on one reading, religious belief and practice have fared rather well at the hands of the bioethics community. Religious choices, as they become clear as genuine choices, are honored. For example, bioethicists defended Jehovah's Witnesses when they refused blood or blood products and today no one argues that physicians should not respect the wishes of adult Jehovah's Witnesses when no one depends upon them. In addition, bioethics centers and programs sponsor seminars on cultural differences, and among the differences religious ones are always noted. Bioethicists may be children of the Enlightenment, at least in their academic origins, but they insist that physicians and other medical care personnel respect the choices that people make. Among those choices are choices that flow from the religious commitments of persons who seek medical treatment.

The clinical side of the bioethics community might even speak up more strongly. Not only were they not formally involved in the Enlightenment project of trying to get past religious divisiveness to develop an ethic that would be universal, but clinicians generally have noted the religious differences of their patients and the effects of those differences. Further, many hospitals in this country have a religious community in their background, and a respect for religious beliefs and practices has long been a part of the clinic. Even many secular hospitals have pastoral care departments that are involved intimately in the care of patients. As a "lurker" on the Medical College of Wisconsin Bioethics Bulletin Board, I must say that I am often impressed with the sensitivity with which the religious beliefs of patients are often treated (there are exceptions) and the realization that the sensitive treatment of those beliefs sometimes increases the difficulty for the medical caregivers.

In addition, the influence of bioethicists upon medical and nursing personnel has been considerable—much of it positive. As a person who started "hanging around" hospitals 15 years ago, I can attest that physicians have become more sensitive to informing their patients and more careful to listen to their patients. Realistically, one might attribute some of these changes to the influence of patterns of litigation and state and federal legislation, but this does not explain all of these changes. In short, bioethics has had an influence upon the practice of medicine that, some would say, is praiseworthy. At the same time, some of the problems with contemporary bioethics flow from these very successes.

There are thinkers who are members of religious communities who are satisfied with bioethics as it is currently being practiced in this country. So the question of what this chapter and this collection might be about would be reasonable.

I cannot speak for other writers in this present collection of essays. Nor can I, in what follows, pretend to speak from anywhere. I cannot claim to be other than a teacher of religious studies who does Christian ethics informed by a particular understanding of the Roman Catholic tradition. From within that perspective, let me give voice to my worries about bioethics, in particular a philosophical bioethics that relies primarily upon principles. Many of the points that follow have been made by persons with religious commitments different from mine or persons with no religious commitments whatsoever. The following concerns are seen as growing out of one interpretation of a particular community's vision of what a good life might be and what role medicine might play in that good life. One might make the same judgments from another starting point. At the same time, one might have very different reasons for these judgments.

HOW BIOETHICS CAME INTO THE CLINIC

Bioethics came upon the scene when American medicine was losing its way. In particular, medicine had lost its service orientation. No longer intimately connected to the communities of service that had sustained it earlier in the United States, medicine had become technologically sophisticated and socially powerful. It also had become the place of arrogant behavior toward patients.

The field of bioethics began to develop in that context and it appeared to be "prophetic." Many writers in bioethics reminded physicians of who they were and what they should become. In that setting, many welcomed bioethics as a corrective to what was happening in medicine. One example of a thinker influenced by his own religious tradition who was important in early bioethics was Paul Ramsey. Ramsey was clear that he expected better of physicians, that they should treat the "patient as [a] person," to paraphrase the title of his influential work.[1]

At the same time, other thinkers were not interested in restoring medicine to the service orientation it once had; they wished to rethink the relationship between physician and patient in the new circumstances of late 20th-century medicine. This reformulation usually took place under the rubric of patient rights and a contractual relationship between physician and patient.[2] Both philosophical and legal analysis would be applied to the rights of patients.

It was in this context that the case became important as a focus of discussion in bioethics. Cases here should be understood in two ways, medical and legal. Briefly, the legal matter first.

In the Anglo-Saxon philosophical tradition, there is an interest in law and legal regulation. In addition, in American culture, contentious events often turn into legal issues. Bioethics simply reflects these two phenomena. The consequence is that it is assumed that one should know the relevant law as part of one's expertise in bioethics and, in particular, one should know the case law. Significant cases such as *Dax, Quinlan, Cruzan,* and *Wanglie* all are part of the knowledge base of bioethics. This attention to legal cases is simply reinforced by the use of medical cases in the clinical setting.

What then happens in the clinical setting with respect to cases? The typical case that is constructed for teaching purposes usually has a number of individuals who are involved around a patient. The patient may or may not be able to make decisions for her- or himself; what is relevant is that something must be decided for and/or with this patient. How to proceed is the question of the day. The conflicts in the case come in at a number of different levels. The patient or the patient's spokesperson may desire care the medical team thinks is inappropriate. Then again, the patient or spokesperson may wish to discontinue care that the medical team thinks is vital. An industry has grown up around the process whereby cases are resolved, and it is a requirement for of the Joint Commission on Accreditation of Healthcare Organizations that hospitals have in place a process for the resolution of such conflicts.

Now it is not surprising that much of modern bioethics is preoccupied with cases so constructed. Many persons in bioethics work in or around teaching hospitals, and they were sometimes brought to those hospitals to help clinicians think about the difficulties of their work. The case is a typical device for teaching in medicine and nursing; it is useful for a discussion of the ethical issues that arise in the practice of modern nursing and medicine. What it is important to realize here is that, for clinicians, cases are one of the ways in which they learn.

It was in the context of cases that claims about physicians' arrogance were articulated. It was by using cases to show how physicians proceeded with their patients that bioethics made its mark in the modern period. The enemy was the paternalistic physician; the object of the paternalistic behavior was the presumably competent patient whose wishes, especially wishes about the discontinuation of treatment, were being ignored. Bioethics became important by providing tools for analyzing cases where the paternalistic physician played an important role. Not so incidentally, in terms of hospital culture, bioethics became allied with various forces within hospitals that wished to limit physicians' power and authority. The choice of the patient was put over against the claims of the physician.

In many important ways, the introduction of bioethics into the clinical setting has been to the good. Physicians' behavior is probably less arrogant than it was in the past. More often than before, physicians and patients have conversations about what is important to the patient and what physicians think their obligations are. Still, it is not often enough.[3]

Note, however, what is not discussed in such a situation. What is not discussed is how the individual came into the healthcare system in the first place. What is not discussed are the ethical issues surrounding the care, or lack of it, for the patient before he or she came into the hospital. The social context within which decisions about the patient have been made are, generally speaking, not part of the conversation. Of course, one does not need to be working out of a religious tradition to make this observation.[4]

The tool that bioethics has used in order to make a difference in the clinic was its understanding of choice. Choice became a key concept of modern bioethics. Physicians claimed that they wanted to seek the good of patients, as the physicians understood that good. Without denying that physicians sought the good as they saw it, many bioethicists focused on the centrality of the patient's choice as determining what should be done. Much of what has happened in modern bioethics can be understood as the attempt to think out the implications of making choice the central datum in medical care. Religions were seen as one more choice that a patient might make.

THE METAPHOR OF CHOICE

RELIGION AS CHOICE

Thus the place to begin this inquiry is with the assumption that one can understand religious belief or religious commitment primarily as a lifestyle choice. Treating religion as a choice might be a positive development for clinicians in that they are supposed to respect patients' choices and, if one is consistent, one recognizes that consequences flow from those choices. Sometimes these consequences are of the type that clinicians are trained to resist and reverse. This is what happened in the discussion of the refusal to accept blood and blood products by Jehovah's Witnesses. Although many perceive this choice as irrational, and the risks of mortality or morbidity are sometimes high, it is argued that this choice should be respected. Note that it is not *religious* choice that is to be respected, but religion as *choice* that is to be respected.

Now it is not surprising that the bioethics community respects religiously based choice insofar as this community is part of American culture. Bellah and colleagues document how many people in the United States think that they can not only choose but constitute their own religious system.[5] But that is only part of the story of religion in American culture.

For many religious believers, their primary experience is not one of choices but of being called or being chosen. The important choice is not theirs but the deity's. Thus, the experience of some believers is that they cannot do other than they now do. To treat religion primarily as a choice is to misconstrue believers' understanding of who they are and what they are called to become. What is perceived by many on the outside as a choice is seen by the believer as being chosen. Jon Levenson does an excellent job of presenting this issue and the political implications of it, in a discussion of "covenant" in the *Harvard Divinity Bulletin*. He points out that to understand the covenant between God and the Jewish people solely as the consequence of the choice of the Jewish people is to distort the textual evidence. This is not to say that choice was not involved; it is to say that it was a choice with no realistic alternative.[6]

The point here for Levenson is that the experience of choice is presumed to be one in which there are options. I might have bought car *A* instead of car *B*. This type of experience is simply not the experience of many believers. They are called or chosen to be who they are. They may refuse that call, but the choice is not neutral. To refuse the call is to be unfaithful. It should be obvious that this discussion is based on "Western" religious systems, ones dependent upon Judaism. Stanley Hauerwas has made this point in the context of speaking about bioethics from a Christian perspective in reviewing the work of H. Tristram Engelhardt, Jr.[7] But this is not only a Western religious view. The point could be made about adherents to other religious traditions. Buddhists know that one "could" choose otherwise than to affirm the Four Noble Truths. To do so for Buddhists, however, is to continue in illusion.

CHOICE AND THE POOR

The difficulties of the model of choice in modern bioethics do not end with its failure to comprehend the experience of many believers. This model of choice is not the experience of people of limited education and income. For many persons in the United States, their lives are shaped not by their choices but by forces around them that they do not understand and of which they are (often rightfully) suspicious. To thrust them into an environment in which choice is presumed to be dominant is to put them in a situation where they will be hostile. Why should they trust anyone offering them choices? Physicians and bioethicists are perceived to be from the community of the educated and the powerful, which has been taking choices out of their hands for years.

For example, persons in poverty know that they do not have choices about the kind of medical care they will receive. There is a "system" of healthcare available to them that is not as good as that available to individuals who have employer-paid healthcare. Anyone who has spent time in the clinics that serve many of the poor people in this country knows that, if the poor had a choice, they would not be there in those clinics.

Given that many people in poverty do not have any choices about the kind of healthcare they receive, they wonder why they should believe they are being given a choice at some critical juncture in the care of themselves or a loved one. Choice, as they understand the world, is simply not the most important reality, and to pretend that it is to misunderstand their lives. This is one of the reasons that sometimes there is so much miscommunication between physicians and ethics committees and poor people. In the circumstances in which these parties often meet, the care of a loved one at the end of life, the only real choice of the poor is to resist. Often that means to refuse to do what the physicians are recommending, especially if the physicians are recommending discontinuing treatment. That recommendation may appear to all in the medical community as not only reasonable but required in order to minimize the patient's pain and suffering. However, for the child or the spouse of the patient, that recommendation appears to be one more way in which their lives are declared less meaningful.

CHOICE AND DISEASE

Disease is another area in medicine where the metaphor of choice is not helpful. The discussion that follows does not deny that persons can make choices that are deleterious to their health. What is being argued here is that often these are not the most important factors.

Some of us are born genetically predisposed to certain diseases. A woman with a family history of breast cancer has certain choices, to be sure; however, her experience is not that of someone who is empowered to make choices but that of a person who has to deal with factors she did not choose. To focus on her possible choices is to miss an important part of her experience. But our genetic inheritance is not the only place where metaphors of choice are not helpful. Disease often comes to us because of causal factors over which we have no control. This lack of control may be due to causes that are unique to the individual, such as an airborne virus, or because of social arrangements that the person did not choose and from which he or she cannot escape, such as living next to a former toxic landfill site. In both cases, individuals have choices. Yet when choice becomes the central organizing feature of the discussion, much of what is important is missed. How one deals with tragedy, how one lives with events over which one has no control, the stance one takes toward these events—all of this is pushed into the background if choice about what to do about a particular matter becomes central. Further, how one might organize and join with others to effect change is often ignored. Yet, in the case of a toxic landfill, for example, changing those circumstances will probably have more to do with good health than any medical intervention.

In summary, the choice model that is assumed to be normative and supportive of religion turns out to lead to misunderstandings of the situation of many believers. Further, this understanding of choice often is a function of class and power. Finally, choice as the central metaphor is not true to the experience of disease for those who are ill.

RELIGION AS A "PRIVATE" CHOICE

The model of choice is part of a larger project, that of the Enlightenment, within which certain phenomena are identified as "public" and "rational" and others as "private" and "a-rational." John Milbank has made this point in *Theology and Social Theory*.[8] Not surprisingly, medicine belongs to the public world and religion to the private one. This construction of reality privileges medical discourse.

Milbank points out how new religious claims are introduced *sub rosa*.[9] The consequences of this for bioethics are quite important. First, bioethicists are unable to appreciate and critique the functioning religious commitments of the Enlightenment project itself. Insofar as bioethicists participate in that project, they are unaware of their own religious commitments. Second, religion is pushed into the sphere of the private. Because bioethicists imagine themselves involved in public discourse, religious language must be excluded because it is not a language of public discourse. An important corollary is that any statement coming out of a religious perspective is perceived to be public and relevant only if the thinker chooses to make it so, and on other grounds. By thus compartmentalizing religious language, religion is thus protected and at the same time neutralized.

In another place I have commented upon the marginalization of religious voice in academic bioethics.[10] The general issue here remains the construction of the public and the private spheres of discourse. Religious voices—whether they are the voices of an individual or of a religious organization or institution—have been marginalized when they are assumed to be private voices that are allowed to have their say as long as they do not influence public discussion. The Enlightenment forefathers of bio-ethics imagined a world in which there were "positive" religions (by which they meant Christianity and Judaism) that were "particular," and a "universal" religion that could be the basis of a civil religion. That entire construction of religion has been subject to critique in the work of thinkers like Nicholas Lash. One point stands out. The Enlightenment thinkers did not realize that they themselves were particular, that their constructions were just as historically limited as were the religions that they wished to overcome. But if that is the case, there is no reason to marginalize religious discourse to the realm of the private on the grounds that there is some language that is not particular but universal. Without that assumption, much of modern bioethics has to change its view, not only of religion, but of itself. Persons working in bioethics would have to attend to the historical circumstances in which they find themselves now and the implications of those circumstances for their task at hand. In short, they would have to enter into history instead of pretending to be above it.[11]

This is not to assert that arguments that rely upon assumptions not widely shared should win the day in public discourse simply because they are religious arguments. However, everyone's assumptions need to be understood, and everyone's voice should be part of the conversation. When voices are excluded simply because they are religious, there has been a confusion between the process of public discussion and the justifications for arguments in public discussion.

RELIGIOUSLY BASED
CRITIQUES OF HEALTHCARE

It is at the level of the public world that members of religious communities have generated critiques of the healthcare system in this country. One example from the Roman Catholic community would be Andrew Lustig's essay on healthcare reform and healthcare rationing. Lustig reports that what is often taken as conventional wisdom on healthcare in this country has come in for critical comment from the Roman Catholic bishops.[12] He points out that the Roman Catholic bishops have articulated a position on what we owe one another in terms of healthcare that is markedly different from that of the U.S. healthcare community. Insofar as the bioethics community participates in that larger healthcare community and does not critique that community on this point, the bioethics community becomes marginal to the discussion of how healthcare should be organized in this country. One does not have to be Roman Catholic to make this point, of course. Indeed, at least one thinker proposes that religious communities have not done enough here. Yet the silence of the bioethics community has been noted.[13]

There is, of course, an alternative interpretation. Bioethicists have benefited greatly from the current medical care system. In their unwillingness to engage in systematic critique of that system and to use religious language here, the bioethics community begins to look like priests who are celebrating the beliefs of the powerful, and the religious communities begin to look like the outsiders. But that religious critique is generally not heard or attended to within the bioethics community.

Why might this be so? When discussion comes from the religious community directed to the larger community, it is difficult for members of the bioethics community to understand it. This is because bioethicists generally share the assumptions of the Enlightenment about religious discourse. First, such discourse can lead to great conflict. This assumption is, of course, true. Second, religious discourse can be a mask for self-interest. That, of course, is also true. Yet these two truths become translated into an attitude that manages to marginalize all sorts of religious critiques of the larger society and of modern medicine as part of that society.

Let us start with the second assumption first, that religious critique can be a mask for self-interest. Modern bioethics owes part of its heritage to the Nuremburg trials; one cannot talk about modern bioethics without talking about the Holocaust. It appears that much of what passes for reflection on the Holocaust is reflection from the perspective of those who did not suffer from it. This does not make it invalid. What it does, however, is to limit the influence of the victims, the majority of whom were Jews. If Jewish communities speak about experimentation upon human beings, for example, they speak out of the memory of this experience. The speech may have elements of self-interest, in that they do not want to see future persecutions of Jewish communities. But the speakers may see themselves as doing a service to the larger community, a service that the larger community may or may not desire. A perspective that can only hear that speech as self-interested or irrelevant for public discourse is going to miss important elements of that speech.

All of this flows with the difficulty of taking religious systems seriously as potential resources for discussion. It is obvious that they can be barriers, but the possibility of using religious systems as a resource is rarely explored. In following a recent discussion of caring and the altruistic caregiver and the ensuing debate on the Medical College of Wisconsin Bioethics Bulletin Board, I was reminded of debates that have occurred within many religious traditions concerning how one sustains persons who care for others so that they do not become self-righteous. One commentator said something like, "Being a child of or a spouse of a super-altruistic person would be very difficult." The proposal being made was that one had to switch to a model of caring in which there is explicit attention to the needs of the caregiver. This, of course, is not news to most religious traditions, which have long worried about how one sustains care in the face of adversity without either being overcome by the adversity or becoming absorbed in the care of some to the detriment of one's obligations. The solutions of the past are not recommended here. However, a familiarity with the literature might give us food for thought, as we struggle today to think about how to care for the sick and for those who care for them.

It is the responsibility of scholars of religion to remind persons in bioethics that these resources exist and might be used as part of the conversation. It is a hopeful sign that some scholars in bioethics appear to be willing to consider what thinkers who proceed out of religious commitments are saying.

One final example. Bioethics has had difficulty doing anything about the lack of universal healthcare in the United States. Although a small number of persons have worked on this issue, it does not seem to exercise the bioethics community as a whole.[14] There seems to be a kind of passivity among bioethicists that has received some notice. Given the fascination with choice as the central organizing metaphor for ethics, the importance of the case for medicine in general and with its choice dilemma for bio-ethics in particular, and the individualism of our culture, it should not be surprising that there is relatively little interest in the issue of universal healthcare. In this sense, bioethics simply reflects the culture instead of commenting critically upon it.

I am suggesting that there are grounds for a critique of the bioethics community from within the religious community where I stand. As I observe those who call themselves bioethicists, it is not clear to me that this critique is even known; the more worrisome alternative is that it might be known but it is being ignored. I have waited, for example, for a lively discussion of the debate going on within American Catholicism over the selling of formerly not-for-profit, religiously affiliated hospitals to for-profit hospital chains. That conversation, which could be a lively one, has largely not occurred. Where it has occurred, it has been around the issues of rights and not of social justice. Rights are important, but fascination with them leads to a minimalist account of healthcare. Such a minimalist account is incapable of raising the more important issues of social justice.

SOME FINAL REMARKS

This essay is only an introduction to the issues within religion and bioethics. Other thinkers working out of the Christian tradition have made more radical claims about the nature of modern bioethics. Stanley Hauerwas of Duke University thinks of medicine as part of the Baconian project whereby humans pretend that they are gods and are in control of the universe. Medicine's power is hidden from us under the guise of its supposed neutrality and its scientific authority. Hauerwas's view is that medicine assists the "liberal project," which involves helping people put off death as long as possible. It is that liberal project that should be critiqued. Unfortunately, in Hauerwas's view, bioethics as it is currently constituted simply affirms that project.[15]

Gilbert Meilaender takes a different but every bit as radical a stance. Bioethics as it is practiced in the United States, according to Meilaender, has forgotten that human persons are beings with bodies. Modern bioethics is the latest form of dualism in Western thought, drawing, as it does, such a clear distinction between being a person and having a body. Meilaender claims that bioethics has in fact become "angelic ethics" and needs to return to the concept of person that is rich enough to include the histories of persons as we know them, from fetus to old age.[16]

There are other critiques of bioethics that arise out of religious perspectives, as well as celebrations of bioethics that arise out of religious perspectives. What is needed now is some attention to these critiques and celebrations. Without that attention, the bioethics community will continue to be entirely too self-referential and will fail to take seriously perspectives that offer fundamental challenges to it. Ironically, that is what some in that community might have said about historic religious communities. Often, in fact, that observation is on target when speaking about religious communities. It is becoming more and more true of the bioethics community as well.

NOTES

1. P. Ramsey, *The Patient as Person: Explorations in Medical Ethics* (New Haven, Conn.: Yale University Press, 1970).

2. R. Veatch, *A Theory of Medical Ethics* (New York: Basic Books, 1991).

3. J. Teno et al., "Do Formal Advance Directives Affect Resuscitation Decisions and the Use of Resources for Seriously Ill Patients?" *The Journal of Clinical Ethics* 5, no. 1 (Spring 1994): 23-30.

4. S. Benetar, "Just Healthcare Beyond Individualism: Challenges for North American Bioethics," *Cambridge Quarterly of Healthcare Ethics* 6, no. 4 (1997): 397-415.

5. R. Bellah et al., *Habits of the Heart: Individualism and Commitment in American Life* (Berkeley, Calif.: University of Californian Press, 1985).

6. J. Levenson, "Covenant and Consent: Biblical Reflections on the United States Constitution," *Harvard Divinity Bulletin* 3, no. 3 (1995): 1-4.

7. S. Hauerwas, *Wilderness Wanderings* (Boulder, Colo.: Westview Press, 1997).

8. J. Milbank, *Theology and Social Theory* (Oxford, England: Basil Blackwell, 1990).

9. Ibid.

10. S.E. Lammers, "The Marginalization of Religious Voice in Bioethics," in *Religion and Bioethics: Looking Backward, Looking Forward*, ed. A. Verhey (Grand Rapids, Mich.: William B. Eerdmans, 1996), 19-43.

11. N. Lash, *The Beginning and End of Religion* (Cambridge, Mass.: Cambridge University Press, 1996), 183-98.

12. A. Lustig, "Reform and Rationing: Reflections on Health Care in Light of Catholic Social Teaching," in *Secular Bioethics in Theological Perspective*, ed. E. Shelp (Dordrecht, The Netherlands: Kluwer, 1996), 31-50.

13. D. Fox, "America's Ecumenical Health Policy: A Century of Consensus," *Mt. Sinai Medical Journal* 64, no. 2 (1997): 72-4.

14. S. Miles, "Is Bioethics One of Kitty Genovese's Neighbors?" *Bioethics Examiner* 1, no. 2 (1997): 1-2.

15. S. Hauerwas, *Suffering Presence* (Notre Dame, Ind.: University of Notre Dame Press, 1986).

16. G. Meilaender, *Body, Soul, and Bioethics* (Notre Dame, Ind.: University of Notre Dame Press, 1996).

9

Religions' "Bioethical Sensibility":
A Research Agenda

Ronald M. Green

INTRODUCTION

Religion plays a major role in forming people's attitudes toward questions of bioethics. Religious teachings about the body, about sexuality and reproduction, and about the meaning of illness and death shape peoples' and cultures' ethical views about biological matters.[1] Whether we are trying to understand the forces that mold an individual's or family's decisions or the considerations that influence social policy and legislation, we must take the religious factor into account.

But which features of religious traditions should draw our attention? For example, if we wish to understand the role that Roman Catholicism plays in shaping thinking or conduct in specific areas of bioethics, at what should we look? One candidate might be the formal moral teaching of the church hierarchy and recognized theologians and ethicists. These teachings, which include such matters as the prohibitions on contraception, abortion, and active euthanasia, form the curriculum of many books and courses on Catholic medical ethics. Other religious traditions have similar bodies of normative teaching that might qualify as the essential reference for those seeking to understand the tradition's bioethical stance. Contemporary commentators seeking to understand Jewish views on specific biomedical questions, for example, have frequently turned to Judaism's classical body of legal and ethical norms, the Talmud, and the subsequent tradition of rulings by rabbinic scholars based on talmudic sources.

One problem with this approach is that the formal normative teachings discussed under headings such as "Catholic medical ethics," "Jewish bioethics," or "Hindu bioethics" often have little connection with the actual beliefs and practices of millions of people who call themselves Catholic, Jewish, or Hindu.[2] Despite explicit condemnations of abortion in classical Hindu and Buddhist texts, adherents of these religions resort to abortion at rates as high as or higher than members of other, less prohibitory traditions. Formal Jewish teaching contains some of the sternest edicts against any kind of active euthanasia or cessation of aggressive care at the end of life. Yet there is evidence that individuals of Jewish background are among the most accepting of any religious group of measures aimed at hastening the death of terminally ill people.[3]

Of course, we can conclude from these discrepancies that many religious adherents simply ignore the bioethical teachings of their tradition. This would suggest that religions actually play relatively little role in shaping people's thinking in this area, and it might draw our attention to other factors—class, education, or nonreligious cultural considerations—that are more decisive. But this conclusion would be premature. Religious traditions are important influences on people's bioethical attitudes and practices. The very fact that Jews have a *more* permissive attitude than other religious groups regarding euthanasia suggests that something in their shared religious background other than their faith's formal normative teachings may be contributing to their thinking. Is there, then, something within religious cultures that influences people's thinking about basic questions of biology and ethics but that is independent of and sometimes dissonant with the heritage of formal moral instruction?

I believe there is. For want of a better word, I will call it a tradition's "bioethical sensibility"—the pattern of religiously informed beliefs, attitudes, and valuations that guide choice and conduct with respect to biologically related moral issues. A tradition's bioethical sensibility is formed by many things. The most basic theological and ethical teachings of the tradition are important. These include but are by no means limited to formal bioethical norms. Ritual practices play a role, providing models of conduct and signaling important values. A religious community's shared experiences also enter into the mix, especially decisive aspects of the community's economic, cultural, and social history. Thus, a tradition's bioethical sensibility is the outcome of a complex process in which the tradition's teachings, practices, and experiences interact to produce novel, and sometimes unexpected, attitudes and values that in turn influence bioethical decision making. How this process evolves and whether it has common features across religious traditions is a further question. For now it is important to note that this bioethical sensibility may be of greatest interest to those who wish to understand the religious contribution to thinking about specific ethical issues.

This essay focuses on the presence and importance of aspects of the differing bioethical sensibilities of four religious traditions: Judaism, Catholicism, Hinduism, and Buddhism. This account is by no means complete, either in terms of developing the full content and range of the bioethical sensibility of each tradition or in regard to its application to all matters of bioethical interest. Rather, it focuses selectively on how these traditions' bioethical sensibilities shape important aspects of decision making at the beginning and end of life. The goal is to show how complex aspects of a tradition's teachings and experience interweave to produce beliefs, attitudes, and values—a sensibility—with powerful normative implications.

JUDAISM

In recent years, scholars and rabbis rooted in classical Jewish thought have made available to a larger audience attractive volumes published in English meant to serve as compendia of "Jewish bioethics."[4] Most of these studies report a fairly uniform set of Judaic teachings with regard to decision making at the beginning and end of life. Starting with the principle of the nearly absolute sanctity of life, however poor its quality or brief its duration, these writers report a general opposition to the practice of abortion or infanticide. In the words of J. David Bleich, "Judaism teaches that human life is sacred from the moment of generation of genoplasm in the gonads until decomposition of the body after death."[5] This same principle is held to support Judaism's historic insistence on efforts to fight for the life of seriously ill persons as well as strong aversion to any hastening of death, whether in the form of mercy killing or cessation of aggressive treatments. Even fully voluntary efforts to end one's own life in order to put an end to mental or physical suffering are condemned. Suicide is regarded as a sin beyond repentance, earning those who commit it exclusion from burial in ritually hallowed ground.

This picture of the tradition's bioethical teachings is not entirely unchallenged. Scholars like David Feldman and others have pointed to a less prohibitory series of teachings with regard to reproductive issues.[6]

According to these teachings, abortion is actually required by talmudic authorities if a pregnancy threatens a woman's life or seriously risks her health. This position follows, in part, from the same emphasis on the sanctity of life that otherwise animates the tradition, in this case with the mother's life being given priority over that of the fetus. But even those who acknowledge this feature of Judaic teaching tend to be negative about abortion for lesser reasons.

Similar challenges are also offered to the stern view of Jewish teachings about decision making at the end of life. Some contemporary students of Jewish bioethics note that there are motifs within traditional Jewish teaching moderating the view that unsparing efforts must be made to preserve life whatever its quality or duration.[7] They point, for example, to passages in the Talmud where prayers to hasten the death of a dying person are greeted with approval, and they ask whether cessation of pointless aggressive efforts is not consistent with some classical motifs emphasizing solicitous care of the dying. Yet even here, any kind of active termination of life, by self or others, is condemned, and a picture of formal Jewish teachings emerges that is as restrictive as can be found in any major world religion.

If these formal teachings dictate Jewish responses and attitudes toward these issues, how can we explain the fact that Jewish women all over the world have been among the most eager adopters of birth control? How can we explain the strong presence of Jewish individuals and groups in the cause of abortion rights or the willingness of Jewish women to undergo prenatal testing (and abortion) to avoid the birth of children with genetic disorders like Tay-Sachs disease?[8] And how can we explain the suggestive evidence that in more recent debates over physician-assisted suicide and various forms of active euthanasia (including neonatal euthanasia in the case of severe birth defects), individuals of Jewish background often champion the most permissive positions?[9]

Answering these questions forces us to think about the Jewish bioethical sensibility in these areas. One component of this sensibility is the "matricentric" focus of Jewish thinking about reproductive matters. Although Jewish norms about sexuality and reproduction were usually formed by male scholars, in arriving at decisions these teachers acknowledged the centrality of female interests in reproductive matters.[10] Recognizing that conception, pregnancy, and birth most affect women's lives, the rabbis avoided unilaterally imposing hardships on women and allowed them to refrain from reproduction—using various methods, sometimes including abortion—whenever a pregnancy proved unduly burdensome.

A second important component in forming the Jewish bioethical sensibility in this area is the tradition's reserved attitude toward prenatal life. By and large, Jewish teaching does not support a notion of souls that we are obligated to bring into being, and nothing within the Jewish tradition led to a sentimentalization of the fetus.[11] The rabbis appear to have viewed pregnancy and birth as a developmental process in both spiritual and physical terms. Before 40 days of development, the fetus was characterized as "like water." Later in pregnancy, it was uniformly regarded in Jewish law and less formal ethical teachings as "a limb or part of the mother."[12] Finally, on the assumption that any newborn might be premature or not viable, the rabbis withheld full ritual recognition of a birth (including full mourning rites) until the child had survived for at least 30 days.

This matricentric focus and reserved moral attitude toward nascent life are deeply rooted in the Jewish tradition. They have shaped (and continue to shape) Jewish thinking about reproductive matters. They certainly account for the alacrity with which Jewish women adopted female contraceptive methods such as the diaphragm. (Earlier in this century thousands of immigrant Jewish women in New York City, most of whom who were still deeply rooted in their Orthodox heritage, were among the staunchest supporters of Margaret Sanger's pioneering birth control movement.) They help to explain why Jews have been so quick to accept prenatal genetic testing. And they may explain the relative tolerance in this tradition for at least passive euthanasia in cases of infants born with severe birth defects.[13]

The willingness of many Jews to expedite dying, in direct contravention of formal moral teachings about the preservation and sanctity of life, summons up another feature of the Jewish bioethical sensibility: the tradition's aversion to suffering in any form. It may seem unremarkable that people should be opposed to suffering, but anyone familiar with religious traditions knows that they are often theologically compelled to place a positive value on suffering. For example, monotheistic traditions committed to the belief that God rules all of creation must find a place for suffering in God's purpose, and this can lead to a host of theodicies converting suffering from a negative into something that human beings must appreciate and welcome.[14] Judaism itself was not entirely immune to this impulse.[15] Nevertheless, Judaism's emphasis on the goodness and

sanctity of life; its lack of an ascetic tradition; and the paucity of historical, theological, or ritual elements validating suffering as something intrinsically good led Jews consistently to avoid suffering and to validate
efforts to minimize it. Foremost among these was the early and ready
acceptance by Jews of the medical arts themselves.[16]

Historically, the Jewish aversion to suffering, the insistence on unsparing efforts to save a life, and the strong formal condemnations of any
form of euthanasia (active or passive) were relatively consistent. Because
of the limited efficacy of most medical interventions, efforts to prevent
death could be urged without incurring the penalty of extended and tor-
mented dying, and the relative briefness of the dying process ensured
that suffering would soon come to an end. Interestingly, it was in cases
where this harmony of values did not exist—where dying was certain,
extended, and painful—that one encounters talmudic suggestions that
more decisive steps are permissible, including the cessation of life-sus-
taining prayers. In the modern period, medical advances have sometimes
driven apart the commitment to preserve life and prevent suffering. In
view of the importance that Jewish bioethical sensibility gives to the
latter value, it should come as no surprise that individuals influenced by
Jewish culture find themselves attracted to more dramatic interventions
to end suffering for terminally ill individuals. Once again, it is the deeper
Jewish sensibility that explains conduct and attitudes in ways very different from the formal ethical teachings themselves.

One can find aspects of the Jewish position, including the reserved
attitude toward prenatal life and some degree of matricentric thinking,
in other religious traditions, especially Islam.[17] Identifying these features
of a religion's bioethical sensibility may help us understand important
similarities and differences among traditions' evolving responses to contemporary issues and problems.

ROMAN CATHOLICISM

If Judaism exhibits a series of tensions between aspects of its formal
normative teaching and deeper components of its bioethical sensibility,
in the case of Roman Catholicism the dominant motif is one of mutual
reinforcement by these two aspects of the tradition. This phenomenon
may help explain the continuing force of many Roman Catholic teachings in these areas both in the lives of individual believers and in the
larger culture.

Where life's beginning is concerned, the Roman Catholic sensibility is characterized by features very different from those noted in Judaism. There is little evidence in Catholic thinking of a matricentric focus; women's experience and needs play relatively little role in shaping the norms governing sexuality and reproduction. This aspect of Catholic thinking, which may be a consequence of the powerful and long-standing teaching role of a celibate religious leadership, illustrates the importance of the interaction between doctrine and historical experience in shaping a tradition's bioethical sensibility.

For prenatal life, Catholicism replaces the reservation we noted in the Jewish case with intense valuation. From conception onward, the embryo or fetus is placed on a moral par with adult human beings or children. Interestingly, this is less a consequence of formal teaching, which over the centuries has varied in its understanding of the process of moral personhood and ensoulment,[18] than of other formative considerations. The New Testament, with its poetic suggestion of John the Baptists's prenatal personality (Luke 1:41), plays a role. Also very important is the centuries-long battle against pagan sexual and reproductive practices, in the course of which the distinctiveness of the Church's teaching on abortion became one hallmark of Christian identity. Together, these and other factors shaped what John Noonan has described as the "almost absolute value" placed by this tradition on the protection of prenatal life.[19] Although this value was not frequently invoked before the modern period, the widespread modern resort to abortion made possible by safe abortion procedures has thrust this issue to the top of the Church's teaching agenda. True, many individual Catholics ignore these teachings, a consequence perhaps of a developing tradition of selective disobedience of formal norms and greater reliance on individual decision making instead of authoritative instruction. How and why individual Catholics arrive at this position alert us to other features of the Catholic bioethical sensibility, including a long tradition emphasizing the importance of individual rational conscience as the final arbiter of moral norms. Nevertheless, the power of the Catholic sensibility in this area continues to be evident in the strength of Catholic intervention in reproductive politics around the world, and in the significant degree of support these restrictive efforts continue to find among the Catholic laity even when individuals do not apply these teachings to their own lives.

Another major component of the Catholic bioethical sensibility links Catholic attitudes regarding the beginning and the end of life. This is the (relatively) welcoming attitude toward suffering. If Judaism is antisuffering at its core, Catholic Christianity may be called "philo-suffering." Here, the central theological and ritual image of Christ is informative—his presence among the suffering and his own career marked by rejection, persecution, and death. Paradoxically, in the course of Catholic history, this important Christian motif led to a positive attitude toward the medical arts that is very similar to that noted in Judaism. Both traditions value medical care. Yet each tradition comes to this common point from a different direction, and each approach shapes the resulting sense of what is most valuable in medicine. In Judaism, it is the aversion to suffering and the sanctity of life that underlie these commitments; in Catholic Christianity, what is important is the presence of Christians *with* those who suffer, the living of a cruciform life, and the imitation of Christ's own compassion. Hence, while Christian medical efforts were always most evidenced by the development of specialized religious orders dedicated to succoring the infirm, in Judaism the healing skills of the physician (or rabbi/physician) were what were most admired. These differences in the path taken to a common point have some importance for other bioethical issues, as well.

To some extent, this emphasis on the positive value of suffering contributes to Catholic attitudes about decision making regarding prenatal life. In Catholic thinking, the prospect of severe genetic disease is not a reason for terminating a life once begun. Suffering is a part of human life to be welcomed and responded to with love and compassion, not merely effaced or eliminated. Remarkably, this basic attitude is carried over by many non-Catholic Christians for whom this feature of the Christian sensibility remains in force. Consider, for example, the following remark by Ronald Cole-Turner and Brent Waters, liberal Protestant theologians, whose recent work focuses on the moral implications of the Human Genome Project:

> Increased use of prenatal genetic testing seems to fit within a larger popular tendency to avoid pain at all costs. We seek not only pain-free dentistry but a pain-free life. We do not know nor do we want to learn how to make painful experiences part of the narrative of our lives. We shrink from these in the fear that they will infect our lives. Is prenatal genetic testing just another way to shrink from the pain of others, in this case by preventing them from living with us? If that is all that prenatal testing is, then it should be resisted as incompatible with the meaning of Christian life in the community of the cross. The aim of the Christian life is not the avoidance of pain but the

faithful following of One who enters into the pain of those who suffer.[20]

This sensibility contrasts dramatically with the Jewish one, for which the avoidance of suffering by morally and religiously permissible means is an expected feature of life. In the future, as our society debates the proper uses of genetic information in the context of prenatal testing, these differing sensibilities will probably play a role in social disagreements. Accustomed to regarding early prenatal life as of little moral weight and schooled in the minimization of human physical or mental distress, individuals of Jewish background will predictably favor the availability of prenatal testing for a variety of conditions such as mild mental retardation or later-onset genetic disorders. In contrast, many individuals of Christian background will feel uncomfortable with such broad uses of this technology and will question whether our society's resort to it indicates a growing intolerance of imperfection and disability. These debates, of course, will not be confined to Jews and Christians, nor will the lines in the debates be drawn in such religiously sharp ways. But the differing sensibilities pointed to here will nonetheless play a role.

One might think that the Catholic acceptance of suffering as an indwelling feature of the Christian life would lead to strong opposition to any form of euthanasia—active or passive, voluntary or involuntary. The cruciform shape of Christian life and the opposition to suicide[21] or murder militate against efforts to end suffering for those in a long or painful dying process. However, another important feature of the Catholic bioethical sensibility somewhat softens this conclusion. This is the deep sense that our terrestrial existence is only a preparation for eternal life. Very early in the history of Catholic teaching about medical matters, this belief led to the teaching that no one need pursue unduly burdensome medical efforts to save one's own life. Later formalized as the distinction between ordinary and extraordinary (or proportionate and disproportionate) means, this teaching has a continuing presence in Catholic medical institutions where it justifies the compassionate cessation of aggressive medical interventions for terminally ill patients. Here again, two traditions with very different bioethical sensibilities arrive at a similar place on the issue of ceasing treatment in such cases. Despite their formal teachings of the utter sanctity of life, Jews' aversion to suffering and their high valuation of existence free from suffering lead them to favor steps to end pain and anguish at life's end. Although Catholicism might be expected to validate such suffering, the sense that our mortal condition is transient and of lesser value than eternal life supports a similar willingness to withhold all means. Of course, in their formal teachings, both traditions remain opposed to any form of direct "mercy killing" (an opposition sharpened in the Jewish case by the Nazi transmutation of euthanasia policy into genocide). How these different strands of sensibility will shape Jews' and Catholics' future positions on physician-assisted suicide and active euthanasia remains uncertain, although these traditions' differing basic attitudes toward pain and suffering may drive a wedge between them.

HINDUISM AND BUDDHISM

On many specific questions of bioethics it would be misleading to treat Hinduism and Buddhism as a single tradition. There are important differences between them on such matters as sexuality, reproduction, and self-care of the body. However, for the issues of abortion and decision making at the end of life, these two traditions have a great deal in common, and the forces that shape their bioethical sensibilities are very similar.

Once again, we encounter a tension between the formal teachings of the traditions and a deeper bioethical sensibility. For example, there is no lack of Hindu or Buddhist condemnations of abortion or suicide. Hinduism's authoritative ancient legal tradition, including texts in the Dharma-Sūtra and Dharma-Śāstra traditions, as well as the biomedically normative Laws of Manu, repeatedly condemn abortion, placing it on a par with the grievous crimes of husband- or Brahmin-killing. As S. Cromwell Crawford notes: "The general picture that emerges from this vast literature is that life begins at conception, [and that] feticide is a major sin."[22] The same is true of classical Buddhist texts, which condemn *brunahatiya*, "the killing of a fetus," as among the most serious of crimes.[23] One authority in the Hindu Dharma-Śāstra legal tradition states that a woman who commits suicide out of pride, love, fright, or anger is consigned to a fetid hell for 60,000 years. In Hinduism, suicides motivated by fear or despair are denied the Śrādda rituals for the deceased.[24] Buddhist rejections of suicide are common. The Buddha himself is said to have labeled as a murderer any monk who preaches suicide to avoid suffering.[25]

Underpinning these formal condemnations are two key doctrines shared by both faiths: *ahimsā* and *karma*. The doctrine of *ahimsā*, or radical noninjury, was made famous by Ghandi, but it reflects ancient traditions of respect for all forms of sentient life. In Buddhism it finds expression as the first of the five basic moral precepts. If the killing of a sentient animal for food departs from the highest Hindu or Buddhist ideals, how can the deliberate killing of a human fetus pass ethical muster? If violence in any form, including violence against oneself, is a sin, how can physician-assisted suicide or voluntary active euthanasia receive approval?

These conclusion are reinforced in several ways by the teaching of *karma*. Since killing is a grave sin, one who kills oneself or others incurs an uneliminable moral debt. Thus, the hope to escape illness or suffering through any form of self-killing is pointless, since it only increases one's karmic burden and suffering in future existences. The idea that each sentient creature has a karmic destiny to fulfill also militates against the premature termination of life through abortion or mercy killing of any sort. Within these traditions, abortion is seen as "thwarting the unfolding of the *karma* of both the unborn and [abortion's] perpetrators."[26] These ideas are frequently repeated in the context of formal prohibitions of these activities.

Nevertheless, despite their pointedness, these formal teachings have far less impact than one might expect on the practices of individuals of Hindu or Buddhist background in India, China, or Japan. The prevalence of abortion in all these countries and the widely criticized practice of fetal sex selection in India and China reveals how allowable abortion is to many individuals in these cultures.[27] Although physician-assisted suicide and euthanasia and are less discussed, there is an openness to these practices among some contemporary students of Hinduism or Buddhism that is unexpected given the formal prohibitions.[28] How can we account for this difference between formal teachings and prevalent attitudes?

Once again, features of the traditions' shared bioethical sensibility provide some explanation. Where decision making regarding prenatal life is concerned, a major factor is the sense of fluidity and formlessness that characterizes life in its earliest stages. This is particularly true for Buddhism, whose concept of life's impermanence and continual becoming is applicable here. But the idea applies as well to Hinduism where each new conception and birth is seen as part of a continuing cycle of transmigration through different physical states of being, and where the lines distinguishing ontological orders of being are not as firm as in Western religions. For both traditions, therefore, the cessation of life at the fetal stage is perceived as far less fateful than it might be in those traditions where an individual has but one terrestrial existence to accomplish religious salvation. William LaFleur describes how this sense of the fluidity of life at its beginnings shapes Japanese popular attitudes toward abortion. In Japanese Buddhist culture, there is widespread belief that the stillborn or aborted child assumes the identity of a *mizuko,* a spiritual being belonging to a realm apart from our world. According to LaFleur:

As a piece of language [the term *mizuko*] connotes something approachable and comfort-bringing rather than awful and frightening. The child who has become a mizuko has gone quickly from the warm waters of the womb to another state of liquidity. Life that has remained liquid has never become solidified. The term suggests that a newborn, something just in the process of taking on "form," can also quickly revert to a relatively formless state. In that sense the term tells of a death. But it simultaneously appeals to the *fons et origo* function of the waters and the sea; it suggests with great power that the child or fetus in question will come to life again.[29]

Anyone schooled in Buddhist or Hindu cosmology, where the world itself is regarded as emerging from water and returning to water in each of the endless cosmic cycles, will appreciate what LaFleur is trying to say here about the Japanese Buddhist attitude toward fetal life and its relation to the eternal processes of becoming. Within this cosmological framework, abortion is perceived as involving not so much the termination of a life as its postponement or redirection.

Despite the outward similarities, it would be misleading to confuse the sense of fluidity of nascent life in these traditions with the Jewish (or Muslim) concept that before a fixed stage of development the embryo is merely "water." In Jewish thinking, the formlessness of the fetus means that it is not yet a moral personality; it has not yet crossed over the divinely established line that separates the human from the nonhuman. As LaFleur makes clear, however, the Japanese Buddhist concept of life's liquidity is not so much a judgment about the moral status of the embryo or fetus, as a global perception of the impermanence and "becomingness" of life itself. In the *mizuko* tradition, the fetus is acknowledged to be a moral person, but its fluid position in the sequence of becoming and its ability to return to an earlier stage in the process makes the act of killing it less definitive and wrongful.[30] This subtle difference between religious sensibilities becomes important when one looks at the matter of decisions at life's end.

The cosmological sense of the cyclical nature, the fluidity, and (especially in the Buddhist case) the impermanence of existence dramatically shape the Hindu and Buddhist sensibility where suicide is concerned. In both traditions, bodily existence is a snare, and one's ultimate religious goal is liberation (*mokṣa, nirvana*) from the perpetual cycle of karmicly determined phenomenal existence (*saṃsāra*). To foster this goal, control of one's mental state and the maintenance of consciousness at the moment of death are important.[31] In Hinduism, this impulse contributed to development of a hermetic tradition of retreat from the world; it was acceptable for a forest-dwelling ascetic, facing the debility of old age or serious illness, to undertake the "Great Journey" (*mahāprasthānagamana*) by throwing himself into water or starving himself to death.[32] Buddhism, too, made an exception to its usual opposition to suicide for those who were motivated, not by ignorance or fear, but by a quest for liberation from *saṃsāra*. Indeed, several stories within classical Buddhist sources evidence an attitude of acceptance directed at accomplished monks who kill themselves with swords to escape pain, illness, or debility.[33] In Jainism, a similar set of ideals and beliefs underlies the practice of death by fasting (*sallekhanā*). In all these traditions, the deepest sensibility is that our condition as the bearer of liberation must ultimately prevail over empirical existence. Life in the narrow sense must not be allowed to stand in the way of Life in a larger, spiritual sense.[34]

It is uncertain what the implications of this very complex sensibility might be for contemporary policy formation and individual or familial approaches to decisions at the end of life. Some spokespersons for Hindu thought have come out forcefully against any form of active euthanasia or physician-assisted suicide.[35] Although cessation of aggressive treatments by caregivers might be allowed, no active steps against self or another are viewed as consistent with the teachings of *ahiṃsā* and *karma*. However, there are statements attributable to Gandhi that justify even active voluntary euthanasia for consenting individuals near death and active nonvoluntary euthanasia for individuals (such as terminally ill children) in great suffering who are unable to give consent.[36] In view of the established traditions of expediting death by means of fasting, one might expect the withdrawal of food and fluids to appeal to people of Hindu and Buddhist background.

CONCLUSION

The preceding discussion illustrates the importance of taking a religious tradition's bioethical sensibility into account as we try to understand responses to contemporary issues and choices by those belonging to the tradition. An approach that focuses only on formal normative teaching but that misses this deeper sensibility often fails to predict real attitudes and behaviors.

As noted earlier, a bioethical sensibility is a set of beliefs, attitudes, and values that results from the complex interaction between a tradition's theology (including its cosmology and eschatology), its gamut of ethical teachings, its ritual practices, and the historical experiences of the community. Some of the main questions that a faith's bioethical sensibility answers include the following:

- What is the meaning of suffering in the context of human life and cosmic reality?
- How should we regard the physical body and its functions?
- What is the meaning and role of gender differences, sexuality, and reproduction?
- How are we to understand and respond to birth, aging, and death?
- What constitutes the self, and how is selfhood to be assessed?
- How are sin and moral culpability understood? What makes something sinful and how is sin relieved or absolved?
- What are the tradition's specific bioethical teachings? How authoritative are they, and who is regarded as their proper interpreter?

Other questions like these remain to be identified and asked with respect to religious traditions if we are to understand their respective bioethical sensibilities. Once those questions are asked and answered, the more complex task remains of seeing how these sensibilities actually affect bioethical thinking and choice. This involves the further comparative enterprise of seeing how similar and different components of religious sensibilities contribute to concrete patterns of conduct. For example, Catholicism, Hinduism, and Buddhism share a view (which is far less present in Judaism) that terrestrial existence should be subordinated to the goal of transcendent salvation. This agreement at the level of sensibility appears to produce similar views about some bioethical issues (passive euthanasia) but not others (abortion and active euthanasia). How, then, do various components of a sensibility interact to produce these diverse results? The concept of a religion's bioethical sensibility thus suggests a research agenda. We must be able to better identify and understand those aspects of a religious culture that really shape adherents' thinking and choices.

Throughout the world, formal religious teachings about bioethical issues may not play as much of a role as they once did (although we should never underestimate the impact of formal teachings by religious authorities on private choice or social policy).[37] But religious bioethical sensibilities live on, often shaping adherents' responses to complex new issues of biomedical choice. The sudden eruption of a great deal of religiously shaped opinion on the issue of cloning provides an example. Facing a novel and disturbing issue, even relatively secular people took positions that tended to reflect their background religious tradition's deeper bioethical sensibility.[38] In the future, attention to these bioethical sensibilities is one important contribution that religious ethicists can make to bioethics.

NOTES

1. D.S. Davis, "Introduction to a Review of *The Encyclopedia of Bioethics*," *Religious Studies Review* 22, no. 4 (October 1996): 280.

2. This point is forcefully made by Davis. Ibid.

3. P. Baume, E. O'Malley, and A. Bauman, "Professed Religious Affiliation and the Practice of Euthanasia," *Journal of Medical Ethics* 21 (1995): 49-54.

4. I. Jakobovits, *Jewish Medical Ethics*, rev. ed. (New York: Bloch, 1975); F. Rosner and J.D. Bleich, ed., *Jewish Bioethics* (New York: Sanhedrin, 1979); J.D. Bleich, *Judaism and Healing* (New York: Ktav, 1981).

5. J.D. Bleich, "Survey of Recent Halakhic Periodical Literature," *Tradition* 24, no. 4 (1989): 71.

6. D.M. Feldman, *Marital Relations, Birth Control and Abortion in Jewish Law* (New York: Schocken Books, 1974).

7. B. Brody, "Jewish Casuistry on Suicide and Euthanasia," in *Suicide and Euthanasia: Historical and Contemporary Themes*, ed. B. Brody (Dordrecht, The Netherlands: Kluwer, 1989), 39-75; R.M. Green, "Contemporary Jewish Bioethics: A Critical Assessment," in *Bioethics and Theology*, ed. Earl Shelp (Dordrecht, The Netherlands: D. Reidel, 1985), 245-66.

8. For a discussion of Jewish women's particular sensibilities in this area, see K.H. Rothenberg, "Breast Cancer, the Genetic 'Quick Fix,' and the Jewish Community: Ethics, Legal, and Social Challenges, " *Health Matrix* 7, no. 1 (1997): 98-125.

9. See note 3 above; A.I. Edelman, "Care of Critically Ill Newborns: The Israeli Experience," *Journal of Legal Medicine* 16 (1995): 247-61.

10. D.M. Feldman, "Abortion: Religious Traditions: Jewish Perspectives," *Encyclopedia of Bioethics*, 2nd ed. (New York: Macmillan, 1996), 1: 26-9; D.S. Davis, "Beyond Rabbi Hiyya's Wife: Women's Voices in Jewish Bioethics," *Second Opinion* 16 (1991): 10-31.

11. In the Babylonian Talmud, Tractate *Eruvin* 13, a formal debate among the rabbis on the question of whether it is better for human beings to have been created than not to have been created ends with the conclusion that it would be better for human beings if they had never been created.

12. See note 6 above, pp. 271-5.

13. Edelman, "Care of Critically Ill Newborns," see note 9 above, pp. 247-61.

14. R.M. Green, "Theodicy," *The Encyclopedia of Religion* (New York: Macmillan, 1987), 14: 430-41.

15. There are motifs in some later Hasidic sources that do not merely try to comprehend suffering but see it as a goal of the religious life. However these motifs are late and relatively anomalous within the Jewish tradition. See J. Dan, *Jewish Mysticism and Jewish Ethics* (Seattle, Wash.: University of Washington Press, 1986), 61.

16. Jakobovits, *Jewish Medical Ethics*, see note 4 above, chap. 1.

17. Islam, too, appears to privilege women's experience in the reproductive area. Perhaps reflecting this sensibility, many Muslim women in Great Britain express keen interest in early prenatal diagnosis of genetic disease. See B. Modell, "Fetal Diagnosis in the First Trimester: Introduction and Historical Perspective," in *Chorionic Villus Sampling: Fetal Diagnosis of Genetic Disease in the First Trimester*, ed. B. Brambat (New York: Marcel Dekker, 1986), 14.

18. J.F. Donceel, "Immediate Animation and Delayed Hominization," *Theological Studies* 31 (1970): 76-105.

19. J.T. Noonan, "An Almost Absolute Value in History," in *The Morality of Abortion*, ed. J.T. Noonan (Cambridge, Mass.: Harvard University Press, 1970), 1-59.

20. R. Cole-Turner and B. Waters, *Pastoral Genetics Theology and Care at the Beginning of Life* (Cleveland, Ohio: Pilgrim, 1996), 139.

21. St. Augustine, *The City of God*, trans. G.G. Walsh et al. (New York: Image Books, 1958), 52-7. In Dante's *Divine Comedy*, those who tried "to escape scorn by death" are found in the seventh circle of hell where "the foul Harpies make their nests." See *The Divine Comedy of Dante Aligheri*, trans. C.E. Norton, in *The Great Books of the Western World*, ed. R.M. Hutchins (Chicago: Encyclopedia Britannica, 1952), 21: 17-8.

22. S.C. Crawford, *Dilemmas of Life and Death: Hindu Ethics in the North American Context* (Albany, N.Y.: State University of New York Press, 1995), 25. See also J. Lipner, "The Classical Hindu View on Abortion and the Moral Status of the Unborn," in *Hindu Ethics*, ed. H.G. Coward, J. Lipner, and K.K. Young (Albany, N.Y.: State University of New York Press, 1993), 42-69.

23. S. Tachibana, *The Ethics of Buddhism* (London: Curzon Press, 1926), 81.

24. *Parāśara Samhitā* 4.1-6, in *The Dharma Shastra: Hindu Religious Codes*, trans. M.N. Dutta (New Delhi, India: Cosmo Publications, 1979), 3: 553, 554. For a review of these prohibitory teachings, see P.V. Kane, *A History of Dharma-Śāstra*, 2nd ed. (Poona, India: Bhandakar Oriental Institute, 1974), 2: 926.

25. L.D. La Vallée Poussin, "Suicide (Buddhist)," in *Encyclopedia of Religion and Ethics*, ed. J. Hastings (New York: Charles Scribner's Sons, 1922), 12: 24-6.

26. Lipner, "The Classical Hindu View on Abortion," see note 22 above, p. 57.

27. V. Patel, "Sex-Determination and Sex-Preselection Tests in India: Recent Techniques in Femicide," *Reproductive and Genetic Engineering* 2, no. 2 (1989): 111-9.

28. R.W. Perrett, "Buddhism, Euthanasia and the Sanctity of Life, *Journal*

of Medical Ethics 22 (1996): 309-13.

29. W.R. LaFleur, *Liquid Life: Abortion and Buddhism in Japan* (Princeton, N.J.: Princeton University Press, 1992), 24.

30. In Hinduism, where ideas about the destiny of the fetus similar to Buddhism's prevail, this may explain why, despite firm ideas of ensoulment at conception, abortion has not been regarded as negatively as it has in the Roman Catholic tradition. For an account of Hindu concepts of ensoulment, see Lipner, "The Classical Hindu View on Abortion," note 22 above.

31. K.K. Young, "Euthanasia: Traditional Hindu Views and the Contemporary Debate," in *Hindu Ethics*, ed. H.G. Coward, J. Lipner and K.K. Young, (Albany, N.Y.: State University of New York Press, 1993), 90.

32. Laws of Manu 6.32, in *Sacred Books of the East*, ed. F. Muller (New Delhi, India: Motilal Barnarsidass, 1984), 25: 204.

33. The *Samyutta* iii.123 reports the suicide in the Buddha's presence of the disciple Vakkali, who killed himself with a sword to put an end to a painful course of disease. The Kathā vattu i.2 reports a similar episode with another disciple, Godhika. For a discussion of these passages, Young, note 31 above, pp. 90, 104.

34. Crawford, *Dilemmas of Life and Death*, see note 22 above, p. 71.

35. K.K. Young, "Euthanasia: Traditional Hindu Views and the Contemporary Debate," *Hinduism Today* (August 1988): 108-10.

36. "Should my child be attacked with rabies and there was no helpful remedy to relieve his agony, I should consider it my duty to take his life. Fatalism has its limits. We leave things to Fate after exhausting all remedies. One of the remedies and the final one to relieve the agony of a tortured child is to take his life." M. Gandhi, *Young India 1919-1922* (New York: B.W. Huebsch, 1923), 395.

37. The work of the National Institutes of Health's Human Embryo Research Panel, on which I served in 1994, was profoundly affected by the opposition of a coalition of Evangelical and Roman Catholic groups opposed to federal funding of embryo research.

38. For example, the Jewish sources and testimony used in the report of the National Bioethics Advisory Commission's (NBAC's) report on cloning are more open to the possible reproductive and medical uses of cloning than are most of the Protestant or Catholic sources. See *Cloning Human Beings: Report and Recommendations of the National Bioethics Advisory Commission* (Rockville, Md.: NBAC, June 1997), chap. 2. This report is available on NBAC's website: < http://bieothics.gov/pubs/cloning1/cloning.pdf >.

10

Religious Ethics, Bioethics, and Public Policy: Cost or Contribution?

Michael M. Mendiola

INTRODUCTION

The role and function of religious ethics within the field of bioethics—what its distinctive perspectives and approaches might be—has received considerable scholarly attention in the recent past.[1] This essay adds another voice to those who argue that religious ethics has something distinctive to contribute to bioethics. Although religious ethics is often perceived as most (or only) relevant to clinical decision making at the bedside, it may offer some of its most important contributions to bioethical considerations of public policy.

At the bedside, the religiously trained bioethicist may be very helpful in interpreting ethical quandaries and issues to patients, families, and staff in a manner that is faithful to the patient, family member, or staff member's religious tradition.[2] Classic examples of such usefulness readily come to mind—the Jehovah's Witness and the use of blood products or the Roman Catholic and extraordinary medical care. Thus the relevance and helpfulness of religious ethics at the bedside, while in a sense limited,[3] is nonetheless real.[4] It is, however, at the level of public policy that religious ethics is often perceived as most problematic and, hence, least relevant.

CONCERNS ABOUT THE ROLE OF
RELIGIOUS ETHICS IN PUBLIC POLICY

Kathryn Tanner offers a helpful characterization of this perceived problem in her consideration of "public theology"—that is, theological efforts to "draw out the implications of Christian symbols and doctrines for issues of general socio-economic and political moment."[5] *Public*, as Tanner uses the term, refers to "a specifically discursive space of interchange in civil society, one that is in principle open to all citizens and that occurs whenever and wherever matters of common concern come up for general discussion."[6] Thus, public theology would include the attempt to bring religious ethics to bear on matters of public policy.

However, such efforts toward a public theology give rise to three central worries or feared costs regarding the use of explicitly religious arguments in public. The first is a concern about fairness—a concern that substantive commitments shared by a specific religious group will be foisted unfairly upon those who do not share these commitments. The second objection is that religious arguments in public will come at the expense of the kind of social solidarity required for well-ordered, cooperative activities such as public debate. The third is that religious arguments hamper constructive outcomes in public discussion, as all participants do not share the premises upon which religiously based recommendations regarding public matters are made. Thus, religious arguments seem futile and obstructive.[7] In short, the public sphere, as a realm of common, general concerns, seems to render religious argumentation and assessment—because it is *particularistic*—highly problematic, leading to unfairness, divisiveness, or futility. It is this perception that religious ethics is excessively problematic, and thus of little useful relevance for bioethically related public policy, that is challenged directly in this essay.

Even some religious ethicists writing in the field of bioethics show reticence about the role of religious ethics in relation to public policy. Essays by James M. Gustafson and Courtney S. Campbell provide illustrations.

Gustafson proposes four types of moral discourse, each of which lifts up a different range of morally relevant considerations, evident in the wide scope of medical moral literature: ethical, prophetic, narrative, and policy discourse. *Ethical discourse*, drawing on the kinds of concepts, distinctions, and modes of argument developed in the disciplines of moral philosophy and theology, focuses on how one is to act in particular circumstances. *Prophetic discourse* is concerned with an often passionate critique, taking the form of either indictment or utopian revisioning of the macro-systemic levels that are the formative context of individual decisions. *Narrative discourse* seeks to remain close to human experience; much like parables in biblical literature, it seeks to illumine the narrative context—with its implicit ethos, virtues, and values—that shapes all discrete decisions. *Policy discourse* is shaped by a concern for the possible, focusing on the enabling and limiting conditions that ground human courses of action (such as what resources exist and how they can be organized).[8]

Gustafson suggests that an exclusive focus on any one form, to the exclusion of the others, leads to an impoverishment of moral reflection on medicine.[9] He sees each form as appropriate to "different 'moments' in medical morality."[10] The concern here is not to engage critically Gustafson's central argument or his typology,[11] but to question the absence of any sustained consideration of the function of religious ethics within the types. Religious ethics, *qua* religious, seems strangely muted in Gustafson's considerations, even though he is himself a theological ethicist.

In fairness, Gustafson does allude to religious perspectives: the emergence of ethical discourse from both moral philosophy and theology, the similarity of prophetic discourse to biblical parables, and the formative influence of religious ethics in the development of narrative ethics. However, he offers no sustained methodological consideration of the role or function of religious ethics within medical morality, even though he begins his essay with a series of questions about the scope of medical ethics and the boundaries of the various disciplines that contribute to it.[12] This lack is all the more glaring, however, considering that the ethical, the prophetic, and the narrative forms are to provide correctives to the policy form and vice versa.[13] Without a serious consideration of religious ethics *per se*, it is not clear that religious ethics has any role to play regarding ethics and public policy.[14]

Unlike Gustafson, Courtney S. Campbell addresses directly the matter of religious ethics and public policy. At heart, he challenges the impact of what he terms the "ideological tyranny of pluralism,"[15] which has led to the marginalization of religious reflections on bioethics in the public forum. He writes: "It is commonplace to hear or read arguments to the effect that it is inappropriate to appeal to religious convictions in a public forum because those convictions assume a substantive account of human flourishing that is not generally shared and in any event must not be 'imposed' on others. . . . [Such a view] entails that the moral price for freedom of religion is that in matters of public policy, including those pertaining to bioethics, religious perspectives will be on the outside 'looking in.' "[16] In other words, religious perspectives are effectively silenced in areas of public concern—a matter that Campbell considers a serious loss.

But Campbell also argues that there is a cost to the tyranny of pluralism for secular bioethics itself—a loss of moral substance. The appeal of secular bioethics has been its *generality* and hence its purported utility for bioethical reflection in fostering consensus across various traditions and communities of discourse.[17] However, Campbell suggests, this generality has been purchased at the price of moral substance. "Secular bioethics gives us a world with minimal moral meaning."[18] Such moral minimalism is suspect because, as a matter of fact, social consensus has not always been achieved on the basis of secular bioethics. For Campbell, the loss of meaning and substance as the moral price for public acceptance "begins to look like a vice."[19] As a corrective, Campbell argues for the inclusion of religious perspectives in bioethics in the public square—not to supplant secular bioethics but to supplement it.[20]

I agree wholeheartedly with Campbell's argument for the relevance of religious ethics for bioethical assessments of public policy. However, I challenge the manner in which Campbell frames his critique: a contrast between a content-full/substantive religious ethics and a content-minimal/general secular bioethics. It is on the basis of this contrast that he offers one of his major criticisms of secular bioethics—that it provides only minimal moral meaning. As argued below, philosophically based bioethical considerations of public policy are anything but minimalistic. They are replete with deep, substantive presuppositions that require articulation and assessment. Hence, the proper contrast is between a content-full/substantive religious ethics and a content-full/substantive philosophical or secular ethics. As Robert Veatch has argued regarding theories of justice, both theologians and philosophers draw on "faith statements" or deep presuppositions grounded in faith as starting points for their ethics. According to Veatch, "When philosophy pushes back far enough, it eventually reaches the point where reasons can no longer be given."[21] Thus, every philosopher "will have to acknowledge that, by assumption, by intuition, or by faith, he has certain starting points, which, by definition, cannot be defended with further reasons."[22] Thus, theologians and philosophers accept on faith certain assumptions or premises which lead some toward equality, others away from it.[23] As Veatch so well illustrates, both religious ethics and secular ethics proceed on the basis of substantive commitments, assumptions, and premises. Neither is content-minimal.

This matter is more than simply a needed conceptual clarification; it also has important implications for ethical considerations of public policy. Campbell seems to assume that secular bioethics can address issues of public policy in a neutral manner that can speak to anyone and everyone. Note the following statement: "I would affirm that the pluralistic parameters of our society are such that a public policy outcome ought to be articulated and justified on such grounds as persons with diverse and conflicting moral visions can agree on. This means that secular bioethics, in both its procedural methods and substantive norms, will play the dominant role in justifying moral conclusions."[24]

Now one can agree wholeheartedly with Campbell's first statement on the need for publicly accessible moral justifications, yet disagree wholeheartedly that it is the province of secular bioethics to provide them in a dominant fashion. Here Campbell undercuts his own argument. He seems to accept the very presupposition—that public policy discourse must take the form of a moral *Esperanto*[25]—that rendered religious ethics problematic to begin with. In the end, it seems that, even in Campbell's otherwise excellent essay, secular bioethics still rules the day in the realm of public policy.

THE POSITIVE CONTRIBUTIONS OF RELIGIOUS ETHICS TO PUBLIC POLICY

In sum, religious ethics is largely suspect in public policy discussions. Religious ethicists themselves have not addressed this complex issue with the comprehensiveness or clarity that it requires. This essay takes up that challenge directly, arguing that religious ethics does have a positive contribution to offer to bioethical considerations of public policy. It proposes three central ways in which religious ethics can so contribute, illustrating these contributions to a matter of pressing public policy—physician-aid-in-dying.[26]

IT INFLUENCES MORAL CONVICTIONS

First, religious beliefs and commitments have exercised historically and continue to exercise today a formative influence on moral convictions and viewpoints. As Ronald Thiemann notes: "Given the historic significance of religion in shaping our national political culture, the removal of religion from the 'public square' would seem to violate our most ancient traditions."[27] Margaret Pabst Battin reflects a similar approach in her consideration of suicide:

> It is Western, Christian-influenced attitudes toward suicide that have historically led to the development of modern psychological, sociological, and legal views of suicide; these now form the basis for the "scientific" and professional study and treatment of suicide throughout the world, even in culturally quite diverse areas. . . . In a secular society, this is often the approach taken: the argument that suicide is wrong because life is a gift from God, for instance, is often said to be unsound because there is no God. But to discard the religious arguments in this summary way is to ignore what is interesting and significant about them, and to fail to see why they remain so strongly influential in supporting prohibitions and in forming public attitudes about suicide.[28]

As both Thiemann and Battin suggest, religious convictions and their moral correlates are formative of and thus relevant to matters of public policy. Thiemann correctly asserts: "To inquire concerning the moral basis of public policy is inevitably to engage the question of the role of religion in public life."[29]

But attending to this formative context is more than simply a matter of historical or sociological interest or accuracy; it is also of *hermeneutical* significance. Particular principles and norms can only be understood and interpreted adequately when they are situated within the nexus of religious, philosophical, and empirical beliefs, affirmations, and judgments that gave rise to these principles and norms and that accordingly give them full intelligibility. Principles and norms, however, have a way of coming "unhinged" from this formative nexus and, so to speak, "taking on a life of their own." This point is best made by a brief illustration.

Consider, for example, the principle that has gained such ethical weight in contemporary bioethical reflection—the principle of respect for autonomy. This principle—or at least the range of the morally relevant issues it is meant to point to—was first formulated relative to bioethics by the National Commission for the Protection of Human Subjects of Biomedical and Behavioral Research. However, the commission designated this principle as "respect for persons."[30] Given that both religious and philosophical ethicists served on this commission, it is not implausible to suggest that a religious viewpoint lay behind and informed, in part, the articulation of this principle and its emphasis on persons. Basic Christian ethical affirmations, such as the dignity of the human person created as *imago dei*, readily come to mind as relevant background beliefs.

What is critical to note, however, is that what was first a principle of "respect for *persons*" has now come to be "respect for *autonomy*." One aspect of persons (albeit an important one), their autonomy, has been selected out and given priority over other relevant aspects of personhood—for example, the social-relational aspect so often affirmed in religious ethics.[31] In other words, this notion of autonomy has come unhinged from its origin in a much wider, more expansive notion of persons—not to the betterment of bioethics. A return to the grounding principle of respect for persons, thoroughly but not exclusively explored in religious ethics, might address some of the limits of the contemporary overemphasis on respect for autonomy and its oft-noted "trumping" tendencies. Again, the effort here is to illustrate the hermeneutical significance of efforts to exclude religious perspectives from public policy debate. Not to consider religious perspectives in ethical discussions of public policy is to run the risk of misusing or misinterpreting particular ethical principles and norms brought to bear on those discussions.

Courtney Campbell takes the argument one step further, arguing that the loss of religious perspectives in bioethics is of deep *ethical* import. He draws an analogy between the process and effect of secularization suggested by Max Weber in *The Protestant Ethic and the Spirit of Capitalism*[31] and the process and impact of secularization on bioethics. Weber argued that, although the Protestant work ethic survived, the theological context that gave it meaning did not. This triumph of secularism resulted in a loss of "personalism in our relations because personal self-interest has become the overriding 'spirit' of the work ethic."[33] We are trapped in an iron cage, "in which genuine human relations are no longer possible, and a social ethic of moral strangers prevails."[34] Under the influence of secularism, contemporary bioethics has embraced a similar ethics of individual self-interest and a morality of strangers in its emphasis on contract as the central model of relationship.[35] In contrast, Campbell draws on the religious model of covenant as a corrective to the contractual model, arguing that it offers "an ethic and a spirit of responsibility that transcends the individualism of contract on the one hand and the tyranny of Hippocratic paternalism on the other."[36]

Campbell illuminates what is at stake substantively in the loss of religious ethics in the public square of bioethics; it leads to a very particular—and in Campbell's opinion, truncated—construal of bioethics. But Campbell also illustrates the potential of religious ethics to exercise a critical role in relation to the dominant philosophical forms of bio-ethics. It is to this critical potential that the discussion now turns.

IT BRINGS A CRITICAL PERSPECTIVE
TO ETHICAL ANALYSIS

Religious ethics can also bring a needed critical dimension to the ethical assessment of public policy. It can do so specifically in reference to the worries about religion in public ethical discourse raised by Tanner above—unfairness, divisiveness, and futility.[37]

It is necessary for fairness to be the first casualty of religious ethic's participation in public policy assessment? Do religious views on how life should be lived inevitably lead to the unfair imposition of these views on those who do not share them? I argue that the inclusion of religious ethical perspectives need not lead to the feared unfairness. To be sure, religious believers, Christian and others, are sometimes guilty of per-petuating the grounds for the charge of unfairness. Religious believers, to the degree that they promote their own viewpoints as absolute truth—whether on the basis of biblical revelation or tradition—may indeed be a primary cause of the charge of unfairness brought against them. It is not the purpose of this discussion to deny or cover over such realities, but to challenge the logic of the worry—that is, that religious ethics alone is problematic because it leads of necessity to the imposition of substantive commitments on others.

The problem with this concern is that it seems to hold that there is some neutral sphere of discourse that is appropriate for public policy because it is free of such substantive commitments. If religious ethics is inappropriate because it imposes viewpoints on others, then, so the logic seems to go, there must be a form of ethical discourse that does not impose such viewpoints because it is devoid of them. Otherwise, ethical assessment of public policy would be an ethical impossibility, always unfair. In other words, fairness (as the nonimposition of substantive view-points not generally shared) seems to require a neutral sphere of ethical discourse and presuppose that it is achievable.

However, as Lisa Cahill cautions, we should not proceed on the as-sumption that "there exists some independent realm of secular or philo-sophical discourse, privileged as more reasonable, neutral, or objective, and less tradition-bound, than religious discourse."[38] Rather, "The pre-eminent and supposedly neutral vocabulary of public policy debates in the U.S. today (liberty, autonomy, rights, privacy, due process) itself comes out of a rather complex but distinct set of political, legal, philosophical, moral, and even religious *traditions*."[39] Even the supposedly neutral standard of liberty—that we each are free to pursue our own sense of how life should be lived—is hardly neutral or tradition-free. Such a standard only makes sense within a vision of life in which liberty is given primacy, as that which renders human life truly valuable.[40] As Allen Verhey has argued, the very language of freedom is not the universal moral language some think it to be; rather, it depends on particular accounts of the moral life for its meaning.[41] The point here is that, under the general notions of autonomy, liberty, and freedom, a substantive commitment—a view of how life should be lived—is imported into ethical reflection under the guise of neutrality toward such commitments. Such unclaimed and imported commitments raise a more serious problem of fairness than the charge raised against religious ethics. At the very least, religious ethics makes its substantive commitments clear and explicit.

Thus, to deny religious ethics a place in public policy discourse because of unfairness itself unfairly singles out religious ethics as alone guilty of imposing particularistic views of the good. All ethical assessment of public policy, whether religiously or philosophically based, involves a vision of the good life for human beings. Indeed, public policy as the realm of practical human concern must involve such. Thus, religious ethics is no more (and no less) guilty of unfairness in public policy debate than is philosophical or secular ethics. Both forms of ethical discourse involve substantive, and at times competing, visions of the human good. What is required in public policy discernment is the articulation, analysis, and comparison of these competing visions of the good; only in this way can we adequately assess and know what is at stake in matters of public policy.

In light of the analysis above, the second and third worries—divisiveness and futility—are more easily dealt with. Both turn on the presupposition that religious perspectives alone involve substantive beliefs and premises that are either in fact or in principle nonshareable, and conversely that secular/philosophical ethics can provide the needed neutral, common grounds. But neither religious nor philosophical ethics is devoid of substantive commitments. Both can contribute to consideration of public policy either in a positive and fruitful manner or in a divisive and futile way. As recent ethical and legal debates about matters of public policy such as healthcare reform and physician-aid-in-dying make patently clear, neither divisiveness nor futility arise from religious quarters alone. It has been under the influence of secular bioethics, and not religious ethics, that the failure to ensure adequate healthcare or to achieve a social consensus about physician-aid-in-dying in the United States have occurred.

To be sure, these worries raise a large and perduring challenge to the religious ethicist—how to remain faithful to the insights of one's religious tradition, while rendering those insights accessible to those who do not share them in public policy discussions.[42] But this challenge faces the philosopher as well relative to his or her own traditions. What is equally important is the character and quality of the discourse and the attitudes of the interlocutors in discussions of public policy. Cahill summarizes this point well.

> It follows that it is best to construe "public discourse" not as a separate *realm* into which we can and ought to enter tradition-free, but as embodying a *commitment* to civil exchanges among traditions, many of which have an overlapping membership, and which meet on the basis of common concerns. The language of "secular" and "publicly accessible" serves exactly to exhort persons from traditions to adopt a stance of dialogue and openness, of mutual critique, of commitment to consensus and to hammering out the institutions and policies that will affect the common life for "the better," as defined by the broadest consensus we can achieve.[43]

Thus, what is at stake in ethical assessment of public policy is not the achievement of a neutral universality, but rather "intelligibility and persuasiveness within a community of communities broad enough to encompass the society to be ordered."[44]

In sum, religious ethics can offer needed critique in the realm of public policy by countering the very arguments and concerns that seek to exclude it from the realm of public policy. But does it have anything positive or constructive to bring to ethical assessment of public policy? I argue that it does.

IT EMBRACES "RELATIONALITY" AND "INTERCONNECTEDNESS"

A comprehensive attempt to define the constructive contributions of religious ethics to public policy is far beyond the scope of this essay. Indeed, such an attempt would require a full exploration of primary religious themes within a given tradition, their general ethical implications and correlates, their implications relative to specific issues of public policy, and so forth. My efforts here are rather more modest. I seek only to illustrate my point briefly, indicating the lines of development such constructive efforts might take in relation to public policy.

Christian ethicist Beverly Harrison offers a helpful starting point through her reflections on "relationality." She proposes a central theological principle: "Everything in life is related to everything else."[45] Because our lives and actions are set within webs of historical processes and relationships, "an analysis is theological if, and only if, it unveils or envisions our lives as a concrete part of the interconnected web of all our social relations, including our relations to God."[46] Note carefully Harrison's point: theology is not "theological" simply by the fact of being "God-talk." It is only theological to the degree that it proceeds from an understanding of and affirms the interconnectedness of all things. This means that relationship to God cannot be conceived of or lived out in separation from our social relations with other people and with the world in which we live, and vice versa. We see here Harrison giving profound expression to a core theological affirmation of Christian faith—the unity of the love of God and neighbor.

Clearly such a theological position entails a normative dimension for Christian ethics. Moral actions must entail some concrete, other-directed engagement, some responsiveness to the neighbor in the concrete and full dimensions of human being. But it is also of epistemological importance for ethics. If, as Harrison asserts, everything is related to everything else, then moral discernment and our efforts to gain moral insight must proceed in a manner that acknowledges this relationality. Thus, ethical analysis must attend to the various dimensions of human being, activity, and agency in their connectedness. Karen Lebacqz, drawing on feminist thought, offers a central methodological principle very akin to Harrison's theological principle. *"The constant assertion of feminists over the last two decades has been that there are connections:* connections between what happens in one medical arena and in another, connections between what happens in medicine and what happens in sex roles in society at large, connections between the 'personal' experiences of women and the 'political' arenas of policy and social institutions."[47]

Thus, Christian ethics embraces the idea of the interconnectedness of human beings, human agency, and human activity, and the concomitant epistemological principle that flows from it—making the connections as an essential aspect of ethical reflection on public policy. Hence ethical analysis is not complete if it focuses *solely* on the individual, whether a person, a situation, or a case.[48] In addition, this approach provides a strong corrective to the heavy emphasis on the autonomy of the individual in contemporary bioethics. Albert Jonsen, although not writing explicitly from a Christian perspective, provides a helpful example of this approach in regard to physician-aid-in-dying.[49]

Physician-aid-in-dying is often framed and justified, in part, as a matter of respect for autonomy.[50] Such respect requires that human beings be free, within safeguarding limits, to determine the manner and timing of their own deaths, particularly in the face of great pain and suffering.[51] But Jonsen argues that much more is at stake than individual self-determination *simpliciter*. Advocates of physician-aid-in-dying, for example, often restrict its practice to a physician and a competent patient in the context of terminal illness or intractable pain. He notes:

> If qualifiers such as terminal condition or intractable pain are introduced, it may be asked why these empirical states are added to self-determination pure and simple. They seem to be limitations of freedom and, in the nature of things, call for assessment by someone other than the self-determining party who requests to be killed. Thus, if we say that intractable pain is a condition, a physician who is asked to kill a patient must make a professional judgment that pain is present and is indeed intractable. This appears to introduce another self-determining party who could veto the self-determining request of the patient. If so, we appear to have something more than a principle of self-determination as the basis of the paradigm.[52]

Thus, what is often touted as fundamentally a matter of respect for autonomy of the individual actually presumes a particular social and institutional context. Public policy proposals for physician-aid-in-dying presume and require at the very least a relationship between a physician and a patient, with all the historically and socially constructed expectations that inform that relationship. They also presume some societal concern to limit the practice; why otherwise would pain and suffering be posited as conditions of eligibility? Indeed, Jonsen suggests that what is intended in current public policy proposals regarding physician-aid-in-dying is a *social practice*.[53]

If we view physician-aid-in-dying as a practice—that is, if we begin to "make the connections," the social and institutional complexities become quickly evident.[54] Yet, the primary justification, respect for autonomy, oversimplifies the matter and deflects ethical analysis away from the level of social practice. Only by making the connections that the social practice of physician-aid-in-dying entails can we begin to assess the ethical sufficiency of respect for autonomy as a justification for physician-aid-in-dying as public policy and undertake a comprehensive ethical assessment of the practice itself. A Christian ethical approach, faithful to its primary theological affirmations and their normative and epistemological implications, can aid—indeed pushes for—just this kind of ethical analysis. It challenges us to make the connections.

CONCLUSION

Religious ethics can contribute positively toward and hence is relevant to bioethical considerations of public policy in a number of ways. First, religious ethics has exercised a formative influence upon our moral convictions, viewpoints, and ethics itself. To exclude it from bioethical assessment of public policy is to run the risk of misconstruing and distorting that ethical enterprise. Second, religious ethics can bring a needed critical perspective to bioethical considerations of public policy, by challenging the very arguments used to ban it from the public policy realm. Religious ethics offers a powerful corrective to any pretenses of achieving a neutral, content-minimal bioethics for public ethical discourse. Third, religious ethics can contribute constructively to bioethical analysis and reflection, as illustrated in this essay by examination of the maxim (theologically construed): "Make connections."

Underlying these arguments lies the conviction that religious ethics, like its philosophical-secular counterpart, is a repository of accumulated moral wisdom and insight. To be sure, the inclusion of religious ethics within ethical considerations of public policy raises many challenges. In the end, however, given the complex and pressing, bioethically related matters of public policy that we face as a society, we do not enjoy the luxury of bypassing moral wisdom and insight, wherever they may lie.

ACKNOWLEDGMENT

I wish to thank Karen Lebacqz for her invaluable assistance in the development and completion of this essay.

NOTES

1. Examples include S.E. Lammers and A. Verhey, ed., *On Moral Medicine: Theological Perspectives in Medical Ethics* (Grand Rapids, Mich.: William B. Eerdmans, 1987); A. Verhey, ed., *Religion and Medical Ethics: Looking Back, Looking Forward* (Grand Rapids, Mich.: William B. Eerdmans, 1996); P.F. Camenisch, ed., *Religious Methods and Resources in Bioethics* (Dordrecht, The Netherlands:

Kluwer, 1994); E.E. Shelp, ed., *Secular Bioethics in Theological Perspective* (Dordrecht, The Netherlands: Kluwer, 1996). The Parkridge Center in Chicago also publishes a most helpful series on health and medicine from the perspectives of various religious traditions. For example, see R.A. McCormick, *Health and Medicine in the Catholic Tradition* (New York: Crossroads, 1987).

2. K. Lebacqz, "Faith Dimensions in Medical Practice," *Primary Care: Clinics in Office Practice*, ed. M.S. Victoroff (Philadelphia: W.B. Saunders, 1986), 263-70. See also L.J. O'Connell, "The Role of Religion in Health-Related Decision Making for Elderly Patients," *Generations* 18, no. 4 (Winter 1994): 27-30.

3. The relevance of a particular religious perspective seems limited to situations in which the bioethicist shares a religious tradition with the patient, family, and/or staff—or at the very least is knowledgeable about the patient's, family's, or staff member's religious tradition. However, even when no shared tradition or knowledge exist, the religiously informed bioethicist is particularly sensitive to the religious dimensions of the patient, family, or staff member's ethical stance and viewpoint.

4. J.J. Fins, "Encountering Diversity: Medical Ethics and Pluralism," *Journal of Religion and Health* 33, no. 1 (Spring 1994): 23-7.

5. K. Tanner, "Public Theology and the Character of Public Debate," in *The Annual of the Society of Christian Ethics*, ed. H. Beckley (Chicago: Society of Christian Ethics, 1996), 79. Tanner draws the term *public theology* from the work of David Hollenbach.

6. Ibid., p. 80.

7. Ibid., pp. 81-2.

8. J.M. Gustafson, "Moral Discourse about Medicine: A Variety of Forms," *Journal of Medicine and Philosophy* 15, no. 2 (April 1990): 127-41.

9. Ibid., p. 127.

10. Ibid., p. 141.

11. However, a serious question can be raised in regard to Gustafson's construal of the "ethical." He seems to limit ethical discourse to an analysis of and moral justification for particular acts, in circumscribed circumstances, involving a limited number of agents (ibid., p. 129). However, from the perspective of social ethics, the "ethical" cannot be so narrowly construed. Ethics proper includes a consideration of the larger systemic contexts, which Gustafson denotes as prophetic and narrative, as well as a concern with the possible that he restricts to policy discourse. The realm of discourse he terms "ethical" might more adequately be termed "casuistic" (ibid., p. 127), thus freeing the category "ethical" from the overly narrow range of application to which Gustafson confines the term.

12. See note 8 above, pp. 125-6.

13. Ibid., p. 141.

14. In a more recent work, Gustafson has explored (more adequately in my judgment) the possible role of religious moral perceptions in science and medicine. He notes, for example, the role of "background beliefs," such as beliefs

about human nature, in shaping attitudes toward genetics. These beliefs influence not only theologians but also scientists. "The regulative idea of the nature of the human, a background belief not derived from science alone, is a critical factor not only for theologians but also for geneticists, as it affects their moral outlooks and judgments." See J.M. Gustafson, *Intersections: Science, Theology and Ethics* (Cleveland, Ohio: Pilgrim Press, 1996), 95. Thus, he proposes that scientists have "aesthetic appreciations and moral beliefs and assumptions" that are grounded only in part in science, and that function, in the eyes of a scholar of religion, "much like myths, doctrines, and practices of religion in various human cultures" (p. 96). Gustafson's analysis offers a helpful tool for a consideration of religious ethics and public policy. However, the analysis noted here only renders more curious the absence of any analogous consideration in his work on forms of moral discourse.

15. C.S. Campbell, "Bioethics and the Spirit of Secularism," *Secular Bioethics in Theological Perspective*, ed. E.E. Shelp (Dordrecht, The Netherlands: Kluwer, 1996), 5.

16. Ibid.

17. See M.M. Mendiola, "Bioethics and Impartial Rationality: The Search for Neutrality," in *Religious Methods and Resources in Bioethics*, ed. P.F. Camenisch (Dordrecht, The Netherlands: Kluwer, 1994), 147-64.

18. See note 15 above, p. 13.

19. Ibid.

20. Ibid., p. 15.

21. R.M. Veatch, *The Foundations of Justice: Why the Retarded and the Rest of Us Have Claims to Equality* (New York: Oxford University Press, 1986), 93.

22. Ibid.

23. Ibid., p. 95.

24. See note 15 above, p. 16.

25. J. Stout, *Ethics After Babel: The Languages of Morals and Their Discontents* (Boston: Beacon Press, 1988), 5.

26. The term *physician-aid-in-dying* is ambiguous in its current usage, denoting assisted suicide or active euthanasia or both. For purposes of this essay, I do not enter into the debate regarding what exactly the term should entail. Rather, I utilize physician-aid-in-dying as an illustration because it is a matter of public policy today.

27. R.F. Thiemann, *Religion in Public Life: A Dilemma for Democracy* (Washington, D.C.: Georgetown University Press, 1996), 3-4.

28. M.P. Battin, "Prohibition and Invitation: The Paradox of Religious Views about Suicide," in *The Least Worst Death: Essays in Bioethics on the End of Life* (New York: Oxford University Press, 1994), 205-6.

29. See note 27 above, p. 11.

30. National Commission for the Protection of Human Subjects of Biomedical and Behavioral Research, *The Belmont Report: Ethical Principles and Guidelines for the Protection of Human Subjects of Research* (Washington, D.C.:

U.S. Government Printing Office, 1978), 4-6. The commission did frame its considerations of this principle in terms of autonomy. This is understandable given its focus on issues such as voluntary participation in research. Nevertheless, it is significant that the principle was given expression under the wider rubric of "respect for persons."

31. M.M. Mendiola, "Overworked but Uncritically Tested: Human Dignity and the Aid-in-Dying Debate," in *Secular Bioethics in Theological Perspective*, ed. E.E. Shelp (Dordrecht, The Netherlands: Kluwer, 1996), 129-43. See also J.F. Childress, "The Place of Autonomy in Bioethics," *Hastings Center Report* 20, no. 1 (January-February 1990): 13.

32. M. Weber, *The Protestant Ethic and the Spirit of Capitalism*, trans. T. Parsons (New York: Charles Scribner's Sons, 1958).

33. See note 15 above, p. 10.

34. Ibid.

35. Ibid., p. 11.

36. Ibid., p. 12.

37. In her essay, Tanner also addresses strategic responses to these worries on the part of religious thinkers. However, given the limits of this essay, I cannot take up her full discussion here. Rather, I concentrate on my own critical response to these worries.

38. L.S. Cahill, "Can Theology Have a Role in 'Public' Bioethical Discourse?" *Hastings Center Report* 20, no. 4 (July-August 1990): 11.

39. Ibid.

40. See note 27 above, p. 79.

41. A.D. Verhey, "Luther's 'Freedom of a Christian' and a Patient's Autonomy," in *Bioethics and the Future of Medicine: A Christian Appraisal*, ed. J.F. Kilner et al. (Grand Rapids, Mich.: William B. Eerdmans, 1995), 84.

42. C.S. Campbell, "Religion and Moral Meaning in Bioethics," *Hastings Center Report* 20, no. 4 (July-August 1990): 5.

43. See note 38 above, p. 12.

44. Ibid., p. 13.

45. B.W. Harrison, "Theological Reflection in the Struggle for Liberation," in *Making the Connections*, ed. C.S. Robb (Boston: Beacon Press, 1985), 240.

46. Ibid., 245.

47. K. Lebacqz, "Feminism and Bioethics: An Overview," *Second Opinion* 17, no. 2 (October 1991): 19-20.

48. Here the weakness of Gustafson's proposal discussed in note 11 becomes very clear. His construal of the ethical is so restricted that it fails to include what I argue is central to good ethical reflection—making the connections to the wider arenas of moral concern indicated by the prophetic and narrative forms.

49. A.R. Jonsen, "Criteria That Make Intentional Killing Unjustified: Morally Unjustified Acts of Killing That Have Been Sometimes Declared Justified,"

in *Intending Death: The Ethics of Assisted Suicide and Euthanasia*, ed. T.L. Beauchamp (Upper Saddle River, N.J.: Prentice Hall 1996), 42-53.

50. Concern for human well-being generally and the relief of pain and suffering more specifically also are seen as justifying physician-aid-in-dying. However, even here, autonomy exerts its influence, for what is proposed is well-being and/or intractable pain and suffering *as defined by the individual*. See, for example, A. Buchanan, "Intending Death: The Structure of the Problem and Proposed Solutions," in *Intending Death: The Ethics of Assisted Suicide and Euthanasia*, ed. T.L. Beauchamp (Upper Saddle River, N.J.: Prentice Hall, 1996), 34-8.

51. See, for example, M. Angell, "The Supreme Court and Physician-Assisted Suicide—The Ultimate Right," *New England Journal of Medicine* 336, no. 1 (2 January 1997): 50.

52. See note 49 above, p. 51

53. Ibid. See also D. Callahan, " 'Aid-in-Dying': The Social Dimensions," *Commonweal* 68, no. 14 (9 August 1991): 476-80.

54. For a helpful overview of these social and institutional complexities, see E.W.D. Young et al., "Report of The Northern California Consensus Conference for Guidelines on Aid-in-Dying: Definitions, Differences, Convergences, Conclusions," *Western Journal of Medicine* 166, no. 6 (June 1997): 381-8.

11

Religious Studies in Bioethics:
No Room at the Table?

Karen Lebacqz

INTRODUCTION

What is the place of religious studies in bioethics? Using John Robertson's argument in *Children of Choice*,[1] I shall argue that those very commentators who are most inclined to shut out religious views are, in the end, dependent upon fundamental presuppositions that reflect deep value commitments. These commitments may not be explicitly and self-consciously derived from religious roots, but they function in a manner akin to faith convictions, they reflect underlying religious traditions that have shaped cultural practices, and they are as dependent on tradition as are religious statements of faith. In short, there is no way to keep religious convictions out of the public arena of policy making in bioethics, for religious convictions determine the very questions we ask and the assumptions that undergird our answers.

ROBERTSON'S VIEW OF THE ROLE OF
RELIGIOUS CONVICTIONS IN BIOETHICS

Lawyer-turned-philosopher John Robertson deliberately and explicitly reflects the liberal philosophical system on which contemporary American law is based. In *Children of Choice*, he mounts an argument regarding the development and use of new reproductive technologies such as in vitro fertilization, genetic screening, and cloning. His intention is to argue for the primacy of liberty as a determinative value in the development and use of new technologies.

Robertson argues that we have three "rights" associated with children: the right to have—or not to have—children; the right to choose the characteristics of our children; and the right to use any technologies that assist us in securing either of the first two rights. The right to have children derives from the centrality of bearing children to our sense of personal fulfillment and happiness. The right to choose the characteristics of our children derives from the fact that our decision about whether to have children at all may depend upon the characteristics that those children would have. The right of access to technologies also derives from the instrumental role of these technologies in fostering our right of procreative liberty. Thus, for example, Robertson argues for a right of access to abortion, in vitro fertilization, and genetic testing—all of which may determine whether we are able to secure our right to have (or not to have) children.

These rights are not absolute; they can be overridden. However, because the right to have children is understood to be a fundamental right, only a "substantial harm" to the "tangible interests" of another can trump one's procreative rights. Robertson dismisses objections to abortion, in vitro fertilization, and other procreative practices if they appear to derive from "symbolic" concerns such as what constitutes proper reproduction.[2] Noting that in a pluralistic society there will be differences of opinion about such matters, Robertson explicitly eschews the use of such concerns as a base for public policy on reproductive technologies.

This argument would appear to rule out of court religious concerns that derive from explicit faith convictions. For example, Christian ethicist Gilbert Meilaender argues against in vitro fertilization on grounds that have large "symbolic" elements.[3] Meilaender argues that procreation should occur only within marriage. Additionally, he suggests that love making and baby making should not be separated—that there is something important in our physical embodiment and its procreative possibilities such that to sunder making love from creating new life is to violate something about what it means to be human. Thus, for Meilaender, children are "begotten," not made, and procreation needs to be seen not merely as a right, but as the "internal fruition of the act of love."[4]

Although Meilaender invokes religious language sparingly, he draws the crux of his argument from H. Richard Niebuhr's threefold typology of "man the maker," "man the citizen," and "man the answerer."[5] What makes us human, argues Meilaender, is not simply what we can do or make, but how we live our lives together as citizens and whether our actions are "fitting" to (or "answer") the circumstances. Thus, there are constraints beyond our freedom to choose to do or not do something. For those who know Niebuhr's work, the presence of God in such a claim is very clear, for "man the answerer" is first and foremost answering to what God has already done and is doing in the situation.

It is precisely these kinds of religiously based arguments, often compelling only to those who adhere to specific faith traditions, that Robertson claims cannot be taken as a base for public decision making in bioethics. Meilaender's symbolic concern for proper procreation would not be shared by society as a whole, as the widescale acceptance of in vitro fertilization makes clear. Nor would Meilaender's restriction of childbearing to those who are duly married be acceptable to all. For Robertson, where there is contested ground about such practices, we do not have a firm enough foundation to limit procreative liberty. Only where there is general societal consensus, clearly embedded in common practices and possibly articulated in law, are there grounds for limiting procreative freedom. For example, Robertson notes that some people would find paid surrogacy offensive, but others would not. Where there are such "splits in perception," he argues, "symbolic concerns alone should not override the couple's interest in having and rearing biologic offspring."[6]

It appears, then, that religious views are relegated by Robertson to the arena of "private" decisions. They may still be compelling for individuals and couples making their own choices, but they are not allowed to enter into or to taint the public arena. Thus, the role of religious studies in bioethics would appear to be minimal at best—perhaps allowing the trained ethicist to be sympathetic to members of religious groups and their symbolic concerns when it comes to their private decisions,[7] but not allowing religious considerations to determine the direction of public policy. At the table of public policy, there is no room for religious ethics.

This, in very brief summary, is Robertson's argument for procreative rights and against the intrusion of symbolic concerns. But does it hold? Is Robertson's presumably secular argument less infused with symbolic dimensions than is Meilaender's religious argument? Can Robertson's own argument for rights be mounted without any reference to symbolic concerns and religious backing? Can religious concerns be neatly relegated to a private arena and shut out of the public? Can they be written off as "symbolic perceptions that do not justify infringing core procreative interests"?[8]

It would be a tall order to develop fully an answer to any of these questions. A sketch of possible answers is all that space permits here, but perhaps that sketch will suffice to demonstrate that religious bioethics is a necessary participant at any public policy table where honest conversation is intended.

THE SYMBOLIC DIMENSIONS IN ROBERTSON'S ARGUMENT

Let us begin with the question of symbolic dimensions in Robertson's own argument. What is the grounding of the presumed right of procreative liberty? Robertson reviews roughly a 50-year history of legal decisions to demonstrate the strength and scope of the right of procreative liberty.[9] This history represents an embodiment in law of underlying presuppositions that derive from liberal culture; at the same time, it represents a new departure from previous practices, in which, for example, procreative matters were not considered so "private."

On the one hand, one might ask why such a short history should be taken as definitive of what reproduction means and how its scope should be understood. If the movement to see procreation as a private matter is relatively new, why should it be taken as definitive? On the other hand, one might ask why the history of liberal philosophy should determine the scope and strength of rights and whether it bears alone all the weight that Robertson wishes to give it. If procreation is a fundamental right because it is centrally bound up with our understanding of who we are as people, surely this understanding is deeply infused with religious values that give childbearing and childrearing special status. Robertson neglects the long religious history of respect for reproduction as central to human life, but religious tradition has surely contributed to the meanings that emerge in liberal tradition. Robertson's attempt to ground procreative liberty in a relatively recent legal tradition neglects the symbolic dimensions of procreation and the ways in which those symbolic dimensions are carried in religious traditions that undergird cultural practices and individual meanings. The recent legal tradition on which Robertson depends has compelling force only because it reflects traditions of longer standing—both the liberal tradition of philosophy and the religious traditions that shape practices and understandings of childbearing in the West. Either way, the grounding of reproductive rights reflects symbolic concerns of liberal society. Robertson cannot eschew symbolic concerns and the traditions that they reflect, for such concerns are central to his own use of recent legal developments in liberal tradition.

For example, attention to symbolic concerns is needed to ground Robertson's argument that only substantial harm to tangible interests is sufficient to trump procreative liberty. What constitutes "substantial harm"? Any answer to this question will surely enter the arena of value judgments and symbolic matters. If my healthcare premiums rise because people in my workplace choose to have children, knowing that their children will have serious genetic problems and will need significant healthcare throughout their lives, have I suffered substantial harm to my tangible interests? Certainly my economic interests would appear to be tangible rather than merely symbolic concerns. Is the harm to these interests that I would suffer sufficient to override the other person's procreative liberty? When is there enough harm for it to be substantial?[10]

In order to know whether a rise in healthcare premiums constitutes a substantial harm, we must have some grounds for knowing what makes something "substantial." There is no way to determine this apart from symbolic meanings of what counts as substance in our lives. Underneath Robertson's seemingly straightforward and legalistic language (the terms *substantial harm* and *tangible interests* have a distinct legal ring and rest on a legal tradition), there are philosophical assumptions about the priority of liberty and about what constitutes substance and what does not. For instance, Robertson's argument would refuse to allow mental anguish to count, because it is not a tangible interest. But who is to say that mental anguish is not fully as important as economic loss? Robertson's assumptions cannot be separated from the symbolic arena, since liberty itself has strong symbolic overtones and since he must make value decisions at every point about what counts as harm and substance in our lives.

In his emphasis on the priority of liberty and his refusal to allow anything other than harm to tangible interests of others to trump that liberty, Robertson appears to have adopted, without explicitly recognizing it, an argument drawn from John Stuart Mill's defense of liberty.[11] For Mill, the strongest society will emerge when personal choices and idiosyncrasies are protected from interference by others. Hence, Mill argued for liberty of thought, speech, and action—unless one person's actions would directly harm another. Robertson's language and the structure of his argument bear strong resemblances to Mill's classic approach. Both support negative rights of noninterference, but do little to provide for any positive rights of support in securing one's ends. To suggest that we may not be interfered with but that we also have no claim to positive support to secure our ends is indeed to enter the symbolic arena.

Thus, *all* arguments regarding reproductive rights and the use of new technologies will of necessity include huge dimensions of symbolic judgment. Robertson cannot escape the symbolic arena, and it is disingenuous of him to suggest that symbolic concerns cannot be the base for social policy. All social policy rests on decisions made in the symbolic arena.

PHILOSOPHERS AND "BOOTLEGGED" RELIGIOUS ARGUMENTS

To the extent that such judgments also border on religious concerns, religion may be a necessary—albeit sometimes hidden—guest at the table. Some years ago, in an argument that appears to have received little fanfare, Robert Veatch proposed that philosophers often "bootleg" religious judgments into their work.[12] Veatch suggested that Baruch Brody's arguments for justice in healthcare depend upon basic assumptions that are parallel to, if not drawn directly from, religious convictions. For example, Brody assumes the equality of all people; that the world's resources at root belong to *all* people, not just to some or to the rich; and that these resources should be used to enhance life for all and to increase equality. Thus, at least three presuppositions are hidden in Brody's argument. Veatch suggested that these three presuppositions bear striking resemblance to three basic affirmations of Jewish and Christian traditions: the equal worth of persons correlates with a belief in an infinite center of value; the suggestion that resources are never just there to be taken correlates with a belief that all of creation belongs to God; and the notion that all people have a responsibility to make the world a better place correlates with classic assumptions regarding stewardship of the world's resources.

Thus, Veatch argued that philosophy, when pushed back far enough, reaches the point "where reasons can no longer be given" and where philosophers are operating "by assumption, by intuition, or by faith" on starting points that are the equivalent of religious convictions; they cannot be defended solely with reason.[13] The convictions of some philosophers—especially those who emphasize equality—are compatible with, if not based upon, faith convictions of Jewish and Christian traditions.[14]

If we look closely at Robertson, we can see that he, too, falls at least partly into the camp of those philosophers who take an egalitarian starting point. The right of procreative liberty belongs to *all* people in Robertson's view, not just to the rich. So do the rights to choose the characteristics of our children and to use available technologies. True, for Robertson, these are *negative* rights—rights against interference—rather than positive rights. Hence, the actual application of these rights can be expected to differ for the rich and the poor. Nonetheless, the rights apply to all.

As would be predicted by Veatch's analysis, Robertson never spells out the grounding for such equality of rights. It appears to be taken on faith. Thus, at least at this level, Robertson appears to assume certain convictions that have the status of faith affirmations; these convictions are based not on reasoned argument, but on prereasoned assumptions. That these assumptions likely derive from the liberal tradition to which Robertson belongs does not undermine the point that they function in a quasi-religious fashion; never challenged or subjected to reasoned argument, they simply set the stage for the claims that are made regarding core values in human life and the parameters of its "rights."

Indeed, it may not be possible to divorce the very assumption of equality from religious faith; the belief that all people have equal worth is a strong tenet of the Jewish and Christian traditions that undergird Western civilization. While it is true that Christians have historically supported slavery and denied women's rights, it is also true that arguments *against* slavery and *for* women's rights have drawn heavily from these faith traditions. Robertson's argument appears to be drawn almost exclusively from the last 50 years of legal tradition, so he does not look to the history of development of equal rights but simply assumes this equality. Veatch's point, however, is that such assumptions of equality have in fact "bootlegged" significant symbolic values from the religious arena. The force of any arguments for equal rights depends in part upon neglected and forgotten religious traditions that still function symbolically for the majority of people.

LIBERAL PHILOSOPHY AND SECTARIAN VIEWS

Regardless of whether philosophers have bootlegged religious traditions and are dependent upon those traditions without realizing it, Western philosophical traditions—such as the liberal tradition on which Robertson depends—are sectarian. As Alasdair MacIntyre notes: "To those who inhabit a social and intellectual tradition in good working order the facts of tradition, which are the presupposition of their activities and enquiries, may well remain just that, unarticulated presuppositions which are never themselves the objects of attention and enquiry."[15] The fact that presuppositions are not examined does not free them from being bound to a particular tradition. Liberal philosophy is only one tradition among many, and its assumptions are as tradition-bound as are the assumptions that accompany religious traditions.

If Robertson is indirectly indebted to John Stuart Mill for the force of his argument on liberty, he is surely indebted to John Locke and the social contract tradition for his argument about rights. Because rights are now deeply imbedded in American law and even in international agreements (such as the United Nations Declaration of Human Rights), it is easy to forget that this tradition of rights is precisely that—a tradition. It is a tradition very alien to some people in the world, who do not think in terms of rights but in terms of community, tradition, or responsibility. The tradition of rights does not derive from reason alone, but from a particular cultural tradition. That tradition has had enough international clout to impose many of its thought structures on others around the world, but this fact does not change the reality that it represents one tradition among many. Liberal philosophical tradition is just as "sectarian" and culture-bound as religious traditions are. The mode of reasoning employed by Kant, and considered universal by him, is no more universal than is the mode of reasoning adopted in traditional Jewish halakic ethics or traditional Roman Catholic casuistry.

Robertson, however, does not assume that he can speak for everyone everywhere. His argument is drawn from and directed to a North American—specifically, a United States—context. The traditions from which he draws may be sectarian, but they nonetheless undergird his argument. If he is tradition-bound, he makes no claim to speak beyond that tradition. Hence, the symbolic meanings that he draws from that tradition feel familiar and acceptable in that context.

Indeed, many of Robertson's symbolic meanings seem so familiar and acceptable that there is much in his argument that resonates with my own position on issues. In spite of my discomfort with the language of rights, I, too, support women's right of access to abortion. I, too, think that women should not be prevented from bearing a child even if that child will have some physical disabilities. Many of the specific arguments that Robertson makes are comfortable for the majority in this culture, precisely because his argument is drawn from majority views that are now embedded in law, custom, and social practices.

Yet because Robertson's views reflect dominant social practices and attitudes, they present two problems. First, these dominant views are not free of symbolic or normative dimensions; their normative dimensions simply tend to be hidden by social consensus. For example, Robertson's argument is carefully crafted to include a right to use in vitro fertilization, which is now widely accepted in our culture. But Robertson stops short of accepting cloning, which does not enjoy popular support. Recognizing that a right to use new technologies that increase choice would imply a right to use cloning when it becomes available, Robertson suggests that perhaps cloning would not be covered by the right of procreative liberty because it deviates too far from the "core" meanings of reproduction.[16] Robertson's support for in vitro fertilization but not for cloning represents a decision with strong symbolic components. Support for one and denial of the other depends on what is taken to be the "core" values of reproduction or the "meaning" of reproduction; these are clearly symbolic matters.

Second, because Robertson argues that we have a right to choose the characteristics of our children and to use any available technologies necessary to do so, one might assume that this right would extend to embrace genetic enhancement, when and if the technological means for choosing such enhancement become available. Yet again, Robertson draws back. To choose enhancement, he suggests, would conflict "with the values that undergird respect for human reproduction."[17] In other words, although his argument is premised on the significance of choice, he operates under a set of assumptions about what values *should* be chosen. Only certain actions fit with the values that undergird reproductive freedom. A set of values embodying symbolic concerns drives the limits of choice in Robertson's system.

For Robertson, those values center in the desire of parents to have normal, healthy offspring. Genetic enhancement may support having healthy children, but it goes against the "normalcy" that is core to reproductive freedom. The scope of reproductive freedom is therefore limited by basic values of health and normalcy. Here, Robertson inevitably runs up against a potential contradiction: Is the primary value *choice* or is it *normalcy*? If it is the former, then on what grounds does one prevent a woman or couple from choosing that which goes beyond normalcy? If it is the latter, then on what grounds is normalcy, which is surely a "symbolic" notion, allowed to trump procreative liberty, when Robertson has specifically said that procreative liberty may not be trumped by symbolic concerns?

In fact, symbolic concerns undergird Robertson's argument at every step. Because he draws on dominant conceptions, however, those symbolic concerns are simply assumed and never lifted up for scrutiny. Robertson retreats into statements about what is "commonly understood" in society. Precisely such "common" understandings present another problem.

The fact that Robertson's views represent majority views makes me uncomfortable. Here is the place where religious views are needed at the table, precisely when and because they are not majority views. That is, Robertson and other philosophical ethicists want to shut out religious voices on grounds that they are sectarian and cannot be used as a base for public policy. In so doing, these philosophers ignore how sectarian their own arguments are. But more importantly, sectarian voices are necessary for public policy making precisely because they will lift up concerns that are neglected by the majority voice. The "tyranny of the majority" is real. Dominant hegemony will force public decisions that undermine people's rights.

If "normalcy" becomes the norm, for example, what will happen to the "right" of Deaf parents to choose to have deaf children?[18] Some Deaf parents are now asking genetic counselors to help them ensure that their children are deaf. On the one hand, Robertson's emphasis on procreative liberty and the "right to choose" the characteristics of our children would suggest that he would support such a request—Deaf parents have a right to use available technologies to try to have deaf children. On the other hand, if the core values undergirding reproduction involve "normalcy," bearing deaf children might be seen as not fitting this core value of reproduction and therefore as not falling under reproductive rights (just as Robertson sees cloning as not falling under reproductive rights because it deviates too far from the core values of reproduction). If prevailing opinion or dominant practice is allowed to set the stage for what rights are recognized and what values undergird reproduction, then the rights and values of minority groups are always in jeopardy. Religious voices are needed not just implicitly but explicitly in the public debate precisely because those voices have a long tradition of lifting up concerns of the marginalized.

CONCLUSION

Robertson wants to have it both ways. He wants to keep symbolic issues out of the public arena, yet uses an argument himself that calls precisely for symbolic judgments at crucial moments. It may be true that there is substantial agreement on the idea that we have a "right to procreate," and that this agreement is well grounded in U.S. law. However, the fact that there is agreement does not mean that rights carry no symbolic force and rest on no value presuppositions. Quite the opposite. The force of rights is a symbolic force. This is why the United Nations Declaration of Human Rights carries force in international law. Robertson cannot get rid of symbolic concerns in the public arena, no matter how much he might wish to.

Robertson admits that "in the final analysis, one's view about the importance of procreative liberty comes down to a normative judgment about the importance of reproductive experience in people's lives."[19] Robertson is correct. The scope and limits of procreative liberty as a right—and even the question of whether it is a right—will be decided on normative grounds. Such normative grounds always involve appeals in the long run to basic value commitments and convictions and to symbolic dimensions of human life. Thus, it is not possible for Robertson to escape from being sectarian and tradition-bound, for his values and convictions reflect those that are embedded in American legal tradition. These are the values and convictions of the dominant groups in America.

What, then, is the role of religious studies in bioethics? If all ethical arguments are at some point pushed back to basic convictions that have the force and effect of religious faith, then the role of religious studies in bioethics must be understood to be central to the establishment of any public agenda for policy making. Robertson cannot defend his appeal to procreative liberty without resorting to basic faith convictions about the worth of human beings that renders them worthy of rights. Although I might share these convictions with Robertson, they are nonetheless convictions that can be understood only in light of a history of religious conviction and faith affirmations. Allowing these convictions to sit unexamined in the background is dangerous, for it runs the risk that only dominant convictions will have a voice in public decision making.

NOTES

1. J.A. Robertson, *Children of Choice: Freedom and the New Reproductive Technologies* (Princeton, N.J.: Princeton University Press, 1994). This argument has been reiterated and refined in J.A. Robertson, "Liberalism and the Limits of Procreative Liberty: A Response to My Critics," *Washington and Lee Law Review* 52 (1995): 233-67; and J.A. Robertson, "Genetic Selection of Offspring Characteristics," *Boston University Law Review* 76, no. 3 (June 1996): 421-82.

2. Robertson, *Children of Choice*, see note 1 above, p. 41.

3. G.C. Meilaender, *Body, Soul, and Bioethics* (Notre Dame, Ind.: University of Notre Dame Press, 1995) This argument bears some striking resemblances to earlier arguments of Paul Ramsey in *Fabricated Man* (New Haven, Conn.: Yale University Press, 1970).

4. Ibid., p. 80.

5. H.R. Niebuhr, *The Responsible Self* (New York: Harper & Row, 1963).

6. Robertson, *Children of Choice*, see note 2 above, p. 141.

7. One thinks, for example, of Jehovah's Witnesses, who refuse blood transfusions on faith grounds. See K. Lebacqz, "Faith Dimensions in Medical Practice," *Primary Care* 13, no. 2 (June 1986): 263-70. Such arguments would fit Robertson's understanding of "symbolic" concerns. Individuals would be allowed to follow practices such as refusing blood transfusions, but public policy would not be made with attention to these symbolic matters.

8. Robertson, *Children of Choice*, see note 2 above, p. 222.

9. Ibid., chap. 2, especially pp. 36-7.

10. Robertson addresses these issues indirectly and rather unsatisfactorily in chapter 4, "Norplant, Forced Contraception, and Irresponsible Reproduction." Here he argues that "the most significant burdens on others" turn out to be rearing burdens and financial costs "on the public treasury" in terms of welfare payments, medical costs, and so forth (ibid., p. 77). This response deals only in diffuse general costs and ignores the *direct* impact on costs that can occur as a result of a rise in healthcare premiums for an employer, for example. Thus, Robertson has not really answered the question as to whether someone else's decision to procreate might be seen as imposing "substantial" harm to my "tangible" interests.

11. J.S. Mill, *On Liberty*, ed. Currin V. Shields (Indianapolis, Ind.: Bobbs-Merrill, 1956).

12. R.M. Veatch, *The Foundations of Justice: Why the Retarded and the Rest of Us Have Claims to Equality* (New York: Oxford University Press, 1986), 80-95. Richard B. Miller has recently made a similar argument regarding the Jewish roots of Michael Walzer's influential *Spheres of Justice*. Walzer's Jewish appreciation of covenant, code, and history, he suggests, "comprise a subtle set of religious attitudes, latent within his rendition of our shared meanings and social practices." See R.B. Miller, *Casuistry and Modern Ethics: A Poetics of Practical Reasoning* (Chicago: University of Chicago Press, 1996), 113.

13. Veatch, *The Foundations of Justice*, see note 12 above, p. 93.

14. Ibid.

15. A. MacIntyre, *Whose Justice? Which Rationality?* (Notre Dame, Ind.: University of Notre Dame Press, 1988), 7.

16. See note 2 above, p. 169. See also Robertson, "Genetic Selection," in note 1 above, p. 438, which suggests that cloning "might fall outside the bounds of reproduction as commonly understood in today's society."

17. Robertson, see note 2 above, p. 172.

18. I use the term *Deaf* to indicate members of a politically active community, and *deaf* to indicate an inability to hear. Not all deaf people affiliate with the Deaf community. For discussion of the politics of the Deaf community, see E. Dolnick, "Deafness as Culture," *Atlantic Monthly* 172, no. 3 (September 1993): 37-53.

19. Robertson, "Liberalism," see note 1 above, p. 236.

12

Religious Beliefs and Bioethics: A Crossed Relationship

Laurence J. O'Connell and Martin E. Marty

INTRODUCTION

In a pluralistic society, religious doctrine and bioethical theory inevitably intersect on the grid of personal, social, and political life. Locked into patterns of inescapable proximity, they crisscross in ways that can be mutually supportive, blithely neutral, or adamantly oppositional. Their stars are fatefully crossed because they both make normative claims concerning the moral dimensions of human life and behavior.

Accordingly, religion is often the wildcard of bioethical debate, while bioethics is regularly the source of anguished reassessment within the lives of religious believers. For example, some religious leaders have already pronounced several reproductive technologies an affront to God's preordained natural law. On the other hand, noted bioethicists have lauded these reproductive technologies as a liberating force for women; in the case of human reproduction by cloning, these biological innovations have been heralded as a pathway to "fluid families" wherein traditional gender and parenting roles would be "deconstructed." Yet, at times religious convictions and bioethical insights have coalesced in common cause against flagrant abuse, such as in their mutual denunciation of medical experimentation on unknowing or unwilling human subjects.

Given the inevitable overlap of religious conviction and bioethical theory, religion and bioethics ought to take each other seriously and welcome the stimulus that searching dialogue can bring. Indeed, such open discussion is indispensable within a pluralistic society such as the United States, which in principle embraces diversity and celebrates individual liberties. The common good hinges upon respectful exchange and civil accommodation of legitimate differences. The common good will best be served when the respective territories of religious belief and bioethical theory are well described, clearly distinguished, and assigned roles that respect their specific differences yet exploit their distinctive contributions to our common moral life.

THE NATURE AND FUNCTION OF RELIGION

A comprehensive discussion of individual religious consciousness or institutional religious expression is impractical in this context. After all, religion is one of those weasel-words capable of many twistings and turnings. Here the discussion must pragmatically focus on the relationship between bioethics and religion.

THE NATURE OF RELIGION

The work of American theologian Paul Tillich provides an ideal focal point. Although religion eludes simple definition, he developed a classic and, for our purposes, sufficiently broad and accessible description of religion. The essential core of religion as described by Tillich serves as the initial span in a bridge to the world of bioethics. After examining Tillich's essential definition of what religion is, we complete the bridge with functional definitions of what religion does, how it functions, and its results. All of this leads to some key questions: How does religion function appropriately within the realm of bioethical decision making? And how do decisions taken in the realm of bioethics appropriately challenge religion?

Unlike other important religious thinkers such as Schleiermacher, Tillich insisted that religion is not a separate faculty or an isolable dimension of the human spirit. Rather, it is the depth dimension of all creative functions of the human spirit. "Religion, in the largest and most basic sense of the word, is ultimate concern" that permeates the entire spectrum of human engagement with the world.[1] As we move toward the deepest levels of meaning—whether in art, science, ethics, or some other expression of the human spirit—we encounter religious space and experience the echo of ultimacy. Religion as "ultimate concern" plunges us toward the core of our being, where we recognize and acknowledge that which matters to us most. It takes us to the level of basic values and fundamental convictions that drive behavior and shape our lives.

Ultimate concern, then, is something that would cause one to sacrifice everything else. It is the ruler by which one measures everything. It is that which is real. There is not the slightest touch of illusion in it. It is at the root of everything; everything grows out of and depends on it.[2]

Tillich sees religion as so essentially a part of our humanity that he understands every person to be religious in some respect. Because ultimate concern of some kind is a universal human possibility, religious experience, even if it goes unnamed, is part and parcel of everyone's life. "Religion opens up the depth of spiritual life which is usually covered by the dust of our daily life and the noise of our secular work. It gives us the experience of the Holy, of something which is untouchable, awe-inspiring, an ultimate meaning, the source of ultimate courage."[3] Tillich would approve of William James's characterization of religion as a person's "total reaction upon life" that prompts us "to go behind the foreground of existence and reach down to the curious sense of the whole . . . which in some degree everyone possesses."[4]

THE FUNCTION OF RELIGION

A functional definition of religion is cast in terms of what it does. What practical purpose does religion serve? What, if any, needs are uniquely fulfilled by the experience of ultimate concern?

John F. Wilson offers a concise answer in his functional definition: "Religion is the means by which a person fulfills *existential* needs"[5]—that is, those needs that are uniquely associated with specifically human existence. Plants and animals do not have existential needs in this sense. They do not formulate existential questions: What is the meaning of my life? Why do I suffer? What is the significance of death? What is beauty and how does it affect me? How may I understand my felt relationship with a divine Other? In fashioning his functional definition, Wilson concludes: "Religion is whatever human beings have used to meet these existential needs. And while many different religions have functioned in this way, they have all functioned to meet the *same* needs."[6] And they have met these existential needs by breaching the confining boundaries of what Herbert Marcuse calls "one dimensionality,"[7] by opening the human spirit to another dimension—namely, a transcendent reality or referent. Religion invites intimacy and an authentic relationship with the divine—that is, "with the supraempirical aspects of reality, be they conceived as God, gods, or otherwise."[8] This is the core operative thrust of religion, which "becomes an essential organ of our life, performing a function which no other portion of our nature can so successfully fulfill."[9]

While the role of religion as described by Wilson serves as a general introduction, the functional theory as explained by Thomas F. O'Dea and Janet Avaid offers a degree of conceptual crispness that sharpens the point and strengthens the bridge to bioethics. They describe the function of religion in a way that emphasizes the concrete conditions that elicit specifically existential concerns noted by Wilson. These conditions are often, if not almost always, embedded in bioethical dilemmas.

Religion, according to O'Dea and Avaid, responds specifically to certain inescapable features of human existence—namely, contingency, powerlessness, and scarcity. Contingency is the unnerving companion to us all, who, despite our best efforts, remain subject to chance and unforeseen effects. The fabric of day-to-day existence is stained through and through with uncertainty and raw chance. But there is more. Powerlessness is also woven into the tissue of human experience as another inescapable fact of life. Helplessness in the face of inevitable death and so much unexplained suffering discloses the magnitude of our existential vulnerability. These two forces, contingency and powerlessness, can and do bring the human spirit to the breaking point—a point where ultimate questions about the human condition arise and demand answers. O'Dea and Avaid observe: "At these 'breaking points,' what Max Weber has called 'the problem of meaning' arises in the severest and most poignant manner."[10] As the human spirit begins to break down under the weight of existential angst, the religious function breaks in, according to the functionalist theory.

In response to the fundamental ambiguity and ever-threatening contingency of the human condition, the religious function springs into action in search of meaning and practical guidance. Various religious traditions have offered rationales and remedies that address our contingent nature, the powerlessness of our plight, and the sting of material scarcity. For example, in the Hindu tradition, the *dharma* (duties and obligations), aims at "keeping the self from falling apart in the everyday world,"[11] where contingency, powerlessness, and material scarcity so often prevail. Existential contingency and powerlessness are not alone in exciting religious sentiment. Without doubt, the existential discomfort they elicit is further exacerbated by the frustrations and deprivations associated with scarcity and material limits. Confronted with obvious disparity and injustice, people reasonably ask: What's it all about? Here religion directs existential inquiry to a broader, transcendent context that grounds and lends stability to the finite human situation of the here-and-now. Religion frames the deprivations and jarring inequities of individual and social existence so that they "may be seen as meaningful in some ultimate sense, and this makes acceptance and adjustment to them possible."[12]

In summary, then, the functional explanation of religion emphasizes its instrumental role in addressing the existential, cognitive problem of meaning and the emotional, practical problem of adjusting to the material limits and frustrations inherent in individual human life and society. For many, it provides a plausible vision of the world and a viable means for getting around in it. In Desai's words: "Religion provides definition beyond the extent of our knowledge, and security beyond the guarantees of human relationships."[13] It meets the deeply felt human need for some reassurance that there is "something which is stable in all change, something unconditioned in all that is conditioned, something absolute in the relativizing experienced everywhere."[14]

The foregoing brief discussion of the nature and function of religion provides a general and schematic introduction to some of the key ideas and controlling dynamics that comprise the world of religious believers. These fundamental features of the religious worldview provide a context for discussing the relationship between religious beliefs and bioethical decision making.

BIOETHICS

Generally understood, bioethics is the systematic identification, analysis, and resolution of ethical problems associated with the biomedical sciences and their application, especially in the practice of medicine. As such, bioethics strives to generate moral insight and offer practical guidance in relevant areas, ranging from the care of individual patients to the development of social policy. In pursuing its goals bioethics champions a central human question: "What are my duties and obligations to other individuals whose life and well-being may be affected by my actions."[15]

In recent years, the field of bioethics has rapidly developed from a fledgling discipline populated by carpetbaggers from several other, better defined fields (such as law, medicine, philosophy, theology, sociology, and nursing) to a moderately mature enterprise. Individuals now identify themselves as bioethicists, and major universities have established programs leading to advanced degrees in bioethics. Moreover, the media and general public expect and seek out expert opinion on sensitive bioethical issues such as human cloning, assisted suicide, and the deployment of healthcare resources. President Clinton has even appointed the National Bioethics Advisory Commission.

RELIGION AND BIOETHICS: SOMETIMES CONTENTIOUS YET COMPATIBLE PARTNERS

Bioethics and religion have always operated in close proximity. They are essentially kindred, yet in some cases competing expressions of the human spirit. Because they both make normative claims regarding fundamental human values and the way these values are weighed, brokered, and acted upon, some conflict is inevitable. This tension does not rule out productive interplay. Indeed, an open and dynamic relationship between religion and bioethics promises to benefit both parties. It will likely promote a more fully engaged style of bioethical reflection while, at the same time, encouraging thoughtful challenges to uncritical religious dogmatism. In short, bioethics and religion best serve our common moral life when they foil each other's tendency to engage in arrogant, absolutist posturing.

ANGLES OF VISION

Any advertisement for the positive value of bioethics is the last thing that those who are engrossed with "religious consciousness" owe those who are involved with the theory of "bioethical decision making." Proponents and theorists of bioethics can and do take care of themselves. In turn, the last thing those involved with the theories of bioethics owe those who are engrossed with "religious consciousness" is any kind of public relations for the virtues of religion. The religionists can and do take care of themselves. And in their more modest moments, those whose vocation carries them further into one field than into the other readily admit that they see too many flaws in the theory and practice of their own discipline to want it simply advertised for its positive values or publicly extolled for its virtues.

Instead, the first thing each owes the other is an attempt to provide some honest accounting of the reality that surrounds their disciplines, their vocations, their expertise, their specialties, and themselves. This means, in the present instance, that they will both have their eyes on the worlds of patients, medical institutions, and the cultures and societies that envelope and set many of the terms for them—worlds that look quite different if viewed without angles of vision and concerns supplied by the other.

DIVERGENT VIEWPOINTS

During the most recent half century, people with religious conscious-ness—here labeled *religionists*—and bioethical decision makers—in this essay simply called *bioethicists*—at first drifted apart into specializations and misunderstanding and then, more recently, have begun to converse and sometimes converge in many of their interests and some of their language. The drifting was not from some original pure spring into sepa-rate and equally pure streams. Which means, if this historical judgment holds up, there were no "good old days" in which the interests of reli-gionists and bioethicists once perfectly coincided. The religionists rea-soned in the context of theology, while the bioethicists' home base was philosophy. In the historic language of the Western world and by refer-ence to two of its sites, this means that Jerusalem and Athens, while both on the same map, were very different kinds of locations. Dwelling intel-lectually in both has never been a simple matter; even commuting be-tween them has caused some tension and strain.

The rise of modern medicine and clinical practice occurred chiefly under the aegis of Athens, of secular philosophies and their scientific issue. (One could argue that "care" developed more under the impulses of Jerusalem.) The attempts to reason about good decisions about the body and the delivery of medicine advanced on the basis of reason and the empirical framework of science alone. In that reasoning, divine rev-elation, particular scriptures, and the language of the diverse religious communities were at best seen as pleasant distractions. More frequently they were irrelevancies. In the end, they could be disruptive of the kind of decision making that has to go on in a constitutional republic rich in religious diversity and whose founders saw nonreligion to be legally on a par with all religions in the public playing field.

Meanwhile, during the centuries in which modern medicine devel-oped, many religionists stayed alert to the demands of critical reason and accepted the gifts of science and philosophy. Not all of them were sectar-ian, fundamentalist, doctrinaire, or inquisitorial. Many championed medicine and cheered the systematic reintroduction of ethical frameworks in medical education and practice. Just as bioethicists have not been con-sistently pure, neither have the religionists tried to keep philosophical ethics at bay.

For those reasons, not long after mid-century, theologians—some of them still active today—did pioneering work in bioethics. But several factors contributed to the drift between the two fields or angles of vi-sion. For one thing, the religious communities did not put much energy into the conversation and paid little attention to the moments and elements of convergence. Some were suspicious of science and the claims of reason alone.

Next, the increasing demand for bioethics and the "supply-side" growth of the bioethics community that had services to offer led the bioethicists to find their three main homes in settings where the secular and pluralist emphases were most congenial: the university; the hospital; and the complex of foundations, research centers, and manufacturers of medical goods. Whether dependent upon tax funds or private investing, and whether in the hands and minds of religious believers or not, these enterprises characteristically kept questions of religious consciousness at some distance, leading some even reflexively to ignore them or to forget to raise them.

RAPPROCHEMENT: A NEW CLIMATE

That situation has been changing in the most recent couple of decades. The conversation between religionists who have bioethical expertise and bioethicists open to many kinds of reasoning and witness has been restarted and is beginning to produce yield. To a pure secularist, which here could at least mean someone who does not admit questions having to do with the transcendent, there is no danger that the religionists will prevail or assume a monopoly. The United States and Canada are not about to be ruled by clerics, hierarchs, or divine intervention. In many parts of the world certain styles of fundamentalists, ethnonationalists, and ideologues who command regimes and all institutions within them—including hospitals and universities—have indeed insisted on a monopoly for religionists and for those of a particular faith community. Not here.

At the same time, certain trends bode well for the religionists as they bring their special gifts to the conversation and practice. First, opinion polls and reporters give evidence that large elements in the public are not satisfied with bioethical thinking that forgets about or insists on excluding religious thought and practice. Ample documentation suggests that many people are conducting a spiritual search. The rise or revisitation of "wholistic," "holistic," "alternative," "natural," and "Asian" or "Native American" accents on healing provides evidence that not all do have faith in pure science or technology. Mention of the many seekers helps account for the new climate in which the conversation between bioethicists and religionists can prosper. There is likely to be ever more of this conversation as bioethical thinking gets applied more frequently than before in home and work situations and in special agencies of human care and cure beyond or short of the hospital.

Second, conversation partners and debaters have begun to see some resources in what the other can bring to the table. Most of the religions were born as healing movements, but their origins were progressively forgotten and the ability to make use of the resources atrophied. In Judaism and Christianity, the majority faiths in North America, the Hebrew and Greek roots for the words *heal* and *save*—two businesses of religion—are similar. Prophets and leaders healed and urged their followers to do the same. They often preached and worked for justice so that the overlooked people of society would have access to care or be remembered by the faithful. In the conversations between religionists and bioethicists, some of these resources have become candidates for reassessment. Similarly, many in the religious and theological community have come to realize that they have often stereotyped bioethicists and their vocational kin in the modern university, clinic, and nation. Not all bioethicists are impersonal worshipers of technology and administration. Many are anything but heartless, soulless scientists. Among them are many who are faithful to "high humanist" concerns, and many who possess an acute sense of the sacred when dealing with the dignity of the human person and systematic care. They are as ready to hear unfamiliar voices as they are unwilling to abandon the philosophical roots of bioethics—roots sometimes described as marked by "secular rationality." So they are open to the conversation.

Third, it has become increasingly clear that patients more often than not bring to their medical concerns and clinical considerations worlds that no one can so neatly define and compartmentalize in uncontaminated containers marked "religious consciousness" and "bioethical decision making." Old definitions of "sacred versus profane," "religious versus secular," and "immanent versus transcendent" have become muddied in the practical life of many inhabitants of the pluralist and secular cultures that make up contemporary society. In dire and creative situations that call for the summoning of all possible helpful resources, few want to rule out *a priori* the potential gifts of "the other."

COMPLEMENTARY PERSPECTIVES, PRACTICAL OUTCOMES

What are the practical dimensions of this new climate? First, it is a practical and efficient matter to be given more accurate pictures of the surrounding reality. It is inefficient and impractical for professionals to live with obsolete, unnecessarily partial, and thus necessarily inaccurate portrayals of the people and cultures in which the specialists operate.

At the same time, it is practical to learn the dimensions of one's own and the other's specialties, because these are likely to lead to a certain modesty of claims. Thus, to hear smug claims that one or another of the specific religious frameworks will ensure the absolute, or true, or only legitimate decision for all who inhabit a pluralistic culture will be a more rare experience when the variety of religionists are at the table, because it becomes immediately evident that they are not a bloc. They do not all agree with one another, even on basic issues. Similarly, the claim that bioethical decisions based on philosophy should alone be privileged and consulted in crucial situations will be qualified; bioethicists who participate in the conversation will learn that, just as doctors and philosophers disagree on substance and method and presuppositions alike, so do religionists. Aristotelians and Platonists, Kantians and Hegelians, Wittgensteinians and Deweyites can make up virtual sects of their own.

Practically, this means that the conversation, encounter, and employment of religionists and bioethicists in ethical decision making will not ensure "solutions" to the problems they deal with. It will mean more likely that the discourse surrounding the decisions will be enriched and capable of offering more options. The religionists tend to accent story, narrative, and the accounting of life courses, against the background of revelation, tradition, and experience. This does not mean that they must be opposed to philosophically principled ethics. It does mean that they are especially attentive to the particularities of cases, the detail of patients' lives. They will be called to be mindful of what the people they serve in dire and dying situations can draw upon, or of what their survivors will have to resort to as they rebuild their own worlds after complex decisions and loss.

Practically, nothing said here assumes that all religionists will become expert at bioethics as a result of their conversations. There are good reasons for specialties in disciplines, methods, employment of resources, and approaches to care, and religionists with imperial claims will soon be dismissed or thwarted. There are just as many reasons to see limits to the tolerance bioethicists must develop for the myriad expressions of faith by religionists. Certainly, they cannot become walking encyclopedias of all that the religionists in their many varieties have stored in their tradition-memory-banks. But through the dialogue and encounter they are less likely than before to be content with scientific or philosophical imperialism and efforts at establishing monopolies.

The conversations between religionists and bioethicists have proceeded sufficiently far by now that they have nurtured among many a fresh sense of awe before the mysteries of faith and science; a commitment to penetrate the mysteries where possible, if such penetration holds promise of better care and cure; an increase in empathy and listening power; and an impulse to pursue discovery in ways that the overly defined and more sterile separate approaches to knowledge cannot do. So one must speak not only of challenges but of promise.

NOTES

1. P. Tillich, *Theology of Culture* (New York: Oxford University Press, 1959), 7-8.

2. J. Wilson, *Religion: A Preface* (Englewood Cliffs, N.J.: Prentice Hall, 1982), 22.

3. See note 1 above, p. 9.

4. W. James, *The Varieties of Religious Experience* (London: Collins, 1963), 53.

5. See note 2 above, p. 27.

6. Ibid.

7. H. Marcuse, *One Dimensional Man* (Boston: Beacon, 1966).

8. T.F. O'Dea and J. Avaid, *The Sociology of Religion*, 2nd ed., (Englewood Cliffs, N.J.: Prentice Hall, 1983), 7.

9. See note 4 above.

10. See note 8 above, p. 6.

11. P.N. Desai, *Health and Medicine in the Hindu Tradition* (New York: Crossroad, 1989).

12. Ibid., p. 6.

13. Ibid., p. 9.

14. H. Kung, *On Being Christian* (Garden City, N.Y.: Doubleday, 1976), 76.

15. D. Callahan, "Bioethics," in *The Encyclopedia of Bioethics* (New York: Simon & Schuster MacMillan, 1995), 1: 251.

13

Every Ethos *Implies a* Mythos: *Faith and Bioethics*

Daniel P. Sulmasy

INTRODUCTION

It has proven difficult to decide what place to assign to religious views about bioethics in a culture marked by religious pluralism and a high degree of academic skepticism about religious belief. Some have wanted to exclude religious views because they argue that such views are based upon faith assumptions that are not accessible to persons who do not share a particular faith. Although all bioethicists would probably agree that tolerance precludes forcing people to give up their religious views, some argued here that only bioethical discussions based upon reason, not religion, should be allowed into the marketplace of ideas in a tolerant, pluralistic society. This view is mistaken. If one understands clearly what tolerance demands and what it means to justify a moral viewpoint, then it does not make sense to exclude religious viewpoints from secular discussions of ethics in a tolerant society.

TOLERANCE

Tolerance of religious differences is an important characteristic of a pluralistic, democratic society. What is meant by tolerance, however, is not easy to explain. It implies, to be sure, a certain sense of forbearance. That is to say, there should be a guarantee of free religious expression and practice without interference by the state or forcible acts by other citizens that limit freedom of religious expression and the practice of religion. This is referred to in the First Amendment of the U.S. Constitution as "free exercise" of religion.

Tolerance also implies, in the language of the First Amendment, a proscription upon the "establishment" of any particular religion. That is to say, the state cannot give any one religious viewpoint or any one church official hegemony in public life. No religion should enjoy a favored status in the eyes of the government or in its treatment by the government.

These two rules of tolerance (permitting free expression and prohibiting establishment) make much practical moral sense in an increasingly pluralistic society. However, the principle of tolerance raises two problems. The first is the relationship between permitting "free exercise" and prohibiting "establishment." There is a tension between the two rules. A prohibition on establishment is a restriction upon religious expression. Completely free exercise means no restriction. Consequently, whenever the state permits free exercise of a religious expression by any particular group, there will be some who readily interpret this as establishment (for example, when a nativity scene is erected in a public square at Christmastime). On the other hand, some will interpret attempts by the state to prohibit establishment as undue restriction upon free exercise (such as when a group is prohibited from erecting a nativity scene in a public square at Christmastime). It can be hoped, of course, that this tension is creative and dynamic and that a genuine Aristotelian mean will be struck between the twin vices of establishment and restricted expression. But it is a tension nonetheless, and one that is far too infrequently recognized in discussions about religious tolerance, which seem to treat the two rules as perfectly compatible.

The second problem raised by the principle of tolerance, perhaps even more profound than the first, is deciding what counts as "religion." Obviously, a tolerant society that wishes to foster free exercise of religion will cast a wide net in defining religious beliefs and practices that ought to enjoy free exercise. On the other hand, the definition of what counts as religion cannot be purely subjective. Citizens who would shirk their responsibilities for paying taxes, for instance, have sought to define themselves as clergy in private religions. Tolerance for this sort of practice ultimately undermines the meaning of religious tolerance. And so, there is an ambiguity that needs to be addressed. It is not easy to address the question of what sorts of beliefs and practices are to count as "religions" that ought to enjoy free exercise and also be precluded from establishment.

Gerald Dworkin has suggested drawing the line as follows: all questions of belief and practice that touch upon life's ultimate meaning and importance ought to be classified as religious beliefs and practices and therefore enjoy the protection of religious liberty.[1] Appropriately, Dworkin wants to narrow the range of what can count as religion. One should not be able to claim, for instance, that having sex with as many minors as possible is an idiosyncratic tenet of one's own personal religion that is protected under the U.S. Constitution. It remains to be seen, however, how Dworkin's definition can exclude such a practice from counting as religious belief. Sex is important. Sexual relationships have a lot to do with life's ultimate meaning and importance. Sex is about such important aspects of human existence as relationships, love, and the reproduction of the species. For better or for worse, religions always have a lot to say about sex.

So, Dworkin's definition may not be narrow enough. These fundamental questions of meaning and importance are at least "religion-like" in character, but perhaps Dworkin's definition needs to be tempered with further restrictive clauses. Space limitations preclude a full justification of these further restrictions. However, to be granted religion-like protection, these very fundamental systems of belief must be more specific, comprehensive, and coherent than simple claims about "life's ultimate meaning and importance." The range of religion-like systems of belief formally covered by religious tolerance should be restricted to those systems that include beliefs about human nature, the meaning of good and evil, the meaning of suffering, the nature of human freedom, the relationship of body and spirit, and the proper relationship between individual human beings and their communities. Religions address these issues (along with plenty of other things). Qualified religion-like systems of belief must address them as well. Finally, respect for the principle of tolerance demands that the scope of tolerance should not be limited solely by harm to others; it should also exclude anything that would contradict or undermine the principle of tolerance itself.[2]

The following is therefore proposed as a working theory of religious tolerance: (1) Religions and religion-like systems are those that set forth life's ultimate meaning and purpose in and through beliefs about human nature, the meaning of good and evil, the meaning of suffering, the nature of human freedom, the relationship of body and spirit, and the proper relationship between individual human beings and their communities.

(2) In a tolerant society, the free expression of religious or religious-like practice may only properly be limited by (a) the prohibition of establishment, (b) harm to others, or (c) the determination that the practice contradicts or undermines the principle of tolerance itself.

EVERY *ETHOS* IMPLIES A *MYTHOS*

The meaning of the unusual title of this essay must now be explained. First, it is important to explain the use of the term *myth*. It is not used here in the pejorative sense that has become its popular meaning, referring to a story or an explanation that is not empirically true and can be refuted by science. Nor does it refer to a story or explanation that could not possibly be empirically verified and subjected to scientific scrutiny. *Myth* is not used here to refer to popular misconceptions, and its use is not restricted to reference to a class of stories associated with primitive religions. Rather, the term is used in the sense articulated well by Fries.

> Myth is characterized by the fact that it sees the empirical world and its happening, and above all, man and his action, in the light of the reality that constitutes them, and makes them a unity, and at the same time transcends them. . . . It is mostly in narrative form, a story which is "sacred word" and hence traditional and authoritative. . . . The events in the myth are "the origins of a given condition and the model for further developments, and myth as such is explanation." It follows that myth was not regarded as fiction and fancy, but as a hereditary experience of reality, as word about true being and the all-sustaining event, not merely in the causal sense, but in the sense that it gave meaning and purpose to all actual being and happenings.[3]

As Raimondo Panikkar has put it: "Myth is that which we take for granted, that which we do not question; and it is unquestioned because, de facto, it is seen as unquestionable."[4] Or, for those who would shun the usage of theologians, one could equally well, for the purposes of this essay, accept the definition of myth offered by anthropology as "the collection of notions a people has of how reality is at base put together."[5]

The maxim "Every *ethos* implies a *mythos*" actually comes from literary criticism and, in particular, is an interpretation of Aristotle's *Poetics*.[6] In literary criticism it means, more or less, that all character development (*ethos*) requires an underlying plot (*mythos*). However, this essay takes liberties with literary criticism in order to extend the meaning of this maxim slightly. For the purposes of this essay, the proposition means that every normative ethics (*ethos*) requires an underlying myth (*mythos*), as defined above.

With respect to Western moral philosophy, Panikkar has argued that there has been a concerted effort to debunk all myth, particularly the mythology associated explicitly with organized religions. Western moral philosophy has tried instead to extract from ancient Western myths the moral lessons that can be gleaned from them. The project of Western moral philosophy, according to Panikkar, has been to strip Western mythology of all narrative elements and turn these myths into pure, abstract principles. But Panikkar makes an interesting observation and poses a very interesting question when he writes of contemporary Western moral thinking, "We have killed the myth. Now we shall demythicize morals. After all, aren't morals just another myth?"[7]

All ethical discourse depends upon mythic narratives of one form or another. Without such mythology, there is no morality. These profound, orienting stories are the source of the premises from which ethical reasoning emerges and progresses. Underlying every *ethos* one finds a *mythos*. No matter how hard an ethicist tries to deny it, disguise it, or cover it up, lurking beneath every ethos that any ethicist might present, there lies a mythos.

This is because logical reasoning requires a set of starting premises. And moral reasoning, as even Kai Nielsen has observed, requires "a set of background beliefs," because "finally, morality does rest on a commitment."[8] These background beliefs, necessary to justify any system of ethics, constitute a myth. Inescapably, every system of normative ethics requires a commitment of faith in some conception of what it means to be human, some conception of the good, a view about the meaning of human suffering, some view about human freedom, a view about the relationship between body and person (or body and soul), and a view about the proper relationship between individual human beings and their human communities. None of this comes from logic. It is the stuff of mythology. These are the questions myths answer. Morality follows from these starting points. And not only logically. What can be abstracted from these fundamental myths as premises and then logically deduced is only part of morality. The myths continue to inform and to shape and to put flesh upon logical conclusions.

This is not to say that there is no place for reason in morality. Far from it. Reason is important, but it is never pure reason. It is always reason that begins in myth and is shaped by myth.

This is not to say that one myth is as good as another. Not every narrative is morally good or morally right.[9] What some narratives have to say about the meaning of human life, the nature of the good, the meaning of suffering, the nature of freedom, the relationship between body and person, and the relationship between individual and community can be morally appalling. Narratives are not self-justifyingly true, and this discussion is not a defense of pure "narrative" ethics.

Reason can help one to decide which narrative to accept or reject. Nonetheless, one must be humble in this endeavor. To assert that some narratives are morally good and some are not does not imply that it is easy to decide. Since there is no sure-fire way of proving which narrative is correct, one must cultivate a spirit of epistemic moral humility and be tolerant about the originating myths that underlie various ethical systems. However, some moral mythologies can be readily recognized as wrong. Together, we can at least draw boundaries around some of these fundamental moral narratives and declare that some are clearly off the moral radar screen. We know, for example, that the Nazi moral narrative was wrong. It was not "just as good as" any other story about human nature and the nature of the good, and the proper relationship between individuals and the community.

EVERY BIO-*ETHOS* IMPLIES A *MYTHOS*

A central argument of this essay is that the *ethos/mythos* thesis is true of every system of bioethics as much as it is true of every system of general normative ethics. Every bioethical system must make assumptions about the meaning and scope of the good, particularly as it relates to biomedical good; about the meaning and purpose (or purposelessness) of human life; about the meaning of suffering; about human freedom; about the nature and purpose of healing; about the relationship between human bodies and human persons; and about the proper relationship between individual human beings and their communities.

In the section that follows, five prominent, formidable systems of bioethics are explored to provide some glimpses of the underlying mythic structures. This endeavor has certain limitations. First, since philosophers often do their best to demythologize their morality, showing that they have failed to purge their moral systems of mythology is sometimes difficult. Some individuals will deny that what is shown here is mythological, but this denial can only be true if these individuals deny the definition of myth employed in this essay. Second, this short list of bioethicists' writings is obviously not exhaustive. It is, however, representative of a wide range of systems of bioethics. These systems serve as case examples to help demonstrate that there can be no bio-*ethos* without an underlying *mythos*.

ENGELHARDT AND THE MYTH OF THE AMERICAN FRONTIER

H. Tristram Engelhardt, Jr. argues strenuously that religious systems of thought have no place in public discussions of ethics. Religious ethics has a content, so he contends, and since there can be no agreement on the content of ethics given the fact of widespread moral disagreement, public moral discourse ought to be limited to procedural questions. Notwithstanding the observation that Engelhardt might violate the naturalistic fallacy by moving from the fact of moral disagreement to a normative claim about the conduct of moral discourse, one must raise the question of whether the secular bioethics he offers is truly free of content.

There is a content underlying the bioethics of Engelhardt. There is a *mythos* in his bio-*ethos*, called here "the myth of the American frontier." The following passage, buried in the middle of a long footnote, illustrates Engelhardt's mythology: "This description somewhat foreshadows the American frontiersmen who moved on further when the smoke of too many neighbors' houses could be seen, or the old Texas view that 'your neighbors are too damn close when you can't shoot in all directions without fear of hitting someone.' "[10]

This passage illustrates many of the fundamental assumptions underlying Engelhardt's system of bioethics. This sort of narrative tells the reader a great deal. Freedom is the most important part of the meaning of being human. Human beings are meant to be rugged individuals. Mind your own business. Get away from people. Be self-reliant. Life is a great frontier to be tamed by powerful individuals. The weak may fall by the wayside as the wagontrain heads West, but they will simply need to be left behind. This is, of course, unfortunate, but one cannot call it unfair.[11]

Engelhardt's bioethical myth has its foundation in the mythology of a general theory of ethics. Engelhardt extensively quotes from the libertarian philosophy of Nozick, and Nozick has his own mythology.[12] According to Nozick, we are all wandering along the beach, where we all encounter beautiful grains of sand.[13] We get to keep the ones we want, and there is enough for everyone. Property is extremely important to being human, as is freedom. We are all unique and more unlike one another than alike. We get along by agreeing on ways to settle our disputes. Life is an empty beach. Life is an open frontier.

One can argue for such a vision, but it absolutely cannot be claimed that such a mythology has been proven to be the truth. This vision is offered as a vision about the most fundamental moral truths. It is a mythology—a powerful American mythology. Followed to its logical consequences in healthcare (and Engelhardt carefully follows it all to its logical consequences, no matter how absurd), one arrives at a view of healthcare that is very particular to the myth of the American frontier.

According to this myth, in healthcare—as in everything else—Americans value freedom more than they value equality.[14] Government should have almost no role in healthcare, because it should have almost no role in people's lives. Healthcare is property—like land on the frontier or grains of sand on the beach to be leased, bought, and sold. We need a minimal number of procedural rules to figure out how it will be exchanged. Free enterprise and the market should govern American healthcare policy. Health decisions are extremely private. Everyone should mind his or her own business and ought never dare to tell anyone whether to take a certain pill or to undergo a certain procedure. The only limit on the freedom of individuals to engage in healthcare contracts should be harm to others (that is, avoid the stray bullets by making sure your neighbors aren't too damn close). Everyone should be self-reliant, in healthcare as in everything else. It's up to the individual to decide whether to have health insurance. It's a free country. But if one should decide not to have health insurance or not to wear a motorcycle helmet, one should be prepared to pay the consequences. This is the myth of healthcare on the American frontier.

VEATCH AND THE MYTH OF
THE PHYSICIAN AS STRANGER

The central myth in the writing of Robert Veatch is called here "the myth of the physician as stranger."[15] According to this mythology, life is not a great prairie, but a city marked by anonymous relationships among strangers. We cling to privacy as a refuge from the intense interpersonal contacts of our working lives. Thus, we prefer that our physicians should be strangers. For Veatch, staying strangers is not a negative situation. "The anonymous patient-physician relationship offers privacy not available with more personal professional relations."[16] We are all alone, each in an isolated urban apartment, all the while dependent upon one another, however reluctantly. As Veatch sees it, "some personality types seem to favor maintenance of more compartmentalized lives."[17]

Why might this be so? It is because if people know us they will have power over us. And whoever has power invariably uses it to dominate others. To be sick is to be weak, vulnerable, and powerless. This is information we can hardly afford to let others know. As Veatch writes, many persons "would not want their 'friends' to see them in weakness, which sometimes is a condition of patients seeking professional help."[18] We should be wary of one another and trust no one. Each individual is always a rational self-interested maximizer. This is especially true of physicians. In a continual striving for power after power, we should be wary of too much familiarity. One does not want a doctor to get too chummy. Once the doctor even learns a patient's name, he or she has power over that patient that the patient reluctantly concedes for the sake of getting well.[19]

The vision Veatch offers is only a modern, urban medical version of the state of nature as described by Hobbes. Competition and striving against one another is the rule. Life in the state of nature is "solitary, poor, nasty, brutish, and short."[20] Trust no one. Do not believe anyone who claims to be virtuous, and demand instead some explicit rules for one's own protection. Virtues are dangerous, says Veatch.[21] No one is really ever out to help others.

Veatch is quite explicit about the debt he owes to Hobbes, Locke, and Rousseau.[22] And in keeping with the long line of contract theorists in whose tradition he is firmly situated, Veatch offers a way to keep peace in the medical war of all against all; he calls this the "triple contract."[23] This is how one is protected against the self-interested strangers who are out to pounce on unsuspecting citizens as soon as they leave the cells of their apartments and venture out on the street. All citizens enter into an initial social contract of mutually assured forbearance as the first level of protection. Society has a contract with the medical profession as second level of protection. And each individual patient seeking services must negotiate a third contract with each individual practitioner, providing a third level of protection.

This is a particular worldview. It is an originating myth. Veatch proves none of this, but rather he offers it as a story about the way things are. This is a myth about human nature, the relationship between individuals and society, and the nature of the good. It is a story about why we value equality, which is viewed as a mechanism of protection against the irredeemable self-interest of others. By making sure that no one gets the upper hand, all are able to pursue their own interests in relative peace and to protect their own vaunted privacy. Veatch's medical ethics follows from this worldview.

BROCK AND THE MYTH OF
THE LIFE PLAN

In the bioethics of Dan Brock, the central myth is the "myth of the life plan." It is not explicitly named as such, but it is the dominant and pervasive myth that characterizes his writings. In explaining what life and death are all about, Brock writes the following:

> People typically develop, at least by adolescence, more or less articulated and detailed plans for their lives; commonly, the further into the future those plans stretch, the less detailed, more general, and the more open-ended they are. Our life plans undergo continuous revision, both minor and substantial, over the course of our lives, but at any point in time within a life people's plans for their lives will be based in part upon assumptions about what they can reasonably expect in the way of a normal life span. When their lives are cut short prematurely by illness and disease they lose not just the experiences, happiness, and satisfactions that they would otherwise have in those years, but they often lose as well the opportunity to complete long-term projects and to achieve and live out the full shape, coherence, and conclusion they had planned for their lives. It is this rounding out and completion of a life plan and a life that help enable many elderly people, when near death, to feel that they have lived a full and complete life and so to accept their approaching death with equanimity and dignity. The loss from premature death is thus not simply the loss of a unity of a good thing, so many desired and expected-to-be-happy-life-years, but the cutting short of the as yet incompletely realized life plan that gave meaning and coherence to the person's life.[24]

Planning, for Brock, is that which distinguishes persons from animals, vegetables, and minerals. He writes:

> Only humans and not animals can have plans about the future.... It is this capacity to envisage and desire a future for oneself that I believe best explains why killing a normal adult human wrongs that person. I believe the severely demented, while of course remaining members of the human species, approach more closely the condition of animals than normal adult humans in their psychological capacities. In some respects the severely demented are even worse off than

animals such as dogs and horses, who have a capacity for integrated and goal-directed behavior that the severely demented substantially lack.[25]

Planning is so deep a myth that one can speculate about what it would be like to plan into the future indefinitely, provided one were not to suffer physical deterioration as a result of the accumulation of years on the planet. "If individuals were able sufficiently to adjust their life plans to great or indefinite extensions of life, and physical deterioration were arrested, it is unclear either that their quality of life *must* decline or that additional years of life must lose value."[26] Planning without deterioration is paradise.

It follows, of course, that the meaning and value of healthcare depends upon life plans. Healthcare interventions "are of value insofar as they facilitate the patient's pursuit of his or her overall plan of life; the aims, goals and values important to the particular patient."[27] The truly awful thing about the early mortality in developing countries is that the inhabitants are prevented from fulfilling their life plans.[28] The myth can be put simply, "I plan, therefore I am."[29]

Where does the myth of planning come from? Not from Hobbes so much as Rawls. Rawls devotes a long section of *A Theory of Justice* to the concept of a life plan,[30] and Brock explicitly cites Rawls as the inspiration for this concept.[31] Rawls ties this whole mythology together very nicely when he writes: "A person may be regarded as a human life lived according to a plan."[32]

Once again, of course, this is a very particular view about human nature, about what constitutes the good and the right, about the importance of freedom of choice, and about the proper relationship between human beings. Yet for most people, life's most fundamental meaning is not about planning; for them, Brock's myth must seem extraordinarily obscure. For example, for most people in the world, life is simply about being able to eat each day. This often involves some planning, of course, but it often involves a lot more luck. And even for most people in the more secure, developed world (outside of a few isolated and inbred university communities), the important characteristics of a good life are not how one imposes one's will upon and controls the world, but rather about how one reacts and deals with all the things about life over which one has no control. The moral life is often about how one deals with the unexpected—about how one adjusts one's own plans to the plans of others. For many, the moral life begins with a realization that the most important things about life—such as the facts of one's own birth and the inevitability of one's own death—are completely out of one's control. For still others, spontaneity is life's great joy, not the dreary hebetude of a life lived according to a plan.

And so, as a fundamental mythology about human nature and the moral life, the myth of the life plan has its adherents, but it is a mythology nonetheless. It cannot be considered absolutely normative *sub specie aeternitatis*. And the bioethics that follows from it, emphasizing personal autonomy and the role healthcare can play in helping persons (that is, planners) to fulfil their life plans cannot be considered absolutely normative either.

CALLAHAN AND THE MYTH OF THE NATURAL LIFE SPAN

Although Daniel Callahan's bioethics has much in common with the views of Dan Brock, it offers yet another fundamental view of human life. Callahan's view is based on the concept of a life *span*, rather than a life *plan*. Dixon has aptly called this "Callahan's foundation myth."[33] Dixon's use of the term *myth* corresponds to my own. By myth she means underlying justificatory scheme. Sometimes one finds an explicit narrative in an author's writing to capture it and sometimes not, but there is always some sort of underlying story about human nature, the good and the right, human freedom, and the relationship of individuals to communities. Callahan offers a nicely illustrative, brief, personal story at the beginning of *The Troubled Dream of Life*.[34] He writes about his grandmother's quiet death, at home, in her sleep, in her mid-80s, followed by a wake, in her own bed, attended by the same circle of friends with whom she had gathered to gossip and to knit. This story says a great deal about Callahan's mythology. *Setting Limits* begins with a similar familial scene.[35]

Dixon identifies four elements in Callahan's foundation myth.[36] First, she identifies his idea of a "natural life span"—the idea of a whole of life with death as an absolute limit. (She also descries its "cultural standards of human fulfillment cloaked in biology.") Second, Callahan appears wedded to a belief in relatively fixed stages of life, considered as psychological or biological transitions. Third, his idea of a "tame death" is one in which one's life possibilities are accomplished, one's moral obligations have been discharged, and one's death occurs in a way that is not offensive to others. Finally, Callahan's writings contain the important mythic theme that the deepest moral meaning of aging is sacrifice. Dixon provides ample textual evidence to support her interpretation.[37]

One more element can be added to the four that Dixon has identified as part of Callahan's mythology. Callahan also gives community a greater role than many other bioethicists do in defining what is natural and good. He thinks that more individual freedom and control is not necessarily better. Callahan calls us "prisoners of choice"[38] and is convinced that the Western view of the self is distorted by obsession with control over nature and control over our own lives.[39]

As in all the other systems discussed here, a particular bioethics emerges from Callahan's mythological foundation. The mythological substructure leads Callahan to multiple particular conclusions about such topics as age-based healthcare rationing and assisted suicide.[40] These conclusions follow logically from his foundation myth. But once again, it must be recognized that his conclusions are based upon his own mythology.

Callahan's myth has some similarities with Brock's in that both place particular importance on a conception of the whole of life. However, Callahan differs radically from Brock over the question of whether a whole life takes shape most importantly by nature or by will, by the community or by the self. Callahan is more explicit than Brock in telling narratives and in acknowledging that these are fundamental assumptions about the nature of things, but both are equally myth tellers. Callahan's myth has all the important characteristics of an originating moral myth; it tells something about human nature, about the good and the right, about human freedom, and about the proper relationship between individual and community.

None of this is proven. One can argue about which myth is truer, deeper, or better. But once the discussion gets this close to the core of an ethical system, there comes a point at which one makes a leap of faith. One must believe in some moral myth or another, or one has no ethical system. Every *ethos* implies a *mythos*.

JEWISH AND CHRISTIAN AUTHORS AND THE MYTH OF THE PATIENT AS STRANGER

In contrast to Veatch's myth of the physician as stranger, Jewish and Christian authors have turned to the myths of their own traditions and found maxims and stories about the moral imperative to care for strangers. This point of view is illustrated using one contemporary Jewish author and a pair of contemporary Christian authors.

Writing in the Jewish tradition, Laurie Zoloth phrases it as follows: "The theological claim is for the stranger and the powerless who dwell in our gates. Extrapolated into the world of the clinic, this becomes, again, almost dangerous, for it assumes an advocacy that, today, becomes named political. . . . The regard for the stranger as central to the social world offers a much needed corrective to the problem of stranger medicine. Traditional texts and the history itself call for the encounter between the self and the stranger to be the place for ethics."[41]

This point of view stands in sharp contrast with that of Veatch. In this mythological schema, the stranger and the orphan have a special moral claim on everyone else. Making strangers feel welcome and less estranged is a central concern of morality. Making the anonymous feel like personal members of a community and addressing their most pressing needs is a crucial moral duty. And when they are sick, the moral claims that the needs of the alienated make upon others are manifest. This means that the manner in which sick strangers are treated is a central concern of ethics, and consequently, of bioethics.

This mythology is not an invention of contemporary authors. These authors have reached into their scriptural tradition. According to the Hebrew scriptures, failure to care for strangers is equivalent to the evils of fraud or adultery. As it is written in the prophet Malachi: "I will draw near to you for judgment, and I will be swift to bear witness against the sorcerers, adulterers, perjurers, those who defraud the hired man of his wages, against those who defraud widows and orphans, those who turn aside the stranger and those who do not fear me, says the Lord of hosts" (Mal. 3:5).

More than simply avoiding harm, the law commands that pious Jews should address the needs of the aliens who find themselves among the people of Israel: "You shall treat the alien who resides with you no differently than the natives born among you. Have the same love for him as you have for yourself; for you too were once aliens in the land of Egypt" (Lev. 19:34).

Assuming this mythological point of view, of course, makes a great difference when it comes to figuring out what to do with pressing bioethical issues such as the care of the poor, age-based rationing, and assisted suicide. It is a myth that says something about the proper relationship between individual human beings and community. It embodies a theory of the good and the right. It is part of a wider system of mythology with definite assumptions about human nature and human freedom. All this is freely admitted. It is an explicitly religious point of view.[42]

Christian healthcare ethics is often undergirded by a very similar mythology (naturally enough, since Christianity grew out of the Jewish tradition). The Christian scriptural texts seem to amplify the moral importance of attending to the needs of the stranger, claiming that serving such persons is serving Christ himself. At the judgment day, the saved will ask Jesus, "When did we see you as a stranger and welcome you, or naked and clothe you?" (Matt. 25:38). Jesus replies that those who served strangers and the naked served him.

But perhaps the Christian story most important for its influence on healthcare has been the parable of the Good Samaritan (Luke 10:29-37). It is a story that makes a compassionate encounter with a suffering stranger the norm for moral action. The Good Samaritan does not complain about living too close to his neighbor or offer the victim a contract. Nor does the Good Samaritan make discrete inquiries about whether the care he plans to offer fits with the victim's life plan, or check to be sure that his intervention is appropriate to the individual's position within a natural life span. The one who is neighbor is the one who acts with compassion.

Pellegrino and Thomasma are two authors in bioethics whose writings are strongly influenced by their Christian beliefs. The parable of the Good Samaritan plays an important role in their explicitly Christian writings about bioethics. Writing about Christian virtue in healthcare, they argue that "true compassion is more than feeling. It flows over into a willingness, desire, and intent to help, to make a sacrifice, to go out of one's way, as the Good Samaritan did."[43] This insistence that the parable of the Good Samaritan is normative carries over into bioethics in very concrete ways. They write:

> Benevolent self-effacement is a minimum obligation consistent with the virtue of charity. Lesser degrees of the virtue of benevolence and beneficence would be inconsistent with such scriptural exhortations as the story of the Good Samaritan and the Sermon on the Mount and with Jesus' own healing acts. On this view, medical knowledge is not proprietary or simply a means to a living. It is a means of service to others, a mission and an apostolate, a ministry to those who have a special claim on the whole community—especially the vulnerable, the sick, disabled, poor, or retarded. Meeting the claims of the vulnerable is an essential feature of Christian belief. It is not optional or heroic.[44]

Carrying this further, it even means that the principles of bioethics must be reinterpreted. They urge healthcare professionals "to extend the notion of beneficence to the point of effacement of self-interest, indeed to recognize the 'hard' message of the Gospel, the message that some unselfish sacrifice, as in the parable of the Good Samaritan, is required."[45]

Once again, this is a particular point of view. It is a foundational myth about human nature, freedom, the nature of the good, and the relationship between individuals and communities. The bioethics follows from the myth. But these authors, at least in the works cited, are explicit in acknowledging that they are coming to these conclusions on the basis of these particular religious stories. They cite scripture explicitly. They take it as part of the scheme of justification for their ethical system.

ETHOS, MYTHOS, AND CONTEMPORARY AMERICAN BIOETHICAL DISCOURSE

The purpose of the preceding section was to demonstrate that what would seem to be true on *a priori* grounds obtains in reality—that every *ethos* implies a *mythos* and, consequently, every bio-*ethos* implies a *mythos*. Some of these mythologies are explicitly religious, but some are not. Each has important things to say about human nature, the nature of the good and the right, the nature and place of human freedom, and the proper relationship between individual and community. None of these positions is proven. One can make arguments for or against adopting one or another of these mythological positions, but often they are simply assumed to be true. The rest of bioethical discourse within one or another mythological system will be based on these foundational, originating myths.

The important question that arises, however, is whether one or another of these systems of moral discourse can be excluded from the public domain in a tolerant society. In particular, should religious voices in bioethics be excluded from full participation in public discourse in universities; academic publications; popular media; or local, state, or federal legislative or public policy discourse? If so, on what grounds? Should a rabbi, mullah, bishop, or theologian be allowed to testify at congressional hearings or participate in bioethics commissions? If so, should their views be discounted as belonging to a particular religion and therefore not relevant to debate in a pluralistic society? Should referees and editors of medical journals reject articles about bioethics topics on the grounds that the views expressed reflect a religious perspective? Should a university preclude a competent individual from participating on an ethics committee or in a public debate about an ethics issue because that individual assumes a religious perspective in ethics? And, if that individual is allowed to participate, should his or her views be discounted as expressing an irrelevant religious perspective? Based on the discussion above, it is hard to justify such a position.

If tolerance truly means what this essay has taken it to mean, then it is difficult to see on what grounds an explicitly religious voice in ethics could be excluded from public discourse. If a religion or a religion-like system of beliefs covered by the principles of tolerance means anything like what this essay has taken it to mean, then no one mythological system undergirding any system of bioethics can be regarded as any more or less deserving of tolerance than any other. Mythological systems that depend upon some notion of a god or gods cannot be taken as any less accessible to people who do not share the faith than those mythological systems that deny the existence of a god or gods. There would not seem to be any principled way to distinguish these. If both types of systems are religious, or religion-like, then both ought to enjoy freedom of "expression" as well as protection from the "establishment" of one or another (or of some and not others) as the official state religious view. This is what tolerance means. Whether one begins a bioethical discourse by stating "your neighbors are too damn close when you can't shoot in all directions without fear of hitting someone" or by stating, "a man went down to Jericho from Jerusalem and fell among robbers" should not determine whether one's arguments can be part of official public discourse.

In fact, in a tolerant society, each mythology should be free to express itself in the center of the marketplace, not assigned to an inaccessible stall in a dark corner. This is because ethical discourse includes, in important ways, arguments about which mythology provides a better basis for the moral analysis of healthcare. Should our healthcare system be constructed upon the myth of the frontier, or of the myth of physician as stranger, the myth of the life plan, the myth of the natural lifespan, or the myth of the Good Samaritan? Can a healthcare system be devised that is agreeable to most individuals with sufficient accommodations for those who espouse different views for themselves? Or, better still, are there touchstones common to each mythological system that can be employed as the basis for a healthcare system? For instance, Judaism and Christianity share attentiveness to the needs of the alienated as a moral touchstone despite disagreements about such theologically crucial themes as the status of Jesus of Nazareth, the afterlife, and the role of the Mosaic law.

CONCLUSION

There is no principled way to exclude or marginalize religious discourse in bioethics without violating the principle of religious tolerance. All ethical views begin with mythology. Every *ethos* implies a *mythos*. The wide variety of extant moral mythologies employed in bioethics includes some that are explicitly religious in the sense of affirming a deity, but all are religious in the broader sense adapted from Dworkin concerning fundamental beliefs about human nature, good and evil, freedom, suffering, and the relationship between the individual and the community. To state that only those moral mythologies that explicitly deny the existence of a god or gods have a place in public discourse and policy making about bioethics violates both rules of the principle of tolerance. Such a policy "establishes" one set of moral mythologies and also unduly limits the "free expression" of the other set. Tolerance requires respect for every *mythos* and for every *ethos*. More such tolerance would be a genuine service to the bioethics community and the wider society.

NOTES

1. G. Dworkin, *Life's Dominion: An Argument about Abortion and Euthanasia* (New York: Alfred A. Knopf, 1993), 160-8.

2. D.P. Sulmasy, "Institutional Conscience and Moral Pluralism in Health Care," *New Theology Review* 10, no. 4 (November 1997): 5-21.

3. H. Fries, "Myth," in *Encyclopedia of Theology: The Concise Sacramentum Mundi*, ed. K. Rahner (New York: Seabury Press, 1975), 1011-2.

4. R. Panikkar, *Myth, Faith, and Hermeneutics* (New York: Paulist Press, 1979), 4.

5. C. Geertz, *Islam Observed* (New Haven, Conn.: Yale University Press, 1968), 97.

6. Aristotle, *Poetics* (1450a.15-1450b.4) in *The Basic Works of Aristotle*, ed. R. McKeon (New York: Random House, 1941).

7. See note 4 above, p. 45.

8. K. Nielsen, "Hobbesist and Humean Alternatives to a Religious Morality," in *God and the Grounding of Morality* (Ottawa, Ont., Canada: University of Ottawa Press, 1991), 23-39.

9. E.D. Pellegrino, "Commentary: Rationality, the Normative and the Narrative in the Philosophy of Morals," in *Knowledge, Value, and Belief*, vol. 2, *The Foundations of Ethics and Its Relationship to Science*, ed. H.T. Engelhardt Jr. and D. Callahan (Hastings-on-Hudson, N.Y.: Institute of Society, Ethics, and the Life Sciences, 1977), 213-20.

10. H.T. Engelhardt Jr., *Bioethics and Secular Humanism: The Search for a*

Common Morality (Philadelphia: Trinity Press International, 1991), 169, n. 79.

11. H.T. Engelhardt Jr., *The Foundations of Bioethics* (New York: Oxford University Press, 1986), 342-3.

12. Ibid., 395.

13. R. Nozick, *Anarchy, State, and Utopia* (New York: Basic Books, 1974), 174-8.

14. H.T. Engelhardt Jr. and M.A. Rie, "Morality for the Medical-Industrial Complex: A Code of Ethics for the Mass-Marketing of Health Care," *New England Journal of Medicine* 319 (1988): 1086-9.

15. R.M. Veatch, *The Physician-Patient Relation—The Patient as Partner* (Bloomington, Ind.: University of Indiana Press, 1991).

16. Ibid., p. 44.

17. Ibid.

18. Ibid.

19. Ibid.

20. T. Hobbes, *Leviathan*, ed. R. Tuck (New York: Cambridge University Press, 1991), 89.

21. R.M. Veatch, "The Danger of Virtue," *Journal of Medicine and Philosophy* 13 (1988): 445-6; R.M. Veatch, "Against Virtue: A Deontological Critique of Virtue Theory in Medical Ethics," in *Virtue and Medicine*, ed. E.E. Shelp (Dordrecht, The Netherlands: D. Reidel, 1985), 329-45.

22. R.M. Veatch, *A Theory of Medical Ethics* (New York: Basic Books, 1981), 7, 123-4.

23. Ibid., 108-38.

24. D.W. Brock, *Life and Death: Philosophical Essays in Biomedical Ethics* (New York: Cambridge University Press, 1993), 295-6.

25. Ibid., pp. 372-3.

26. Ibid., p. 253.

27. Ibid., p. 149.

28. Ibid., p. 296.

29. D.P. Sulmasy, "Review of D.W. Brock, *Life and Death: Philosophical Essays in Biomedical Ethics,*" *Academic Medicine* 68 (1993): 831-2.

30. J. Rawls, *A Theory of Justice* (Cambridge, Mass.: Belknap Press, 1971), 407-16.

31. See note 24 above, p. 318, n.38.

32. See note 30 above, p. 408.

33. K.M. Dixon, "Oppressive Limits: Callahan's Foundation Myth," *Journal of Medicine and Philosophy* 19 (1994): 613-37.

34. D. Callahan, *The Troubled Dream of Life: Living with Mortality* (New York: Simon and Schuster, 1993), 11.

35. D. Callahan, *Setting Limits: Medical Goals in an Aging Society* (New York: Simon and Schuster, 1987), 13-4.

36. See note 33 above.

37. Dixon provides much of this in her article. See especially Callahan,

Setting Limits, 65-76.

38. See note 34 above, pp. 69-71.

39. Ibid., pp. 120-55.

40. See note 35 above, pp. 76-83; 91-119.

41. L. Zoloth-Dorfman, "One of These Mornings I'm Going to Rise Up Singing: On the Necessity of the Prophetic Voice in Jewish Bioethics," *The Journal of Clinical Ethics* 5, no. 4 (Winter 1994): 351. [Zoloth presents a revised version of this essay as chapter 14 of the present volume.—ED.]

42. Such views do not always need to be religious. Robert Burt has offered a nonreligious, Freudian interpretation of the myth of the care of the stranger, in which he notes particularly that love and violence are often admixed, as reflected in the disquieting ambiguity of a phrase such as, "I'll take care of him." See R.A. Burt, *Taking Care of Strangers: The Rule of Law in Doctor Patient Relations* (New York: Free Press, 1979).

43. E.D. Pellegrino and D.C. Thomasma, *The Christian Virtues in Medical Practice* (Washington, D.C.: Georgetown University Press, 1996), 86.

44. Ibid., p. 75.

45. E.D. Pellegrino and D.C. Thomasma, *Helping and Healing: Religious Commitment in Health Care* (Washington, D.C.: Georgetown University Press, 1997), 97.

14

Faith and Reasoning(s):
Bioethics, Religion, and Prophetic Necessity

Laurie Zoloth

INTRODUCTION

The conversation in this book emerged from an article written by Dena S. Davis that I replied to, along with others—notably the late Benjamin Freedman—in the pages of *The Journal of Clinical Ethics*.[1] Davis and I next organized a panel at the first national conference of the American Association of Bioethics in 1993, invited Stephen E. Lammers and Carole Taylor to join, then the others you will encounter in this book. We have continued the conversation ever since. This chapter is an expansion of this conversation. First, I revisit my response to Davis's article, which is reprinted here (see chapter 1). Then I further explore how Jewish ethics is a conversation partner in the ongoing discourse among bioethicists with scholarly training in the field of religion and theology about the nature and the place of religious studies, and about our passion for the questions of religion and theology in the discipline of bioethics.

In the past, there has been a persistent stance taken at such panels on religion and bioethics, which have become a staple at every national conference in bioethics. Participants ask: "Why is it that the intellectual engine of bioethics seems to be driven by legal or medical theorists rather than theologians?" The tangential, often wistful quality of such panels is an interesting phenomenon in itself. Any serious student of the canon of the Western tradition in the humanities knows clearly that theology and religious practice have been central to any discourse on justice, duty, death, personhood, and well-being—the very core of bioethics. Conversant knowledge of the traditions of canon law, the Church, and biblical literature was assumed to be the basis of all rigorous scholarship. The first arguments of bioethics were largely compelled by the reflections of religious scholars and the first public cases regarding withdrawal of treatment. The 1976 case of Karen Ann Quinlin, arguably one of the first fires to forge and galvanize the field, was shaped in large measure by the sincerity of the quest of faith by the family, physicians, and clergy who were firsthand participants. Now scholars of religion ask how such compelling influence could have been lost.

As a Jewish ethicist most comfortable in the postmodern philosophic tradition of our field, I note this wistfulness with irony. How can one go beyond an admittedly self-serving yearning for the past? Is this all that we are doing when we religious scholars yearn for lost leadership—conducting a quest for the power itself, or for the familiar? I think not. For the delineation of religions and acts of faith as irrelevant—or worse, as irrational—marginalizes not only theologians, but also the far wider world of patients and families, who are often similarly marginalized and pathologized by bioethicists in the very performative gestures—of prayer, of witness, or of belief—that most strongly guide them through clinical dilemmas. Let me reflect on how this came to be the case and offer the subversive suggestion that the pre-Enlightenment insights harbored by religion might present the strongest challenges to a modernity and a medicine desperately in need of such challenge.

BACKGROUND AND FOREGROUND IN MODERNITY

When I was young I learned not to talk about God. At first I thought it was because I was a Jew; I quickly learned not to talk about that in the West Coast suburb where I grew up. (Once, on a vacation in a Southern California beach town, a big blonde man glanced over at my small, dark father, my mother, and the three black-haired children and asked us our name. "What kind of a name is *that*?" he demanded, and my father answered "Russian." Better to be a Communist, even in the 1950s, than a Jew. The otherness that marked us and was our real nomenclature was better passed over).

Now, post-Oprah, I, as author, could talk to readers about anything—sex, illness, or old grudges; but nothing in the midst of an academic argument would make us all so uncomfortable as if I talked seriously about

God. (Californians have a way to deal with this: it's called "spirituality.") But if I want to talk about God, or rather talk about the act of talking about God in the context of scholarly bioethics, it would be heard as confessional. Is such a discourse tangential, soft, marginal, or worse still, merely pastoral (a thing for the patients, but not for "us")—which is to say, not real, not rigorous, not like science, or not defensible and logical like analytic philosophy? Such is the *sotto voce* claim in the field, and such is the reason that there are not panels called "secular humanist views in bioethics." I want to address this claim head on and ask: What is the point of theology in the field of bioethics? When scholars of religious studies speak through their discipline toward the emerging field of bio-ethics, and contend for the power to shape its future, what is it that we insist upon? What is gained by the admission of religious studies and what is lost by its exclusion?

Dena S. Davis's article, "It Ain't Necessarily So: Clinicians, Bioethics, and Religious Studies," asked this very question.[2] She asked how useful was religious theory to the clinician and raised significant questions about both the nature of religious scholarship in applied ethics and the irony of efficacy in the debate. Davis's article had much to agree with and much to quarrel with. In my reply to Davis I attempted to do both, as a way of grounding my larger point about the tasks of religions in the field. I note here for the record that a quarrel is the very nature of the traditional Jewish textual response and that this quarrelsome tradition in and of itself suggests much about any analysis of the field.

Davis made four claims in her article about the tasks of bioethicists who would address religion. The validity of these four straightforward tasks for religious ethics scholars would be difficult to question, although none of the tasks are unique to a theological view. Davis claims that ethicists, whether secular or religious, should (1) explain the role of be-liefs in the lives of individuals and in the culture as a whole, (2) explain how a specific ideology wrestles with a moral issue and describe the ideo-logical position's current teaching, (3) describe how real people actually believe and act, and (4) be helpful and honest about their own positions. That Davis is concerned with religious beliefs does not call religious ethi-cists to a special imperative. It would, of course, be equally important (perhaps more important, since it is less common) for secular ethicists to explain their faith in Kant and the role such a structure of beliefs plays in the lives of individuals and cultures.

Although Davis initially made her claims about the tasks of any reli-gious scholar, the bulk of her original article accounted the failings of scholars in the field of Jewish bioethics. Most particularly, while Davis apparently believes that the second task (relating the specifics of ideology) is important, she clearly is most concerned with how Jewish bioethicists fail to fulfill her third task—describing how the constructs of faith are manifested in behavior that she can witness in the world.

Let me first delineate the areas where I agree with Davis, then offer my opposition, and finally describe the additional, necessary tasks of Jewish bioethics in the conversation of clinical ethics.

FISH ARE JUMPING AND THE COTTON IS HIGH: THE CREATION OF THE PERFECT WORLD

First, it is true that what was initially and, in the words of ethicist Ronald M. Green, "aggressively"[3] published in Jewish bioethics was primarily from only one venue of the wide range of Orthodox Judaism, which is, itself, part of a wider spectrum of Jewish theology that dwells in a community as diverse as the American context. Hence, the range of what we have accepted as Jewish bioethics has been too narrow. To take the most cogent example, women scholars have been largely excluded from the discourse. It is still possible to find a major national conference on Jewish medical ethics that features 15 men and a lone woman who only offers welcoming remarks (something Davis has written eloquently about in earlier articles.)[4] The most accessible authors have been those who write in English for American audiences; thus, many Israeli thinkers, who often have more liberal views even within the Orthodox position, have been excluded from the discourse. The field of these initially published thinkers is small, and obtaining credentials to become an authoritative voice is a complex and tightly restricted process; historically, the field has been limited to men who have studied in traditional academies (yeshivas). Many physicians rely exclusively on such a limited account of the field, unaware that it is the very nature of the Jewish tradition to invite a lively debate. As Davis points out, we need to listen to, read, and honor the insights of other thinkers: all of this is indisputable.

Further, the arena of scholarship featured in many texts is insular. Directed toward those who would care enough to actually purchase a book on Jewish medical ethics, these texts are written for a specific audience living within a particular scholarly tradition, and the language can be difficult for outsiders to understand or evaluate. Many of the scholars do not engage in the multidisciplinary community that is the field of bioethics (Fred Rosner is the exception here), and some are genuinely innocent of the major national societies of bioethics. Just as it is critical that general, secular bioethics learn from the insights and language of the Jewish tradition—particularly from the creative casuistry of the talmudic method itself—so too it is critical for Jewish scholars writing as bioethicists to understand the deeply nuanced and intricate world of bioethics debate and to take the time to go beyond reaction to the debate to engage in the trouble and tension within the field.

I would add that more tragic still is the way that the passionate intensity of the texts themselves has been demurely obfuscated by many authors. Jewish texts are convoluted, deeply intertextual, and culturally referent. Across centuries and geography, across details and stories, the rabbinic authorities shout and interrupt; barely an answer can be given that cannot be refuted. Because of the diversity inherent in this method, it is imperative that today's writers claim their own perspective, open their texts, and not merely give conclusions that, in turn, can be reexamined and critically reviewed. This is too rarely done.

Second, I agree with Davis that all analyses of difference should be located in the actual history and sociology of the difference. In other words, ethics is framed by the parameters of the actual. Such sociology is of great interest in any ethical analysis. It is churlish to note that much of the secular bioethical reflection fails to do this well. Many places offer such reflections on the sociology of the Jewish-American community. Davis is right to note a sort of disconnect in the writing of many authors, an oddity that she would find even more painful if she were to look at the talmudic discourse upon which they draw. Here, she would find the dramas and cases of the time—embodied human narrative and richly detailed stories that are the grounds for the axioms that all too often are presented to modern readers as principles divorced from today's realities.

YOUR DADDY'S RICH, AND YOUR MOMMA'S GOOD LOOKING: THE CENTRALITY OF HISTORY AND TRADITION

This being said, I disagreed with Davis on other significant points. Davis's article, for all of its thoughtful insight about the troubled history of Jewish bioethics, is ultimately propositioned on a fundamental misconception about the role of religious ethics in the clinical and sociopolitical world. It is the historic place of Jewish rabbinic commen-

tary to be at the juncture of the messy details of human and social life
and to argue for an actual response from such a location. But Davis relies
on a truism for her analysis that is the stuff of common angst among the
organized Jewish community: most American Jews, while happy to claim
bagels and early Woody Allen movies as their own, practice little in the
way of their religion, know less about textual or historical tradition, and
are committed to only the briefest moments of Jewish daily observance.
The Jewish identity in the American diaspora has become an amalgam of
cultural nostalgia for a Yiddishist past of a particular era and stock liberal
theory (civil rights, regard for the underdog) that emerged in more or
less a continuous line from the Enlightenment. Such is the nature of
assimilation—the loss of distinctive beliefs and behaviors in an effort to
merge with the cultural norm. That these data might be helpful in understanding the sociology of the Jewish community is undoubtedly true,
but it is not the question asked in queries about Jewish ethical systems or
about what a Jewish tradition offers when confronted by normative problems in clinical ethics.

That differential gaps exist between theory and practice is not news
in either normative or descriptive ethics in any tradition. We can understand this by returning to one of Davis's own stories. Davis imagines
that we are to explore the beliefs and behaviors of, for example, a ballet
dancer. Suppose further that a medical resident wanted to understand
how ballet dancers approach issues in bioethics. To do this, the resident
must understand how various social factors influence the dancer's belief
structure. Is this fellow a ballet dancer who practices daily, who performs publicly, who works in the world as a ballet dancer? Or is he
someone who likes ballet, took ballet lessons as a child, and now dances
a few times a year?

Similarly, when seeking an answer from Jewish ethics about the Jewish view on a particular question, it is important to understand the nature of the question and the intent of the questioner. Is the question
really about how most Jews in America would react to a problem? (Or as
Davis would have it, how real Jews relate to the fantasy world she finds
in the modern theology?) If so, then a descriptive sociology would be
called for. Does the question concern how a religious Jew is urged to
react by authorities in her community? If so, then a response that addresses normative patterns within the tradition is certainly more appropriate than a description of what lots (or even lots and lots) of Jewish
people do. Hence, the questioning medical resident posited by Davis
must be asked further questions if we are to help her. Does she want to

know how Jews who live within the traditional context think about that context? And such a question asks more of us as respondents than a simple excursion into multicultural understanding of the exotica of religious communities. Here we need to make fundamental decisions about the nature of authority in bioethics; what makes texts authoritative is the stake claimed by the participant for use. Davis's article reflects some confusion about the nature and the relevance of such authority. Not only is sociology insufficient, but such quantitative sociology might lead our resident to think that the belief structure, the meaning, and the necessity that religious Jews find in the texts is simply not relevant for her practice. Nothing could be further from the truth.

Bioethics in general, and religion in general, serve both a legitimizing and a prophetic function. This fact is commonplace in any religious tradition. When we ask for explanations of religions we want to know both how they work in the world and how we struggle to make them work in the world. This is not so very different from how we teach informed consent or truth-telling, for example. We quote Kant with the same seriousness as Jewish authorities quote Maimonides; we repeat his notion of universalizability as though it were the golden rule. We argue about the principle of autonomy with a nearly sacred attachment to its reality, all the while undeterred by the fact that many real clinicians lie to patients with alacrity in the clinical context. And few of those clinicians have heard of Kant, let alone structure their lives consciously on his principles. This information[5] does not seem to discourage us. In fact, the reason people turn to bioethics texts for authoritative advice on how they should act is precisely because any sociology, even a reflexive sociology, does not create normative guidelines. Philosophy is not a poll of attitudes. Were this true, no warrant would exist for teaching virtue theory. Hardly a clinician can be found who always acts as we propose in the perfect world of bioethics.

What Davis misses is the nature of the resident's quest. The resident may well meet representatives of the Jewish community who do take talmudic inquiry seriously. Such people are not rare curiosities; she will meet many if she practices in New York. In fact, since honest disclosure is a premise that Davis encourages, I write and practice from within the very tradition. I struggle with the meaning of belief and with commitment to a method, with a history and with a religious legal system of commandedness (*Halakah*) that is central to a vision of a moral journey. To live within such a tradition has meant, for all the thousands of years since its inception, to quarrel, to study, to rethink texts, to reflect on the world around as it changes, to seek a casuistic and nuanced and mutable analysis. When Davis makes the following claim: "There are almost no similarities between the views set forth by the authors and the behaviors and attitudes of most Jewish people. . . . [The resident] almost would have been better off had she done no reading at all,"[6] she is simply missing a key point. It is precisely the people who do read and rely on such texts that the medical resident wants to know about. Surprisingly large numbers of Jews do know and care about the talmudic inquiry. It is abundantly clear even when reading Reform, Conservative, or secular Jewish ethicists. Why? Because in article after article, all cite texts as a way to locate the discourse. It may be the one thing that such diverse Jewish thinkers as Ronald M. Green, Louis Newman, and Fred Rosner have in common. Even in his call for a new approach to Jewish ethics, Green quickly cites, as prooftext, essential talmudic sources. Note that even in refuting the traditionalist approach, he immediately turns to the talmudic text to make his point.

All agree that any rigorous Jewish ethical response must reference the halakic system, the language of such a system, and the cultural context of a particular people.[7] There are valid reasons to start with the talmudic texts, and that common reference point is a strength. Such texts ground the complex reality of the field—a field unthinkable without the history of the Jewish people, the shadows of oppression, the tragic choices, the attention to the texts of long-ago arguments, carefully preserved. The cases and the debate are the rabbinic texts of the Talmud, and any serious investigation of any ethical system must consider its internal structures. Just as it would be important to explain to a new student that what the Pope thinks does actually influence what American Catholics think, even if they disagree, so too it is important to explain that particular texts of the Talmud and the later medieval Responsa literature do have meaning in this context, and that Jewish values do not spring mysteriously from the past. Just as we carefully teach *Quinlan, Cruzan,* and other case law to new students and just as we do not discuss bioethics without actual clinical cases, a grasp of secular law, and a sense of the importance of the U.S. Constitution, so too we cannot teach Jewish bioethics without attention to the internal legal structure of the tradition. As in secular bioethics, it is not an attachment to legalism *per se,* it is that the legal record of our disputes and dicta describes the process by which our thinking about the tangible clinical world has evolved.

Davis is correct in noting the difficulty in descriptive language in the field to this point, yet even as her first article was published in 1994, the discourse was overtaking her argument as more scholars entered the field to reshape it. In this, I want to turn to the challenge that Davis raised: What are the tasks of method and content in Jewish bioethics? In my initial response I described the centrality of the prophetic voice in Jewish medical ethics. In this chapter, I expand both the list of tasks for the field and a justification of why my claim emerges from the rabbinic tradition to offer some critical metaphors for the larger field of bioethics. Here follows what I argue can be counted as some distinctive contributions to the field of bioethics—a justification for the unique tasks of the discipline to an emerging discourse.

RELIGION'S DISTINCTIVE CONTRIBUTIONS TO BIOETHICS

THE SUBVERSION OF THE MASTER NARRATIVE

The widely shared presumption in medical science is that human physical redemption is in fact possible.[8] Medicine "works" on a collective, even if not entirely justifiable, faith in the progressive Enlightenment narrative that reason and science can solve any conundrum. In this narrative, technology is heroicized and, moreover, this technology has a Tayloristic, motion-study stance that is certain, solutional, and hence nearly sacred.[9] Like any other machine, the medical machines and the medical orders that are impelled by a culture shaped by machinist ideology, there is a hierarchy and "one best way." It is a technical challenge to research and to discover but, once known, the right act is inescapable, efficient, with measurable data on the best possible outcome.

Modern medical science trumped a religious apprehension of the world because it could be, in this important sense, proven, whereas the truth claims of faith could not. But modernity faltered at the very moment of its triumph in the 20th century. What could be certainly known and universally experienced became contended, deconstructed by the recognition that the particular vantage of the "reader" defined the meaning, worth, and truth of the text of any endeavor. With the collapse of modernity as an organizing story for this century—and in at least some measure because of the consequences of medicine and technology taken to the most immoral of extremes in the Holocaust—the linear absolute of a liberating secularity that was rational, objective, and therefore truthful was deeply shaken. In fact, even the premise that modernity offered—that full control and hence autonomous choices are directly and linearly related to the constitution of human personhood—was contested.

In particular, the language of bioethics has rested in the notion of a universally held belief that what made one free, and human, were the personal, individual liberty rights that allowed for choice. Yet postmodern critiques question the search for the universal, not only as an imposition of a false unity, but as a false and incomplete totalizing of how the human world is witnessed. The free, choosing self with unlimited and insatiable needs is a fine description of a consumer or contract buyer in the marketplace, but this person might not be the best sort of citizen.

And hence in this view, if the secular is suspect, the religious (usually named as the spiritual or numinous, rather than the transcendent) is figured to supplant it. Religion—because it is particular, culturally bound, and relationally based—offers a particularistic narrative that, simply by existing, serves as a comment on the totalizing effects of the scientific method. At the very least, to acknowledge the particular voice of religion's claims is to acknowledge the multiple voices of the moral horizon. There is, by now in bioethics, nothing new in this critique. Michael Walzer, Charles Taylor, Stanley Hauerwas, and Alaister MacIntryre have fully explored this view. It is a commonplace of the field to note the tension between our attachment to autonomous choice, and to read the documents of the protection of that choice—the advance directive, the Patient Self-Determination Act (PSDA)—with canonical authority. At the same time, bioethics as a field does understand the limits of that language, hence the simultaneously ritualized gestures toward the importance of "nesting"[10] or toward the location of the family. This tension and contention about what is truthful in our experience has marked the history of medical ethics for generations. In this the field recognizes the way that the very existence of a passionately held alternate claim disrupts the authority of the tightly ordered reality of the clinical world.

THE TEXTS OF RESISTANCE

It is an old contention that the disruptive, prophetic quality of religion is what makes religion so historically dangerous to the state, authority, and dominant worldviews. In point of fact, religious discourse and stubborn interpretation of texts and meanings underlie the particularly American idea that religious freedom is a matter of social policy. Religions, particularly populist religious movements, were the historical enemies of modernity. In fact, the stance and formative vocabulary of modernity posited a free individual, born at last free into a venue without prior obligations or nonvoluntary commitments, promises, or passions.[11] Modernity's hegemony rested on universal language and universal notions of the good—in this sense, a "text" of order that was universally held—and in the ideology of equality as similarity. Universalism meant that the liberal and then the progressive thrust was for a democratic egalitarian spirit. It was precisely this spirit that animated modern philosophy and public policy. Religion, in this system, was divisive, destructive of that which could unite all peoples and nations. Religions—as archaic, as ruthlessly embodied—were best discarded, as they were attachments to the irrational, the superstitious, the ignorant.

But we do not live in modernity, only in its explanatory shadow, knowing the darkness behind the buildings of the cities we have made. Hence, in the clinical world, where much has gone astray—where we are already dealing with the outskirts of the expectable, controllable world— we are confronted with both the force and the pluralities of religious explanatory narrative. In fact, it is precisely at the moment of crisis in the clinic that there is the utter recognition that the medical gesture (even the dramas of reproductive technology) is actually a gesture concerning death. This is a moment that Americans see as their most religious, a moment when what is at stake is the relationship between the self and God.

And Americans-as-patients are a very religious people, relative to many other European nations and to most medical staff. Americans attend church or synagogue, or the mosque, and Americans believe in God. In fact, the sober *New York Times* surveys can tell us that a paradigmatically typical American day includes daily prayer. One might argue that Americans just *say* that they pray daily to the Times-CBS poll takers, along with believing in organ donation, but American also *act* religiously (and they do not donate organs willingly). We can witness this behavior at moments of national crisis—the Oklahoma City bombings, for example—when prayer becomes public, and clearly genuine.

Consistently, despite the ubiquitous faith in secularity, pleasure, and science, there is a persistent yearning to see a moral, meaningful trajectory in one's private arena, in one's workplace, and in the social goals of a state. Alasdair MacIntryre and Stanley Hauerwas have reminded us that we learn secular history in discreet sections; secular history does not have an intrinsic thematic importance, an end, a goal, or a good, let alone such a shared good as the group project of Exodus. But religion persists in asking about goal, *telos,* ultimate meanings, and long-term consequence. While religion is not alone in this endeavor, it insists on this, insisting on the question of moral meaning in the way that science insists on the question of replicable physical data. In the context of religion, human persons are entasked or burdened by the obligations that are linked to this goal. This is the mark of the person of faith, as much as the mark of the Enlightenment was to describe the human person as possessive of rights and capable of possessing tangible commodities, another kind of freight.

For MacIntryre, a central aspiration of the Enlightenment was to provide for debate in the public realm of standards and methods of rational justification by which "alternative courses of action in every sphere of life could be adjudged just or unjust, rational or irrational, enlightened or unenlightened."[12] This project of reason, like the project of industrialization, was seen as liberatory; the ascendance of rationality over authority was viewed as despotic, and tradition was viewed as constraint on the human imagination.

But once the modern self is liberated in this way—untied from all precommittments, social position, and communities other than those that are freely chosen from a position of complete autonomy—a new authority has to emerge, an autonomy that must unhesitantly act as guide in a trackless world. Because this world has no intrinsic signposts, and because the maps are out of favor, the authority must be constructed as absolute, yet rational, based in laws of physical science. In this view, unchosen religious faith and inexplicable commands and laws are suspect, wacko, embarrassing, certainly not in the same discursive encounter with the sciences. In this context, MacIntryre reminds us, suffering is absurd and needs to be eliminated, because it is a threat to complete autonomy. Michael Walzer describes a similar development: that hospitals have replaced churches as projects worthy of joint communal action.[13] As reason and science promise restoration and rescue, then the tasks of redemption and witness become less compelling and, hence, less "real."

THE PLACE OF THE SUFFERING STRANGER

Charles Taylor noted that this Enlightenment ideology meant not just new science, but a new view of human dignity—a view in which dignity of persons comes from their ability to be in disengaged, rational control of unruly processes.[14] In fact, the notion that all of life is subject to rational control became the hallmark of early modernity, reflected in art, architecture, and horticulture. The assumption of the Enlightenment is that everything that trespasses on this rational control that is ordered by personal autonomy—including suffering, disease, and loss—can and ought to be progressively eliminated. Ernest Becker traces the increasing denial of the unruliness of illness and death as a development associated with this understanding.[15] Meanwhile, theology as a discipline and a discourse became disassociated from the emerging views of science and gradually eliminated from serious academic inquiry; it came to be regarded as superstition or folk affiliation rather than as a reasonable explanatory or organizing principle. But without the coherency of a moral life project, or an agonistic struggle for meaning, there could be no sensible—certainly no rational—explanation for suffering. Death's framing inevitability becomes denied and avoided.

Thus the new explanation emerges, shifting the explanatory burden from reliance on God's will to the belief in human understanding and power. Then, sickness is utterly meaningless, merely the occasion to be marginalized, powerless, out of control. It is the worst problem imaginable—far worse for humans in the modern age than the problem of divine reward and punishment or the afterlife, because we think of sickness as something we should be able to affect (witness the popularity of bran flakes and now soy products). If we are the ones in autonomous control of our destiny, on an unpredicated terrain, then if we are lost it is our own foolish fault; if the stranger next to us is wandering, ill, or lost, it is not our problem to address. Our most cherished presumption is that we can control the invisible world of foes—an invisible virus or invisible corrupt genetic codes. We then do not need a community capable of caring for the sick, in the words of Hauerwas; we need a personal instrumental rationality made powerful by technological sophistication.[16]

Hence, all illness is pointless. The ill one can play no role; his or her life is an absurdity, a perversion. It is disquieting to see. Thus the call comes to eliminate sufferers from chronic illness if their chronic illness defeats us; is judged too disturbing; or, lately, is judged too expensive. And from this cause comes the flight from this terrible, lonely vulnerability to the only structure for control left intact in modernity—the legal assertion of autonomy; the thinnest and the most desperate of the requests we can truly honor in the clinic is the request to be left alone.

But religious practice insists on far more than this view and, in this, bioethics has a critical emulative model. Even in religious communities that emphasize individual responsibility and individual relationships with God, and surely in the practice of traditional Judaism, the suffering stranger will not be alone. We will always live in a world where people will sicken and die. We cannot cure this, if by cure we mean eliminating the creaturely experience; this is, after all, the point of the story of Eve.[17] But in a society of strangers, doing "stranger medicine," we act as if we expect that each encounter should be successful, that our part in it must "work."

This affects us as ethicists. I too want my every consultation to be successful, whatever this means in bioethics.[18] But living this way, without humility, which is a religious virtue—has its price. The primary cost to us of this amnesia is the failure to connect the position of the stranger with the life course of the self. But this is not the only cost. Another cost results when we turn over the entire problem of a fitting end to human life to unmediated medical science. If there are no moral limits describable, except "medical failure," there is a rising importance of the law in bioethics. Linked to this are the struggles about medical futility, in which teams of people argue about finding a "purely objective medical limit" to life, or the way that many yearn for physician-assisted suicide to sanction a medicalized death. These issues constitute the other side of the coin of the perspective that control ought to be ultimate, and that suffering is a medical failure and can be medically managed.

Hauerwas has reminded us of this problem: "When we have overcome winglessness with airplanes, summer heat with air conditioning—when we can overcome all this, there will be two things that will shatter our illusion that we can make do without coping: death and the evil in our hearts."[19]

THE PROBLEMS OF IDOLATRY

In bioethics we can tend to forget that medicine is about the problem of human suffering and that human loss is not a failure to be managed, but a tragedy. We forget this at our own moral peril, because forgetting one's place and confusion about one's stature is the classic problem in religion, called by the name of *idolatry* in Jewish texts. An attention to classic texts returns us repeatedly to the problems of relationship between the self and the stranger that are at the heart of the clinical relationship in the modern period. There is an oddness about stranger medicine—a moral oxymoron. Here we, as healers and as ethicists who witness healing, have our work, our workplace, our income, and our research project; our work is only possible because of the dark tragedy of others, their brush with death—it is because of their wager with death that they will acquiesce to us—because we are medical professionals. They will submit to the clinic to be rescued from mortality.

But theological speculation is never far from this problem—the making of meaning in the face of suffering and the search for the veracitic nature of the world against the potential for false gods and false passions.

This may be why it is uncomfortable to the field of bioethics to have theologians around, why it is embarrassing to have a tradition of exposure, of skepticism about the local miracles and the fancy artifice. In part it is a linguistic problem. The language of the Golden Calf, the language of the battlefield, the language of the playing field, or more recently the language of the marketplace is undermined by the principle of faith. This is in part because of what I have called the *prophetic imperative* of religious bioethics, and in part because of the moment of faith itself—the way in which that sacred moment, made specific in time and place, fully apprehended and encountered, breaks the totality with which modernity surrounds us.

This is one reason why the issue of whose vision "counts" is important when disagreement about the use of life support in futility cases ends up in the courts. The cases involving Helga Wanglie and her family, Stephanie Harrell and her Baby K, and countless other families whom bioethicists have seen clinically are, paradigmatically, struggles waged by deeply religious people. Only strong and certain faith can offer a serious challenge to the strong faith of medicine; any other resistance appears in the medical context as psychosis. Here the claims of religious faith do create impediments to the system—ones that recall the fragility of medicine's claims. The systemic theology of science is quite powerful, tantalizing not only to the clinician, but also to the ethicist. It takes the serious regard for religion to remind bioethicists that our faith in science can be as abstract as religious commitment, to remind us that prayer works at least as well as, for example, Zantec does for the treatment of pyloric ulcers or fiber does for prevention of colon cancer.

MIDRASHIC IMAGINATION AND
THE ARGUMENTATIVE DISCOURSE

Texts of resistance remind us of this and resonate with the narratives of the clinic. Biblical texts, with their unsettled questions and the dark lacunae and the flawed heroes are a template for the lacunae of medicine and allow for a midrashic, interpretive, and contextual analysis of the medical narratives that we are called on to reflect upon. Walzer notes that the Exodus story has been a resource for challenges to authority for resistant communities for centuries, with its narrative of faith and opposition of the powerless to the technology of Pharaoh. Unlike the narrative of medicine, the central message is of the triumph of the weakest over the certainty of the given order.[20] Such texts serve as the tropes of resistance. Hence, the first and most critical distinction of the religious imagination and sensibility would be the admission of that canon as equally weighted with the canons of philosophy, law, and the history of medicine—all texts before which we stand and argue. Full attention to these texts illuminates far more than the etiology of the rituals and constraints that one encounters in the clinic. Attention to the intertextuality of the narratives offers a methodology for casuistry and debate in bioethics.

But it is not only the way that the complex classical texts are explored, it is the method of adjudication of the law that is drawn from the narratives that can offer bioethics an alternative method of reflection. *Halakah,* the law, is justified by recourse to story, the *midrash,* and the placing of the classic type scenes against the dilemmas of community life that the scholars struggle to adjudicate. The habit of social, textualized argument is one that is central to the system of Jewish ethics itself. Since the texts are in disagreement at many points, and since the midrashic texts are often fanciful and speculative, with much to quarrel with, the tradition is clear regarding respect for the forum of debate rather than regarding the principles of the argument. Such a method—which allows participants to draw from the full range of story, history, and anecdotal evidence—is not only talmudic; Catholic canon law is based on the same argumentative approach. But the talmudic argument operates without a papal authority structure. The community discourse, the logic of the justification, the consideration of the minority, and the privilege of multiple voices all are hallmarks of the conversational method of Jewish ethics. Just as Socratic dialogues suggest a heuristic method, a rabbinic method provides another such template for inquisitive reflective analysis. Not only does the *bet midrash*—the house of study—replace the destroyed Second Temple as the central theological venue for normative Judaism, but also the metaphor of the discourse community is the controlling metaphor for intellectual and ethical life.

A SENSE OF PLACE

Our understanding of the tasks of the scholarship of religion, I argue, can emerge from the cognition that a questioning, conversant community surrounds every gesture of medicine and bioethical reflection. Such a central focus on community is related to yet another argument for the role of religious studies, based on a classic insight from the discipline of cultural studies. The sense of place, history, and tradition; a past that is shared and a future that is anticipated; and a cultural stance that frames the context of health, illness, and death cannot be apprehended without a real understanding of the role that religious praxis plays in the life of the medical provider and the patient. In this way, the work of Dena S. Davis and others draws our attention to the varieties of the religious experience and intensity of culture at the moments of confrontation with vulnerability and chanciness.

But it is not only in the clinical arena that communities of religious meaning play a central role. Americans greet each research advance with a query toward faith commitments, staking out the ground of faith and negotiating the response in light of faith in a reflexive casuistry. When cloning or human embryonic stem cell research is on the agenda, it is apprehended as a religious-moral problem, solved by textual recourse or an interview with the religious expert. This is not a formalistic gesture. When interviewed in the popular media, Americans selected for their ordinariness speak of the problem in religious terms—unease with "playing god" or the "sanctity of life." What makes the sense of violation or at least controversy in these situations is that some boundary has been crossed—a concept that makes rational sense only if one notes a boundary. Yet it is not constraints of philosophic reason that create such a terrain. The parameters of religions, even the lost ones of childhood faith, are the ones cited when discomforture is described.

Without a religious discourse, the issue of brokenness, of evil, of the necessity to heal a broken world irrespective of personal monetary gain— *tikkun olam*—all are lost to bioethics. Bioethics itself becomes "placeless" and can be marginalized by most people as sterile, abstract, or—worse yet—reducible to jurisprudence.

ONE OF THESE MORNINGS, I'M GOING TO RISE UP SINGING: THE NECESSITY OF THE PROPHETIC VOICE

Of all the tasks that religious theorists and theologians must take as central, and one of the most important reasons to have the theological voice about in the field, is the responsibility of the frankly prophetic voice. Religion ought not to be content with sweet pastoral explanation: at its heart theology is a lot of trouble. The stance of the theologian, and most especially the Jewish theologian, to be an outsider, claiming possession of an unpopular truth.[21] That this may seem radical is to be expected. It is a radical claim that one's meaning is important; it is not simply a quaint or polite attraction in the public arena, but a challenge to it.

Jewish bioethicists, for example, must explain how both the "commandedness of the daily," and the sacredness of the daily act, function not only for the Jew who is alert to this role, but for the secularist who is not. Christian bioethicists must explain how the model of the sufferer as healer can work in the modern context. This must be done in a way that is neither triumphant nor apologetic, which suggests that theology is neither extraneous nor privileged.

SPEAKING TRUTH TO POWER

Calling the ethical question in the clinical world is of necessity very difficult. The clinic is steeped in the tradition of the hierarchical relationship; the role of the ethicist is nearly always that of a curious outsider, the scientific enterprise made difficult by the freighted nature of the search for objectivity that is itself embattled. Yet the prophetic tradition can tell us much about the imperative of the outsider who can see an alternate vision. Challenging the "is" with the "ought" leads us to fruitful understandings about the role of the alternate claim, leads us to challenge the givenness of the relationships as presented, and leads to an ironic view of diagnostic certainty. Such language is neither safe nor endearing. That the historical place of the philosopher, as well as the theologian, was to remain the outsider can easily be forgotten. The first task of any theology is to remember that it is the brokenness of the world itself that calls us to the work of repair.

The issue of suffering in medicine is political as well as personal and, in this, the texts and commitments of religious discourse can be critical. What potentiates the suffering associated with illness in the United States is the framing of medical care by the marketplace and by the system of distributive justice that is chosen for healthcare. A story to serve as an example: A child in the pediatric hospital where I have consulted, who has Medicaid coverage, can only get morphine for her terminal cancer pain and cannot get the more effective pain medication that a child with better, private health insurance can get. Addressing such a problem demands an insistence on justice that is as clear as our commitment to autonomy, and only the strongest of justice demands can answer the argument based on cost-benefit analysis. Where can an academic field divine the prooftexts for such an argument, and where can an academic field find the justification for an activist praxis? We can learn, for example, from theologian Gustavo Gutierrez that the ethical question begins with the question of our alliances.[22] From Guiterrez's liberation theology, a literature that is barely mentioned in the footnotes to bioethics, we can know that the voices of the most vulnerable carry with them a power that is unimaginable—a paradox. We can remember to regard claims of medicine as claims of a particular ideology, and use a hermeneutics of suspicion when we encounter them. Guiterrez, and in the Jewish tradition, Emmanuel Levinas, insist that the call of the stranger is not only a normative issue, but an ontological one.[23]

THE CONSTRUCTION OF THE SELF

It is this ontic call of the stranger that allows religious theorists to have a differently apprehended view of the self, and it is this differently apprehended self that demands a rethinking of one of our most treasured concepts of bioethics. In the past, the field of bioethics has turned to scholars of Jewish bioethics and other religions to focus on precisely what was mentioned in the paragraphs immediately proceeding this one. What was sought was a descriptive account of how different traditions do the things that attend birth, illness, and death, and to be taught how to be culturally sensitive to such accounts. But this type of approach only begins our work; it is akin to a multicultural cookbook—a curiosity, but not the way one really eats. An attention to the broader question of what religion's tasks might be in the field of bioethics brings us to a larger methodological problem. What might it mean to construct an ethics in which we speak as both particular persons and as members of a particular community, living in a contending state? An ethics in which we speak to an explicitly postmodern critique, of which religious differences and other differences play a central part?

Such a method will call for a different vocabulary and a careful analysis of our moral location. Who are the subjects and who are the objects of all of the talk we do in bioethics? How are the nature and the vocabulary of the talk reflexively shaping our understanding of the field itself?

When we reflect on the secularized language of bioethics, we find that it asks: "How ought you (implied subject: powerful doctor) treat the other (implied object: powerless patient)? Religious ethics and moral theology ask instead: "How ought I to live?" and asks how a Subject—who is simultaneously an object (I, you, believer)—ought to respond to the Other (who is always both the object of the moral gesture and the powerful Subject).

The power relationships shift dramatically and uncomfortably. Dramatically because the embodiment of the discourse is far from classic reflections of philosophy; uncomfortably because it is only in the worlds of faith and illness in which we are so exposed and vulnerable. Thus, we see the use of the reflexive method that can be implied by religion in bioethics. First because we are embodied, and next because we are both subject and object, as we truly are in the medical encounter. Not only are we, as theorists, providers of healthcare, but we are impending patients. Hence, we are partakers of the complex passion, desire, and moral discipline that characterizes such paradoxical human social order. We live in bodies limited and graced by finitude and fecundity.

Without the radical recognition that this is so, all work in bioethics is singularly managerial in nature,[24] written from the disembodied, professional scientific perspective of the provider or manager of healthcare or the privileged venue of the academic that serves to distance us. Such work is emblematic of the project of the modern age itself, of course, but it bespeaks of a problem far deeper. For example, if we write from the point of view of the manager of healthcare, *we*, in the text of our accounting of bioethics, will never get sick and die. Hence the delineation of order within the analysis of the medical care system becomes a sort of protective mechanism. Think of how much is written about advance directives, for example, and how few physicians and nurses actually have them. Without a reflexivity in the field, without a humility and a sober knowledge of uncertainty and contingency, we can perform as healthy observers; the subjects are the sick ones, who need our guidance to help them in their pathology. This perspective pervades not only the medical literature and the canonical ethics literature, but the contentious task of the bioethicist as well. The tendency to treat the patient as the object of our rescue is the most benign face. Other views of patients include the "demander," the threat to rational allocation plans, the religious fanatic, and the story that we curiously examine.

A CRITIQUE OF AUTONOMY

Because of the near hegemony of the assumption and power of autonomy in clinical ethics, it is important for Jewish ethics to offer some reflection on the tenuousness of that claim. Jewish thought struggles not only with the nature of the self relative to the other and relative to the community, but also with whether the embodied self has what post-Enlightenment thinkers describe as rights at all. The notion of the good in this formulation rests not on the promise of voluntariness, but on the promise of obligation. A Jewish theological approach would explore the debate on the problem of informed consent with a reflection on the difficulty of the model of the unencumbered, disconnected patient engaged in neutral, rational discourse as a template for clinical ethics decision making. Such an approach would insist on the community of others who are dependent on and depended upon on as part of the process, questioning if voluntariness itself is possible or the ground for human freedom. Elsewhere I have argued that the talmudic method itself is one such template.[25] I posit here the talmudic notion that coming to truth is a process of debate, a conversation, and that this method can be extrapolated to clinical ethics review.

A VOICE FOR THE VULNERABLE: THE WIDOW AND THE ORPHAN AND THE STRANGER

Serious conversation and the serious call to prophetic responsibility and justice require a recognition of alterity. Linked to this alterity, or "otherness," is the necessity for advocacy rather than neutrality on behalf of the most vulnerable. As the theological stance of the Jewish text is that of the outsider, the theological claim is for the stranger and the powerless that dwell in our gates. Extrapolated into the world of the clinic, this becomes, again, nearly dangerous, for it assumes an advocacy that, in this era, becomes named as political. But to take seriously either the text, the history, or even the vaguely expressed "value" of Jewish thought means to take a partisan stand in the name of *tzedakah* (righteousness); this will of necessity have ramifications in the clinical world. The regard for the stranger as central to the social world offers a much-needed corrective to the problem of stranger medicine. These texts call for the encounter between the self and the stranger to be the place for ethics. Such a recognition of obligation and responsibility[26] is a problem of a far larger and more interesting order than naming the texts relative to, say, in vitro fertilization as a permitted or unpermitted reproduction tool, but it is precisely tasks of this magnitude that lie behind the daily encounters in the clinical setting.

Neighborliness, not the social contract, is the formative ground for religious reflection. In this, a sense of place allows us to see how a surety, a particularity, might offer a claimed moral terrain. The activities on this terrain might not be enforceable, but they might offer an organizing template for what we can hope for (in Kantian terms) in a larger social order. For example, the principle of neighborliness is that the stranger whom one meets might well be you; that vulnerability is inevitable and sequential in a human life; and that the challenge of autonomy is not how to liberate oneself from the bonds of human necessity, but the unlimited way one can pursue one's obligations without interference by a state.

But philosophy is worried about the stranger *as* stranger. And right relationships between strangers need minimalist, not maximalist, contracts. In a society as deeply divided as ours, it is useful, but *only* useful, to ask first what basic, decent, minimum standard of decorum, and of law, we might rely on. Hence: Rawls—the philosopher concerned with justice between strangers who make minimalist (but fair) contracts—serves as the ground of ultimate meaning. Callahan, Hauerwas, Lammers, and others have noted the paucity of this model in the freighted worlds of the clinical encounter. But religious theorists also note its power. For the Jewish ethicist, it is the necessity of the stranger that frames the obligational relationship itself. For the medical encounter, in which the obligation to the stranger is central, the stranger's call is that which wakes us in the night, the obligation from which we cannot turn.

Perhaps it is the presumption of the neutrality of strangerhood itself that needs to be challenged. It is, paradoxically, part of the power of the dogma, or of the certainty of the claim to truth, that it includes the listener as member. Seeking a faith ground assumes a maximal agreement—a contention regarding the ultimate question of death and veracity, the nature of the good, the ultimate obligation to one another. And the nature of the acts of evil are real, are actually choices. The liberal vision of a well-regulated state fails to capture the passion that binds the stranger; how intense the enmity can be, the xenophobia; and, hence, how deep the response of empathy and reversibility must reach.

Finally, a paradigm of neighborhood allows us to reexamine our assumptions of the field and its sense of appropriate uses of relationships of power and authority. Rawlsian relationships take account of contractual inequity and attempt to address this, but are truly impoverished when addressing the tragic at the heart of medicine. It is not self-evidently true that the relationship between health professionals and patients is best seen as a relationship between free and equal agents sharing in a cooperative venture.[27] We first need to ask in what way are patients "free" and in what ways not? What is the impact of one side carrying all the pain and loss, while the other partner is actually making a living—in many cases a living wildly privileged in proportion to what the patient partner could even hope for—because of the painfulness of the other? The human body is like the "body politic" in few ways but linguistically. The problem of "befalleness" is not only a management problem, it is a crisis of moral meaning, neither adjudicated nor corrected by justice. Patients really are sick. It is their pain, their call, their need, their *caeru* that sociologist Marianne Paget has reminded us that we address when we encounter a patient.[28] Attentiveness to the cry itself is far more than a marketplace interaction, frankly difficult to "deliver" and to "manage."

INTEGRITY IN THE FIELD

Can we hope that the field of bioethics will merely "emerge" as one with an internal integrity? Without a guiding moral theory, and without a mooring in some tradition of accountability, there is no sure counting on a decent response to the starkness of need—not for an ethics with the ability to remember Tuskgekee and Nuremburg, nor for an ethics willing to address the manipulation of HIV-positive blood, the falsification of consent forms, or the hundreds of daily encounters with evil large and small in clinical practice. These challenges to basic internal morality are what allow us to imagine bioethics as the Greek chorus, an idea developed by Kathryn Montgomery.[29] Such a chorus allows us to imagine an ethics that addresses the "text" that is the genuinely moral enterprise (Hauerwas's term) for the clinical encounter. And the reader, or the hearer of the text, or the self-reflective ethicist, will both hear the tragic need and have the tragic need—this will happen as surely as the breaths that we take now, as you are reading this sentence. But without context, the text becomes merely an interesting or arresting story. The premises of religion are what allow us to see that a link between command, authority, and normative action can be liberating as well as oppressive. How might evil be addressed? How can good actions be shaped and morally compelled? Faith traditions display one way in which discipline can be both normatively addressed and fully chosen.

HONORING THE DAILY

It is the attention to the detail of the daily encounter that a commanded religious system names as important. Jewish ethics speaks not only to the ontological and epistemic tasks as noted above, but also to the normative tasks, as well, and it demands an attention to each casual habit of speech, each clinical encounter, desire, and consumption. Such language can offer a changed perception of how clinicians see the interior textures of a variety of human choices, including lives that may appear to have a limited "quality" when measured in terms of economic productivity. Such language moves away from the contractual ground of clinical medicine into the terrain of the mutually obligatory. Such a stand is not hesitant to suggest that this claim is warranted by a conscience attributable not only to the self or even the community, but to a relationship with God. This is, after all, what makes up religious ethics.

Further, if a Jewish bioethics is to be truly honest with its readers, the field must recognize that being Jewish is distinctive from being Italian or Irish or African-American. Although it would be of interest to note cultural preferences among national or ethnic groups, what makes for a religious ethical system is not merely the compilation of (very many) prooftexts, but that such texts are a record of how a people seek for a relationship with the Divine—a subject deftly avoided in some reflections on Jewish ethics, even on religious ethics.[30] Although this creates automatic discomfort in academic conversation,[31] it is important to distinguish theology from social science, and it is a claim of truth based on that faith relationship that delineates the discipline.[32]

Bioethics has focused like media has focused on the big-ticket items—acute illness, rescue medicine, fringe research, decision making at the end of life—rather than on how to address the daily construction of illness, the ill and the well self, the simple actions of medical practice. The canon largely does what it has been asked to do, rather than seeking out new ground or going where it is not wanted. Accordingly, there is more in the literature about the dilemma of the "manager" and less about the "owner" of the enterprise. But focus on the "dailyness" of our decisions recalls for us the ordinary problem. Bioethics is also about and perhaps centrally about the tasks of daily living in a fragile body with foreknowledge of our own death.[33]

Bioethics needs to be praxis based; one might suggest it is tragically based, in narratives that are stopped—catching their breath, as it were—not only by the illness, but by the moral question of the continuance to the meaning of the story in the face of the illness.

This is the subject of religious view. It is this that classic religious ethics seeks to understand—not what is the relationship between me and my patient or my constituent, but what does God ask of me and what does this imply about how I ought to be in relationship to my neighbor? This question is not a marginalized or particular one for most Americans. (It may be marginal for persons who have devoted their lives to a close reading of Kant; of Rawls.) In this concern, the bioethicist who is concerned with these questions takes both their meaning and the fact of the inquiry as centrally important intellectual tasks. Religious inquiry is not reducible to dogma—any more than insistence on autonomy, or even those much-maligned principles are. In turning to these queries, one does not succumb to a loss of either self or reason. But, in part, at least, such a stand would envision a moral agent who believes in the religious paradigm that is centrally important—not an aside, or a quirky habit, or mere preference. To focus on the query is to contend for vocabulary in an academic discipline in which the act of conversation or ordinary talk matters, where talk is the currency of our social capital. If, in such a field, "faith talk" translates with oddity externally, it is at least partly because, in translation, the silence of the ritual act, of the gesture of trust, can seem absurd—an awkward, wingless flight.

THE NARRATIVE OF JUST CITIZENSHIP

The last few years in bioethics have seen an increase in Jonah literature—stories and movies about the physician turned patient who suffers all the indignities of the experience of illness, of being swallowed whole, as it were, and emerging to warn Niniva. But the people of Niniva are only a little more than cattle; as in the biblical story, they cannot tell their left hand from their right. They want to do the right thing, and they are *really sorry.* But all the Jonah stories repeat the tale. The hero will try to warn of the largeness of the task, the clinical world will try to respond, but the power of modernity is daunting. We know the truth of the tale, but the institution remains, and, without the edgy constancy of the prophetic voice, the insights that are gained in these narratives become mythic stories that we repeat over and over.

Without a conscious advocacy, the stories are ignored just as the patients were. But the power of bioethics and its tasks are real, and this will eventually offer everyone in the clinical setting a moment of conscience. The recommendations that we help formulate result in real life-and-death choices. We will find here that history cannot protect us, nor can the language of utility. As bioethicists, we partake of the violence inherent in both the embeddedness of medicine in the society at large and in the fortunes of the marketplace that supports the enterprise. This is precisely why the field's struggle for autonomy is so hard fought and takes so much of our attention. But, as a religious theorist, I believe that autonomy alone is not enough to guide us in this duty. When we investigate, when we "understand" the specifics of the situation of the other, we must be exquisitely aware of the transparency of even this gesture, of how agency sees the agency *as* agency, how our seeing of it constructs it, and how even the options that we bring are limited.

I am not sure how one patrols the borders of the political activity that bioethics creates or how, finally, that watchfulness translates justice and meaning into policy. For moderns, and especially for post-moderns, the insistence on justice and the thunder of outraged prophecy smack of moralism or hysteria. But I cannot imagine that bioethics without that voice can remain credible in a world of injustice. The discipline of religious studies insists that justice will be central to the matter of healthcare, it will name even the personal as political, and it will then claim the whole ground as a circumstance of citizenship.

It is this citizenship, the exchange of the clinical world that is surrounded by the larger social forces, that creates the final argument for religion in the discourse of bioethics. What will count for the reasonableness of argument in an actual world of chaos and competition will be the fullest, richest, and most robust alternate challenge. This is why I might argue for the reimagining of John Rawls's metaphor of justice. Rawls imagines justice and distribution at a table surrounded by veiled strangers, who face veiled strangers. But I picture something else—the kitchen table: the laundry is to be folded; the meal is to be made; the child will interrupt the old guy with the story retold; and me, with my argument from Jewish religious thought, will be interrupted with the argument of philosophy, then the argument of the law, then the argument of medicine, and this is the right metaphor for the social ground of the theory of bioethics. Instability and uncertainty stand at the center of the field, perhaps for an important reason—they stand in for the darkness at the heart of the work of healing, in whose service and whose light we as bioethicists have the privilege of witness.

Because clinical ethics consultation is rooted in the actual and tangible world of the bedside, it is too easily forgotten that efficacy entails vision as well as consequence, faith as well as rational discourse. In this venue, the perspective of the religious theorist has much to remind the bioethicist. There is a caveat to the largeness of the cultural tasks I propose for Jewish ethics and for all of religious ethics. As Davis points out to us, the relationship between the prophetic and the delusional can sometimes be judged by the presence of the congregation. The religious theorist who hopes to comment on the world of clinical medicine needs to find her or his home in the discussion without compromise, but without blindness. The rabbis of the Talmud emphasize that the age of prophecy has passed; that none are now given that ability; and that the role for intellectual leadership is to be teachers, enmeshed in the problems and the questions that come before them from the life of the people. This tradition creates a certain tension in that the role of the teacher is both to analyze what is practiced and to remember that more is possible.

AN ONUS OF MERCY

Finally, the work of the theological voice in bioethics is to insist on the onus of judgment and of mercy. Bioethics is about living within the tension between freedom and command, duty and choices—not simply about the resolution. It might seem obvious, in the breach, hence it needs to be explicitly stated that there is a responsibility that religiously informed bioethicists bear to the pastoral tasks within the clinical context. This is true for each discipline in the multidisciplinary field. Ethicists with medical training pay attention to the details of physiologic parameters, and lawyers have a clearer concept of the law. For religious scholars, the work of the spiritual, the role of the chaplain, and the necessity that the resolution of clinical cases include attention to the existential anguish engendered by illness is imperative. Bioethics' prophetic responsibility in this sense is about the *onus* of moral problems—not only the analysis of moral problems, but the *onus*—of affliction, liability, responsibility, trial, hardship, blame, load, and difficulty.

"He took him outside and said 'Look toward heaven and count the stars, if you are able to count them.' And he added, 'So shall your offspring be.' " (Gen. 15:4-6)

In the language of Israeli poet Yehuda Amichai:
Count them.
You can count them. They're
not like sand on the seashore. They're
not like stars without number. They're
like separate people.
On the corner and in the street.

Count them. Look at them
watching the sky through ruins.
Leave the rubble and come back.
Where can you come back to? But count them, for they
soothe their days with dreams
and walk about freely, and their unbandaged hopes
are agape, and that's how they will die.

Count them.
They learned too soon to read the terrible
writing on the wall. To read and to write on
other walls. And the feast goes on in silence.

Count them. Be there, for they've
used up all the blood and still need more.

Like major surgery, when you are weary
and sorely wounded. For who's to judge and what is judgement
unless it's the full import of night
and the full onus of mercy.[34]

NOTES

1. D.S. Davis, "It Ain't Necessarily So: Clinicians, Bioethics, and Religious Studies," *The Journal of Clinical Ethics* 5, no. 4 (Winter 1994): 315-9; L. Zoloth-Dorfman, "One of These Mornings I'm Going to Rise Up Singing: The Necessity of the Prophetic Voice in Jewish Bioethics," *The Journal of Clinical Ethics* 5, no. 4 (Winter 1994): 348-53; B. Freedman, "Bioethics and the Old-Time Religion: Response to Dena Davis," *The Journal of Clinical Ethics* 5, no. 4 (1994): 353-5.

2. Davis, "It Ain't Necessarily So," see note 1 above; D. Heyward and G. Gershwin, "Summertime," from the opera *Porgy and Bess* (Gershwin, 1935.) It should be noted here that Davis's use of the opera *Porgy and Bess* is (probably an unintentional) intertextual comment on her theme. An opera that is focused on the African-American experience and written by a Jew serves as an interesting parallel to the issues discussed here. Is this a Jewish opera? An African-American opera? What are we to make of such a text? Thus, I have elected to reply to her metaphor in kind.

3. R.M. Green, "Contemporary Jewish Bioethics: A Critical Assessment," in *Theology and Bioethics*, ed. E.E. Shelp (London: D. Reidel, 1985), 245-66.

4. D. Davis, "Beyond Rabbi Hiyya's Wife: Women's Voices in Jewish Bioethics," *Second Opinion, a Journal of Health, Faith and Ethics* 16 (March 1992): 10-30.

5. L. Zoloth-Dorfman, "Must We Always Tell the Truth?" (paper presented at the Washington Academy of Family Physicians Annual Meeting, April 1994). For additional work on the problems in informed consent, see D. Sulmasy et al., "Patients' Perceptions of the Quality of the Informed Consent for Common Medical Procedures," *The Journal of Clinical Ethics* 5, no. 3 (Fall 1994): 189-95.

6. Davis, "It Ain't Necessarily So," see note 1 above, p. 317.

7. See note 3 above; L. Newman, "Talking Ethics with Strangers: A View from the Jewish Tradition," *Journal of Medicine and Philosophy* 18, no. 6 (December 1993): 551. In this important article, Newman discusses some of the problems in the distinctiveness of the method of Jewish bioethics. "Neighbors do not share our moral values, hence the problem is how to speak one's own particular language in a conversation conducted in neutral, secular language." Newman notes that Jewish method derives from obstacles that Jewish theologians and ethicists have faced over the centuries. He is careful to remind us that his account is qualified. Classic sources are differently weighted, and there is controversy among the sources themselves. Further, one "must confront the

hard reality that our moral perspectives are incommensurable and that no ethics can be constructed solely on rational (that is, metaphysically neutral) grounds." See also F. Rosner, *Medicine and Jewish Law* (Northvale, N.J.: Jason Aronson, 1990).

8. M. Walzer, *Spheres of Justice* (New York: Basic Books, 1993).

9. Taylorism was an early response to modern industrialization. Taylor studied the physical actions of factory workers to attempt to eliminate all "wasted motion." The goal was to make workers more perfectly mechanized.

10. S. Wolfe, "Ethics Committees and Due Process: Nesting Rights in a Community of Caring," *Maryland Law Review* 50 (1991): 798-858.

11. Except for nationalism, which still allowed for hatreds.

12. A. MacIntyre, *After Virtue: A Study in Moral Theory* (Notre Dame, Ind.: University of Notre Dame Press, 1997); A. MacIntyre, *A Short History of Ethics* (New York: MacMillan, 1996); A. MacIntyre, *Whose Justice? Which Rationality?* (South Bend, Ind.: University of Notre Dame Press, 1989).

13. See note 8 above.

14. C. Taylor, *The Ethics of Authenticity* (Boston: Harvard University Press, 1999).

15. E. Becker, *The Denial of Death* (New York: Free Press, 1973).

16. S. Hauerwas, *God, Medicine, and Suffering* (Grand Rapids, Mich.: William B. Eerdmans, 1990).

17. Ibid.

18. There is, for example, scant literature on error in consultations. Since this chapter was written, there has been a stronger focus on error in bioethics. See, for example, the author's and Susan B. Rubin's work, *Margin of Error: The Necessity, Inevitability, and Ethics of Mistakes in Medicine and Bioethics Consultation* (Hagerstown, Md.: University Publishing Group, in press).

19. See note 16 above.

20. M. Walzer, *Exodus and Revolution* (New York: Basic Books, 1986).

21. Note, not *the* only truth.

22. G. Gutierrez, *The Making of Modern Theology: Nineteenth- and Twentieth Century Texts* (Philadelphia: Fortress, 1996); G. Gutierrez, *On Job: God-Talk and the Suffering of the Innocent* (New York: Orbis Books, 1985).

23. E. Levinas, In the Time of Nations, trans. M.B. Smith (Bloomington, Ind.: Indiana University Press, 1994).

24. D. Ainsle, "On Managerial Medicine," (paper presented at the Society for Health and Human Values, 1995 Annual Conference, San Diego California). Many of these remarks were made in connection with a response to Ainsle's paper. Ainsle uses his experience as a provider/participant in the acquired immunodeficiency syndrome (AIDS) community as a metaphor for how bioethics fails to address existential human agency. AIDS is a disease in which patients refuse to wholly accept the construction of themselves as ill as their shame, even in the face of the discriminatory response. In all other diseases, the message is clear—it is somehow the patient's fault. Americans use blame as another way to

protect themselves from the inevitability of pain. Ethicists are no exception to this deeply held liberty impulse.

25. See L. Zoloth-Dorfman, *The Ethics of Encounter* (Chapel Hill, N.C.: University of North Carolina Press, 1999).

26. Found for example in the work of Emmanuel Levinas. For a longer explanation of this point, see Zoloth-Dorfman, *The Ethics of Encounter,* ibid.

27. See note 24 above.

28. M. Paget, *A Complex Sorrow* (Philadelphia: Temple University Press, 1994).

29. K.M. Hunter, "Limiting Treatment in a Social Vacuum: A Greek Chorus for William T.," *Archives of Internal Medicine* 145 (1985): 716-9. [Katherine Hunter changed her name to Katherine Montgomery.—ED.]

30. Jewish ethics then is not just Jewish persons writing about bioethics. When I write an article about clinical consultation that makes no reference to the discourse of Jewish ethics, it is not an example of Jewish ethics.

31. For a full account of this, see S. Carter, *The Culture of Disbelief* (New York: Anchor Books-Doubleday, 1993), 3-83.

32. Ibid. Even to write seriously about a faith commitment is tricky; one runs the risk of being considered as a zealot. My intention is not to claim that a Jewish stance is the privileged one, but that it is my moral location, and as such I can claim some critical tasks as my own.

33. Such a canonical managerial approach is limited because it often ignores the deep passion for religion on behalf of the licensed vocational nurses (LVNs), aides, technicians, and others who do much of the invisible housework of the life-world of the patient. I cannot recall any articles in bioethics that focus on the dilemma from the perspective of the nurse's aide or LVN. I was an LVN for many years. I do not normally add this to my résumé, although, paradoxically, this experience—especially the experience (rare in America of extreme social and political solidarity) with African-American women coworkers—has shaped me as firmly as has graduate school. Secular bioethics literature is written from the assumed stance of and for the White, middle-class, university-trained reader. (Our committees too often reflect this, our documents are worse.) Little serious investigation has been done, as well as little analysis of the role of the ancillary staff (ancillary of course to the doctor, and not the patient). Is this because of who offers space to publish? Or is it because of the taint that might occur to one who focuses on the concerns of the powerless (such as salaries for pediatric and daycare center workers)? Given this, it is not accidental that little is know about strikes or opposition to managed care—issues that really concern workers and consumers. Are strikes moral? What is the dilemma of the housekeeper, of the clerk? Do we even know? Do we even ask? Does it strike us as irrelevant, and why is this?

34. Y. Amichai, "The Onus of Mercy."

Conclusion: Articles of Faith

Laurie Zoloth

THE NARROW RIDGE

The following quote from Martin Buber has animated this consideration of bioethics and religious thought: "I have occasionally described my standpoint to my friends as the 'narrow ridge.' I wanted by this to express that I did not rest on the broad upland of a system that includes a series of sure statements about the absolute, but on a narrow rocky ridge between the gulfs where there is no sureness of expressible knowledge, but the certainty of meeting what remains undisclosed."[1]

This book is, we hope, like a good talk with a few good friends or, better yet, a long walk with them on the narrow ridge that Martin Buber speaks of. It is a walk between and among everything that we know—and everything that we do not know, the covenant and the visions, the sacrifices and the blood, the lives cut in half and placed together—counting on the not-knowing to be that blazing scatter of stars that lights the way. Bioethics is not only about the big choices at the crossroads, but about how to live decently always, as though that would be enough. But it is also about, as the authors in this book recall for us, how the account of the community and of the ontology of the choosing self is deepened by a larger narrative—an uncontrollable, but ultimately trustworthy hope for order, which is to say the possibilities of language, the probabilities of compassion, and the deep and persistent yearning for justice that we believe inhabits the world.

The authors in this volume have addressed the large and complex issues of how to speak of the narrow ridge that lies for us directly in the midst of the terrain of bioethics. Why this is the case—that for modern Americans the persistence of faith maintains its hold and its claim of truth is far more easily observed than explained. That is why we can "do before we hear" and why we can maintain a moral imagination and intuition before we can write of the event. The ethicists in this volume are not alone in the event of faith. Many Americans speak of intuition as "just knowing" that something is wrong as new ideas and events in the clinical world unfold, and attribute this to their religious constructs.

As I was writing the conclusion for this book, a colleague dropped by for coffee. He read the paragraphs above, which I had just written, and decided that they made little sense. He had trouble understanding why it was that religion—aside from an abstract commitment to cultural diversity—should matter in a real and actual intellectual sense to the rational task of analyzing bioethical dilemmas. He was particularly amused by the part about "just knowing something is wrong" when Americans believe in such a lot of random passions.

As a child born under into the desert of Los Angeles, I decided that the night sky was a kind of a cover to the world, but a broken one, and that just under it lay the sheer, white, crystal blaze of light, revealed only by the holes in the blanket. We saw them as white fire on black, but they were really white fire through black—a critical reversal. My brother the scientist explained orbits and the arms of galaxies, but I was the philosopher and argued: beyond that, how could he really know? He won, of course, having maps, and finally, John Glenn. As Jeffrey Stout points out, there are things beyond relativistic stances. So perhaps religion is a variant of this idea, a delusion when we are struggling with medical fixatives as predictable as orbits.[2]

A question of modernity is: Of what *use* is religion? And it is tempting, although not sufficient, to answer this question with a modern response. Possible candidates for utility include the need for cultural coherency; the need for obligation beyond the frailty of romantic love; the regard for the stranger; the strength of communities of resistance; and the notion, first carried by science—but now, ironically, far more profoundly carried by faith—of deep skepticism in the givenness of modernity. There is more. There is the way that religion, because of the resistance community, not only resists triviality and the ugly, mundane banality that surrounds us, but offers a serious challenge to evil in the word; religion is not ashamed of seeing evil, naming it, and struggling to oppose it. And, not every time, but very many times in the last 2,000 years, it has been named as evil to oppress the vulnerable, to harm the widow and the orphan and the stranger. It is the basic argument made in my chapter, by Mendiola and Lebacqz, by Campbell, and many others herein.

In this sense, the existence of the strongly located alternate voice has functioned powerfully in the face of the certainties of history. (One thinks here of pharaonic or Roman or totalitarian certainty, and the courageous struggles and great losses to keep truth and human freedom alive.) One thinks of the yoke of faith that inspires the hospice volunteer to spend all night at the bedside of the poor man. Is this enough—that the large order of the universe reminds us, just enough, that the chief of academic medicine is not the final authority? To deconstruct the very ground of being in the hierarchy of the clinical world allows for the voice of the most vulnerable to claim linguistic terrain.

But there are many possible voices that could claim our attention and allow us to understand the multi-vocal nature of the conversation of bioethics. We could, and we should, be claimed by calls about race, class, and gender. So, what is it that is distinctive about what I am claiming about faith and this reasoning of faith done in this book?

RETHINKING THE QUESTION

The question to be asked of the place of religion in the field of bioethics is not whether we theologians and scholars of religion can make ourselves useful around the place or what we can add to the construction project of medicine and science, holding out in our cheerful, faithful way the clever tool to fix a problem. But rather, the question to be asked is the older one: How shall I live? And by this I mean: How is it that I can live, understanding that beneath the floor of this being—the solid stage, this intricate scaffold, and the good wood and sturdy decency of modernity; the technology and the art, and most especially the truth claims of science, buoyed by the big machines of science, Hubbell telescopes, and MRIs—lies a dazzling Reality, only glimpse-able.

In his consideration of this question, Peter Berger uses the term *doppelbodigkeit*, a term derived from the German stage, which refers to a stage with more than one floor. "Those who walk about on the upper floor may at any moment fall through a trapdoor onto the lower one."[3] Berger's argument is that modernity has created in us a credulity in the certainty of our ordinary reasonable existence, while dismissing as absurd anything that points us toward or hints at what philosopher Musil calls "the other condition,"[4] or what Emmanuel Levinas reminds us is the infinity, under the totality of what surrounds. Here I think, we are beginning to hear the right sort of question.[5]

Nowhere is the totalizing stronger, or more necessary, than in the clinical world. It is in the clinical encounter, where both of the participants have, for a moment, fallen through the trapdoor in the floor—You will die! I will die!—that we yearn the most for a way out. We, as good-hearted and well-trained modern individuals, proceed back up to the top floor, we get a grip, we talk of statistics and strategy, we understand the immanence of death, and we turn away from one another to the world of use. If we are healthcare professionals: What is to be done? Or if we are bioethicists: What is to be said?

And because we, as bioethicists, are the kind of moral philosophers who like applications (or we would be still off discussing bears in caves, or lifeboats in the 19th century), we turn our attention to how to make that talk lucid and truthful, and we help write policies that one can check off. If something goes awry in the conversation, we understand how to testify in the lawsuits, and we understand how each law functions for us as a measure of the strength of the structure we build, the moral architecture. These things, the words, and the events, all translate into the Hebrew term *devarim*—the "thingness" of the history.

LAWS OF GRAVITY

The world of words—the *devarim* world—is the world of creation that we are told to repair. It is a broken and unredeemed world, to be sure, so not only is it tempting, it is a good act to arch our moral gestures toward repair, colluding in what Martin Luther King reminds us is the human task: "The arc of history is long, but it bends toward justice." We must live as though there is certainty in such norms as, for example a maximum tolerated dose in Phase I drug trials, or reliable outcomes in genetic testing, or a diagnosis-related group for cancer surgery. But it is—as the members of the conversation in this book remind us—the role-specific duty of the bioethicist to pull the discourse away from the certitudes of social support—what Berger calls the "plausibility structures" that make a certain kind of belief possible (that one has an unconscious that can influence one) and certain kinds of belief impossible (that one has dead relatives that can speak).[7]

In some sense, the stance, the partisanship of the religious in bioethics is the rare claim for absolutes just beyond our understanding. What that means is that against, or rather beyond the idea of relative truths, Berger is asserting the knowledge, based on the feel of the actual world—or in his terms the "honor" one must ultimately give to one's perceptions—that there is a reality beneath us, and that there are these moments when, if we listen, we could hear it, glimpse it, be struck into silence before it, the numinousness of things.

An example of partisanship: I have spent much of this year thinking about the issues of genetics and bioethics. In this, as in so much of bioethics, what is at stake is the extent that we can "play God." But what is meant by that locution (odd in the context of the field)? It is, after all, a claim about power—that the unjustified use of our power will place us over some boundaries that we value. But what boundaries, and what values? Such a problem can only be understood as a secular way to ask the question of theological ethics, such as is struggled with by the authors in this book: What does God want of me? And that question implies that there is a transcendent way that the world must be structured, and it is a sacred order (in both senses of this term); to push beyond it might be arrogance. But the partisanship I am speaking of is not so simple. Jewish thought, for example, is in large part about the need to play God— "play" in the sense of "performing as"—acting as God might act. By this I mean that "play" admits the inevitability of failure, of conjecture and of risk, and that one is not working to deliver a product, but that one is involved in the process, which is everything. Performing the actions of goodness in the world, and of justice in the world, and of loving kindness are the very things we must try out again and again. Would that we would act with wild justice more often—unrealistic, larger than life, not accepting that the battle for the world's progress is a cause long lost.

ALIVE TO PARADOX

Religion, says my interrogator, looks phony. Meaning: the gestures and rules look like another kind of artifice. It is a familiar enough problem. If *real* is what is tangible—the boards beneath our feet—then religion as a premise looks like a stage set. For the more that religious institutions struggle to compete with modern organizations, the odder religion becomes—less believable; those guys on TV are like any other guys on TV. We cannot live on the broad uplands of any certainty after modernity, certainly not after graduate school. We will find the instrumentality of some religious forms a painful loss, dressed up in the trappings and do-dads of the marketplace. The basic idea of modernity is that the surface of the world—its appearance, how one looks, the clothes on the naked body—is what matters. One needs to look a certain way in order to be the object of the gaze; the gaze—the attention to the externality—is everything, and there is no meaning to be derived from the "itness," the surface facticity of the world. In fact, one of the essential premises of analytic secular philosophy is that there is no *ought* to be derived from the *it*.

But the point of faith is precisely that there is a nature *beneath* the nature of things—what it looks like now is only a part of what is possible; the moral action is not always visible. Such an understanding is only possible if one is alive to the complexities that link the physical to the possible—to the text of belief. A paradox.

AFTER THESE
THINGS/WORDS/EVENTS

We live walking along the way, taking comfort, then, in exile. It is only with the admission that we must live in the daily and do emulative and evocative gestures—ones that remind us of a column of smoke that we once saw—that life is bearable. We are, after all, at home in the world. But as Buber reminds us, we can see the spine of the ridge, see the stones and the bones of it under our feet at times. The shudder of a good read, the man who turns to me and tells me of his memory of an act of mercy in Bergen Belson, the silence after we hear of death, the passionate love for our children, the grief we feel at injustice, the times of love as sharp as the blade of a knife's edge, a knife that has been sharpened against stones— these represent the gleam of light, blinding.

It is from the story of Genesis, the Torah written in the rabbinic imagination as black fire on white fire, that these images come. The human project has failed again and again—Adam, Cain, Noah, Nimrod. The image we confront is of the aging Abraham, a man who travels about, acquiring. He has much—the world well-constructed with much cattle, an heir, and many things and many words and events. But after these things, in the midst of this, he falls through the bottom into the fiercest test, the Akedah, in which he is asked to hold that knife to his son's throat and cut it through to the bone.

And waiting at home, Sarah dies, not when she imagines her son's death, according to the classic rabbinic texts, but when he returns alive, and she dies, according to philosopher Aviva Zornberg,[7] of the "unbearable lightness of being"—the restoration of Isaac that in no way forgives what nearly was at the hand of Abraham. What was the test of Abraham becomes for Sarah a measure of how out of control this path can be—the truth of the hair's breadth that separates life from death.

Paul Ricoeur speaks of the "vertigo" that is "the understanding that being already born which reveals to me the non-necessity of my being here . . . the possibility there was of being different, of not having been at all . . . that only my death will one day fulfill the contingency of my birth and will lay bare the nothingness of this non-necessity of having one been born."[8]

The "near-miss" of the Akedah reveals to us the "near-make" of our lives, but reveals the knowledge of our contingency, the vertigo of being, the symmetry of equivalent possibilities. Perhaps what modernity reveals to us, if we look, is the vertigo of the understanding of that ridge without certainty, the height of absurdity, the darkness of it, the world a lost place, and we, spinning as lost ones, infinitely small in the totality of darkness. Certainly the classic rabbinic texts are aware of this; they argue that Isaac is both killed and not killed, and Zornberg reminds us that this dialectical tension prevails in many aspects of the biblical tale. This tension is found in a variety of faith traditions, the tension between the "very goodness" (*ki tov*) of the human person and the evil and destruction that prevail—the vertigo of despair. Zornberg returns to her consideration of Ricoeur to reflect on his concept of de-negation, or the negation of the negation, the understanding that one can emerge—*in spite of* one's finitude—to creation; the recognition that doubt leads to a fundamentally affirmative goal. Sartre understands that doubt, interrogation, absence, and anguish create the possibility of freedom. Ricoeur speaks of "the human being putting his past out of play by secreting his own nothingness."[9] For Zornberg it is this quality of double negative (found in the text) that leads to the possibility of the construction of a "better past."[10]

The primary answer that one could assume here is that, given this terrifying vertigo, a community of faith offers a path toward home again. Serious belief insists that one must ask that question: What is the good life?—and not: What is the happy life? In the face of the contingency reversibility of fate, one must carry this question all the time; one must be marked by it—the sign on the forehead. (To have such a reckoning would make us, at the very least, aware of the fragility and the touching faith of outcomes measures and five-year assessment planning.) Faith communities link us back to the daily world with tasks that protect the marginal and make holy the necessity despite the despair. Negation can be negated by this knitting back of each obligation, each prayer, each charity given.

But Buber hints at something more, and this will be the name of it: the real vertigo, the real terror, is not the darkness but the light: the extraordinary and fled-from, as one knows that, after all of these words, it might be real—that a first cause, and a force, and a power exists: a Presence who could call one to give everything, who could create cosmos, who could hang the stars, slap carbon into being—into us—and it is terrifying that this vastness could involve me. And it is that falling—not from belief, which is only the first floor down, but the next one, the deep belief—that is why we are fearful. For seeing both the contingency and the largeness of the possible universe, and sensing the forces for justice, the force for passion, here call us into the last task we know that we will need to do in a human life, the after-the-thingness, to face with nobility our own death. And a bioethics informed by this vertigo and this struggle is indeed a changed bioethical terrain.

Religion, then, is an approximation of what to do and say after one pulls back a little from the darkness, it is, in the words of Lorrie Moore, how to be a narrator.[11] It means being a narrator who is aware at all times of the way that the death of the other is about the knife at our throat—a hard way to live in the bright disembodiment of the clinic. It means understanding the need to work on the creation of an integrity of a self that is both alone and not alone, that one is both choosing and chosen; it will mean walking around the modern American medical center, with a loneliness met only with the certainty of witnesses of the encounter with the other that will cut against our clarity, and cleave us—the covenant of memory and the hiddenness of the future. It will mean we will not be given the sureness of expressible knowledge, not the explanatory schema of any easy system; it will mean hearing the agonal power at the heart of the world.

NOTES

1. M. Buber, as quoted in the introduction to M. Friedman, *Life on the Narrow Ridge* (New York: Paragon House, 1991), x.

2. J. Stout, *Ethics after Babel: Languages of Morals and their Disconnects* (Boston: Beacon Press, 1990).

3. P. Berger, *A Far Glory: The Quest for Faith in an Age of Credulity* (New York: Free Press, 1992), 129.

4. Musil, as cited in Berger, ibid.

5. E. Levinas, *New Talmudic Readings* (Pittsburgh, Penn.: Duquesne University Press, 1999).

6. Berger, *A Far Glory*, see note 3 above; p. 125.

7. A. Zornberg, *Genesis: The Beginning of Desire* (New York: Jewish Publication Society, 1998).

8. P. Ricoeur, *The Philosophy of Paul Ricoeur* (Bloomington, Ind.: Indiana University Press, 1996).

9. P. Ricoeur, "The Ethics of Memory," in *Questioning Ethics* (New York: Routledge, 1998).

10. Zornberg, *Genesis*, see note 7 above.

11. L. Moore, "People Like that Are the Only People Here," in *Questioning Ethics* (New York: Routledge, 1998).

Contributors

COURTNEY S. CAMPBELL, PHD, is an Associate Professor in the Department of Philosophy at Oregon State University in Corvallis.

RONALD A. CARSON, PHD, is Harris L. Kemperer Distinguished Professor and Director of the Institute for the Medical Humanities at the University of Texas Medical Branch at Galveston.

JAMES F. CHILDRESS, PHD, is Kyle Professor of Religious Studies and a Professor of Medical Education at the University of Virginia in Charlottesville.

DOLORES L. CHRISTIE, PHD, is an Associate Professor of Religious Studies at Ursuline College in Pepper Pike, Ohio.

DENA S. DAVIS, JD, PHD, is an Associate Professor of Law at Cleveland-Marshall College of Law, Cleveland State University, in Cleveland, Ohio.

H. TRISTRAM ENGELHARDT, JR., PHD, is Professor in the Department of Medicine at Baylor College of Medicine in Houston, Texas; Professor in the Department of Philosophy at Rice University; Member of the Center for Medical Ethics and Health Policy in Houston; and an Adjunct Research Fellow at the Institute of Religion in Houston.

RONALD M. GREEN, PHD, is the Eunice and Julian Cohen Professor for the Study of Ethics and Human Values in the Department of Religion, and is Director of the Ethics Institute at Dartmouth College in Hanover, New Hampshire.

STEPHEN E. LAMMERS, MA, PHD, is a Professor in the Religion Department of Lafayette College in Easton, Pennsylvania.

KAREN LEBACQZ, PHD, is the Robert Gordon Sproul Professor of Theological Studies and a Professor at the Pacific School of Religion, Graduate Theological Union, in Berkeley, California.

MARTIN E. MARTY, PHD, is the George B. Caldwell Senior Scholar-in-Residence at the Park Ridge Center for the Study of Health, Faith, and Ethics in Chicago.

MICHAEL M. MENDIOLA, PHD, is an Assistant Professor of Christian Ethics at the Pacific School of Religion in Berkeley, California.

LAURENCE J. O'CONNELL, PHD, STD, is President and CEO of the Park Ridge Center for the Study of Health, Faith, and Ethics in Chicago.

THOMAS A. SHANNON, STM, PHD, is a Professor of Religion and Social Ethics in the Department of Humanities and Arts at Worcester Polytechnic Institute in Worcester, Massachusetts.

DANIEL P. SULMASY, OFM, MD, PHD, is Sisters of Charity Chair in Ethics at Saint Vincents Hospital in New York, and is Professor of Medicine and Director of the Bioethics Institute of New York Medical College in Valhalla.

LAURIE ZOLOTH, PHD, is an Associate Professor and Chair of the Jewish Studies Program in the College of Humanities at San Francisco State University, and Cofounder of The Ethics Practice in Berkeley, California. She is President Elect of the American Society for Bioethics and Humanities (ASBH) for the years 2001 and 2002.